# DATE DUE

# DISENTITLEMENT?

# DISENTITLEMENT?

*The*

*Threats Facing Our*

*Public Health-Care Programs*

*and a*

*Rights-Based Response*

TIMOTHY STOLTZFUS JOST

OXFORD
UNIVERSITY PRESS
2003

# OXFORD
UNIVERSITY PRESS

Oxford   New York

Auckland   Bangkok   Buenos Aires   Cape Town   Chennai
Dar es Salaam   Delhi   Hong Kong   Istanbul   Karachi   Kolkata
Kuala Lumpur   Madrid   Melbourne   Mexico City   Mumbai
Nairobi   São Paulo   Shanghai   Taipei   Tokyo   Toronto

Copyright © 2003 by Oxford University Press, Inc.

Published by Oxford University Press, Inc.
198 Madison Avenue, New York, New York, 10016
http://www.oup-usa.org

Oxford is a registered trademark of Oxford University Press

Library of Congress Cataloging-in-Publication Data

Jost, Timothy Stoltzfus
Disentitlement?: the threats facing our public health-care programs and a rights-based response
Timothy Stoltzfus Jost.
p. ; cm.   Includes bibliographical references and index.
ISBN 0-19-515143-7 (cloth)
1. Medicare—Law and legislation.   2. Medicaid—Law and legislation.   3. Entitlement
spending.   4. Insurance, Health—Law and legislation.   5. Health care reform  I. Title
RA412.2 .J675 2003   368.4'2'00973—dc21   2002032951

2 4 6 8 9 7 5 3 1

Printed in the United States of America
on acid-free paper

*To Robert Ball and Wilbur Cohen*

# PREFACE

THIS book joins the rather crowded field of those that describe the American health-care system and the health-care systems of other nations. In particular, it aligns itself with the many that contend that our nation should follow the path which all other wealthy nations have already taken toward providing universal health-care coverage. The book is different from the others, however, in several important respects, and thus it makes a new contribution.

First, it brings to bear on the problem of comparative health system analysis an awareness of law and of legal institutions. Health-care systems are not simply driven by economic incentives or political forces. They are also structured by law and overseen by legal institutions. Public health-care financing systems are created by statutes, governed by administrative agencies, and overseen by the courts. Private health-care financing systems are regulated by regulatory programs and bodies, with ultimate recourse to the courts. Because they do not focus on law and legal institutions, the disciplines of health politics and policy and of health economics, which form the framework for most recent volumes analyzing national health-care systems, are not sufficient in themselves to fully comprehend the nature of those systems.

Second, this book explores not only the legal structure of our own health-care system but also the legal structure of the two primary alternative foreign models for structuring health-care systems: national health service, general revenue tax–based models (represented by the United Kingdom) and social insurance models (represented by Germany). For each of these models, this book examines the laws that establish the system and the role of the administrative agencies and courts in management, regulation, and oversight. It further considers the influence that the legal structures of these systems have on the key health policy issues of cost, access, and quality.

Third, the book focuses on the notion of entitlements. Although we often speak of our public health insurance programs as "entitlement programs," we attend too little to the meaning of the concept of entitlement. Indeed, a term that is inherently positive, connoting security and collective solidarity, has in some circles taken on a negative cast, suggesting profligate spending and self-interested aggrandizement. Entitlement, however, is ultimately a legal concept, denoting a legal claim. This book argues that we must construct a health-care system based on legal entitlements, and then shape the content and nature of our health-care entitlements to achieve the goals that we want our health-care system to serve, which I would define as universal access, acceptable cost, and adequate quality.

Fourth, the book describes the threat of the current movement toward dismantling the modest system of entitlements that we have already constructed. In the first place, that system provides some level of public health-care coverage for some of the most vulnerable persons in our society—the elderly, children, and the disabled—and, in the second, it encourages employers to provide health insurance for the rest of us. We have left the domain of health policy too much to health economists, and too many (though not all) of them seem to believe that economics is the only tool one needs for understanding humans and their institutions—that the organization and finance of health-care systems, like any other human concern, is simply a matter of economics. This has led to a growing movement, which seems ever more politically powerful, to turn health-care delivery and finance over to markets, and in the process to weaken or destroy health-care entitlements as we and other nations have known them. This book argues against that trend and attempts to elucidate the fundamental flaws in its approach to understanding health-care systems.

Finally, the book attempts to help us comprehend our health-care entitlements not only from a legal and a comparative perspective but also historically. National health-care systems, and health-care laws, are the product of unique histories. It is important to understand how our system came to be and how it has evolved if we are to understand its nature and to discern the paths that are available for our future.

I thank the many people who assisted me in this project. I express my gratitude to the Frances Lewis Law Center (and its directors Scott Sundby and Blake Morant), Dean David Partlett, and Robert L. and Crystal Willett, whose financial support made this project possible. I thank Allison McJunkin, my tireless research assistant, and Vera Mencer, who helped to get this project into order. I am also grateful to many who helped me with locating hard-to-find sources, including Professors Jürgen Wasem, Reinhard Busse, and Ingwer Ebsen, along with Sandra Erben and Justice Rainer Schlegel in Germany; Christopher Newdick and Diane Longley in England; and Linda Newell for the rest of the world. Finally, I must once again thank Ruth, Jacob, Micah, and David for patiently putting up with me as I struggled through this project

*Lexington, Virginia*                                                                    T.S.J.

# CONTENTS

# DISENTITLEMENT?

# 1

# Introduction

$$\equiv$$

O N September 11, 2001, the United States experienced an event un-precedented in the living memory of the American people—a devastating attack on two major population centers, resulting in the loss of 3,056 lives and in untold economic damage. America's political leaders responded dramatically and forcefully: within days, Congress appropriated $40 billion for homeland defense and for rebuilding. President George W. Bush announced a worldwide war on terrorism, and shortly thereafter, American troops were engaged overseas. The American people also responded resolutely and generously, donating over $2.3 billion to private charities for rescue and rebuilding efforts. A great sense of purpose and determination bound us together as a nation, both to sustain those who had suffered directly from the attack and to restore the security that we had previously enjoyed.[1]

Even as America was responding to the events of September 11, however, our nation was experiencing another disaster, even more devastating in terms of lives lost and also deeply threatening to the day-to-day security of many people. Approximately 41 million Americans currently have no public or private health insurance coverage. The number of the uninsured grew by 1.4 million during 2001.[2] Current trends, moreover, indicate that the number of the uninsured will grow rapidly in the near future. The boom economy of the late 1990s, coupled with the slowest increases in health-care costs in recent years, led to a modest expansion of insurance coverage in 1999 and 2000.[3] As this book goes to press, however, the economy remains in the doldrums, while health-care costs and health insurance premiums are increasing at rates unknown in a decade.[4] The number of Americans who are uninsured is likely to continue to increase quite dramatically for the foreseeable future.

In May of 2002, a panel of experts convened by the prestigious Institute of Medicine released a report documenting the effects of this national crisis.[5] This report confirmed and summarized a large and growing literature that has documented the dangers of being uninsured in America. The long-term uninsured face a 25% greater likelihood of premature death than do insured Americans.[6] Uninsured Americans with breast or colorectal cancer are 30% to 50% more likely to die a premature death than those who are insured.[7] Trauma victims, many of them young and otherwise healthy, experience a 37% greater chance of death if they are uninsured.[8] In sum, an estimated 18,000 Americans, six times the number killed in the attacks of September 11, die annually because they are uninsured.[9]

Premature death is not the only risk faced by the uninsured, of course. The uninsured encounter greater risks of disability and diminished capacity, as well as greater suffering from curable diseases. They also face, day by day, the risk of imminent financial disaster. Medical expenses are one of the leading causes of bankruptcy in the United States. An estimated 324,268 families—one in four families filing for bankruptcy in 1999—identified "illness or injury of self or family member" as a reason for filing bankruptcy.[10] About one-third of the families filing for bankruptcy in 1999 had medical debts.[11] Many Americans burdened with medical debt, however, choose not to file for bankruptcy because to do so would cut them off from access to the health-care providers they depend on.[12] Rather, they attempt to pay their medical bills, often using high-interest credit cards or mortgaging their homes and property. As they become overwhelmed by these obligations, they often face loss of employment because of repeated garnishments, as well as humiliating harassment from aggressive collection agencies. Lack of health insurance is among the greatest threats to financial security that Americans currently face.

These risks and dangers are encountered especially by the poor and by minority Americans. Two-thirds of uninsured persons are members of families earning less than 200% of the federal poverty level, and one-half of all uninsured American are members of minority groups.[13] The risks of being uninsured are not perceived by middle-class or wealthy white Americans to be as immediate a danger as the threat of terrorism. But few of us have accumulated wealth sufficient to pay for truly catastrophic health care, and most of us are only a pink slip away from losing our current health insurance coverage. Moreover, the loss to the nation from diminished productive capacity due to disability and premature death of the uninsured is truly immense.

This threat to our national security has not resulted in resolute, unified, and effective national action, however. We have not seen a bold political response to the crisis—no emergency appropriations bills, no outpouring of private charity, and little more than mild interest from the public. Only 10% of Americans mentioned health care as one of the two most important problems facing the nation in a recent survey, compared to 29% who listed terrorism and 37% who chose the economy.[14] This paralysis of action is undoubtedly attributable in part to a general lack of understanding about the scope and nature of the problem, as well as confusion about the best solution. Perhaps most important, our political immobility reflects the fact that a real solution to the problem would threaten powerful economic interests that thrive in our current system.

Our inability to act in the face of this national crisis is all the more remarkable because all the other wealthy nations of the world, and many nations whose wealth does not approach that of our own, have taken effective steps to avert the crisis in which we now find ourselves. Every other developed nation has created a system for insuring its entire population (or, in some nations, all but the wealthiest segment of the population) against health-care costs. In every other nation, that is, residents are legally entitled to coverage of their health-care costs. While these universal entitlements have not succeeded in guaranteeing equal access to health, or even to health care, they have assured that all residents of other developed nations enjoy basic health security and do not experience the physical suffering and financial distress that Americans do because of lack of health insurance.[15]

What is even more remarkable, however, is the fact that provision of universal health-care entitlements has not bankrupted these nations. In fact, all of the other developed nations spend less on health care than does the United States, both absolutely (in terms of dollars per capita) and relatively (in terms of proportion of gross domestic product).[16] Germany spends per capita on health care only about 59% of what the United States spends, and the United Kingdom, our closest ally in the war on terrorism, only about 39%. Yet these other nations enjoy a standard of health care that is roughly equivalent to our own. Residents of other nations, for example, tend to be as satisfied with the quality of health care they receive, and more satisfied with their health care system than are Americans.[17] Figures 1–1 and 1–2 show the breakdown of health-care costs by GDP and per capita in other wealthy countries.

This is not to say that we do not have our own public programs for financing health care. In fact, the United States has developed public programs at the federal, state, and local levels for ensuring access to health care. Indeed, if one counts the cost of tax subsidies and public employees' health insurance, as well as the direct cost of government programs, almost 60% of all health care in the United States is paid for by the government.[18] The largest of our

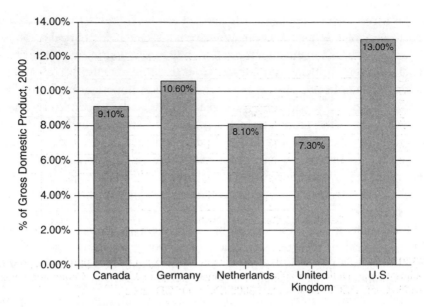

**FIGURE 1–1.** Total expenditures on health: percentage of gross domestic product (GDP), 2000. *Source:* Organization for Economic Cooperation and Development, OECD Health Data 2002 (Paris: OECD, 2002).

programs—Medicare and Medicaid—are entitlement programs. They entitle the elderly, the disabled, and poor children and their families to health-care services. Further, all working Americans are entitled to tax subsidies supporting employment-related group health insurance (if their employers offer insurance). These subsidies have helped make private insurance available to many Americans who are otherwise not eligible for public insurance. But, on the whole, our health-care entitlement programs are more limited than are the programs in other developed nations. In particular, they are limited in the populations they cover. Perhaps most important, the continued capacity of our public insurance programs to ensure health security to Americans is threatened by a powerful movement to reverse the progress we have made—a movement toward disentitlement.

This book is about American health-care entitlements and about disentitlement. In fact, the book has four themes, four stories to tell.

The first theme is that health care is different from other goods and services. In the United States, access to most goods and services is governed by willingness—and ability—to pay. None of us is entitled to receive an automobile, a computer, or fast food unless we can afford to purchase them and, in fact, choose to do so. But many of us are entitled to receive health care regardless of our ability to pay for it. And many more should be. Markets cannot, in fact, achieve universal access to health care.

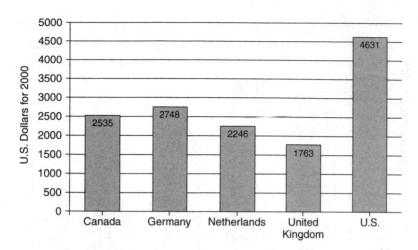

**FIGURE 1–2.** Total expenditures on health: per capita expenditure in purchasing power of adjusted U.S. Dollars for 2000. *Source:* Organization for Economic Cooperation and Development, OECD Health Data 2002 (Paris: OECD, 2002).

Second, I explore the long, slow, and faltering history of the emergence of health-care entitlements in the United States. Although the history of public health-care provision and insurance is as old as the Republic, in one brief historical moment in 1965 the United States dramatically expanded health-care entitlements for its elderly and its most needy by creating the Medicare and Medicaid programs. Continuing on through about 1990, coverage of these programs expanded at the margins, while their character as legal entitlements became more clearly articulated. Parallel to, and antedating, our development of public health insurance programs, moreover, were attempts to use entitlements to tax subsidies to extend insurance coverage to the middle class. The third chapter of this book explores the legal character of these contemporary American health-care entitlements, while the fourth describes how these entitlements came to be and to take on their present legal characteristics.

But national American health-care entitlements have never rested easily. They have always been opposed by powerful economic and ideological interests, and in the past two decades they have faced a particularly vigorous and articulate challenge that seeks both to block further expansion of health-care entitlements and to roll back or to privatize many of the entitlements we currently enjoy. This is the third story told by this book. During the past half decade, these forces have begun to enjoy some success in their push for privatization (replacing public with private insurers); individualization (replacing group and community-based approaches to insurance with approaches based on individual choice within markets); and devolution (devolving authority over entitlements from the federal to state governments, and from government to private entities). In Chapters 5 through 8, I examine proposals and attempts to privatize the Medicare and Medicaid programs through the use of managed care; to privatize Medicare, our most ambitious and successful public entitlement program; to devolve authority over the Medicaid program from the federal to the state governments; and to replace tax-subsidized group health insurance with individual insurance policies. These chapters describe the disentitlement campaigns and explain why they are not only likely to result in decreased access to health care but also to fail in their attempts to control health-care costs.

The fourth story that this book has to tell moves beyond our borders to examine the health-care entitlements of other countries. In Chapters 9 and 10, I look more closely at the legal character of health-care entitlements under the two primary models that have arisen for structuring public health insurance in other nations—the general taxation-funded national health insurance model exemplified by the United Kingdom, and the social insurance model exemplified by Germany. These chapters explore in depth the nature of the health-care entitlements that have arisen in these countries, and they show how the programs differ from each other and from the models that we have developed for our public programs. In particular, I identify characteristics of the programs of these nations that we could embrace to make our own entitlements more sustainable.

The final chapter pulls together the lessons of these four stories, describing what an entitlement-based health-care system could look like in the United States. In particular, I focus on how the legal structure of health-care entitlements affects their acceptability and sustainability. I propose an expansion and strengthening of our health-care entitlements, but also a recasting of their legal characteristics to support their long-term sustainability. By this means we can turn back the threat of disentitlement, and secure for all Americans an entitlement to health care and to all of its benefits.

# Notes

1. "WTC Recovery Effort Concludes without a Word," *USA Today* (May 31, 2002), A2; Lena H. Sun, Sarah Cohen, and Jacqueline L. Salmon, "Much of Sept. 11 Charity Remains to Be Disbursed; $2.3 Billion Exceeds Estimates, Overwhelms Groups," *Washington Post* (June 11, 2002), A1.

2. Department of Commerce, "Numbers of Americans with and without Health Insurance Rise, Census Bureau Reports," available at http://www.census.gov/Press-Release/www/2002/cb02-127.html (cited October 16, 2002).

3. Paul Fronstin, "Source of Health Insurance and Characteristics of the Uninsured: Analysis of the March 2001 Current Population Survey," *Employee Benefit Research Institute Research Brief* (December 2001): 240.

4. See, e.g., Bradley C. Strunk, Paul B. Ginsburg and Jon R. Gabel, "Tracking Health Care Costs: Growth Accelerate Again in 2001," Health Affairs web exclusive, available

at http://www.healthaffairs.org/webExclusives/2106Strunkpdt. (cited October 22, 2002). "HMO Rates Continue to Rise at Double Digit Pace," available at http://was/hewitt/com/hewitt/resource/newsroom/ressrel/2002/06-04-02.htm (cited June 4, 2002).

5. Institute of Medicine, *Care without Coverage* (Washington, D.C.: National Academy Press, 2002).

6. Ibid., 13.

7. Ibid., 8–9.

8. Ibid., 12.

9. Ibid., 162.

10. Melissa B. Jacoby, Teresa A. Sullivan, and Elizabeth Warren, "Rethinking the Debates over Health Care Financing: Evidence from the Bankruptcy Courts," *New York University Law Review* 76 (2001): 387.

11. Ibid.

12. See Hugh F. Daly III, Leslie M. Oblak, Robert W. Seifert, and Kimberly Shellenberger, "Into the Red to Stay in the Pink: The Hidden Cost of Being Uninsured," *Health Matrix* 12, no. 1 (winter 2002): 39–61.

13. Institute of Medicine, *Coverage Matters: Insurance and Health Care* (Washington, D.C.: National Academy Press, 2001), 62, 84.

14. Kaiser Family Foundation, "NPR/Kaiser/Kennedy School, National Survey on Health Care," available at http://www.kff.org/content/2002/20020605a (cited June 12, 2002).

15. See Adam Wagstaff and Eddy Van Doorslaer, "Equity in Health Care Finance and Delivery," in Handbook of Health Economics, vol. 1B, edited by A. J. Culyer and J. P. Newhouse (Amsterdam: Elsevier Science, 2000): 1803.

16. Uwe E. Reinhardt, Peter S. Hussey, and Gerard F. Anderson, "Cross-National Comparisons of Health Systems: Using OECD Data, 1999," *Health Affairs* 21 (May/June 2002): 169–181.

17. See Robert Blendon et al., "Inequities in Health Care: A Five-Country Survey," *Health Affairs* 21 (May/June 2002): 182–191.

18. Steffie Woolhandler and David U. Himmelstein, "Paying for National Health Insurance—and Not Getting It," *Health Affairs* 21 (July/Aug. 2002): 88–100.

# 2

# Why Entitlements Matter

HEALTH care is different from other goods and services. Health care entitlements matter a great deal because health care is different.

To begin, a striking fact about health-care costs is that their distribution is remarkably skewed. In any given year, the 1% of the population that spends the most on health care is responsible for 27% of health-care costs, and the most expensive 2% are responsible for 38%. The top 5% are responsible for over 50% of health-care costs, and the top 10% are responsible for nearly 70%. By contrast, the least expensive 50% of the population accounts for only 3% of health-care expenditures (see Figure 2–1).[1]

This distribution has been remarkably stable for decades. It has not changed significantly under managed care and remains almost identical among health maintenance organization, other managed-care, and indemnity plans.[2] The skewed concentration of health-care costs also holds regardless of age, although health care costs more for the elderly than for younger populations.[3] It also seems to hold true in other countries.[4]

The cost implications of this skewed distribution are dramatic. Health-care expenditures for the most costly 1% averaged $56,459 per year per person in 1996.[5] The most expensive medical conditions, which affect many of these costly consumers, include ischemic heart disease, motor vehicle accidents, and acute respiratory infections.[6] Health-care expenditures for the least costly 50% (healthy

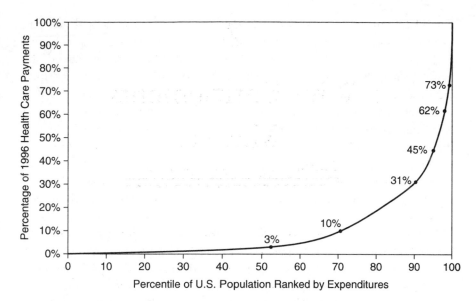

**FIGURE 2–1.** Health-care expenditures by population strata. *Source of data:* Marc L. Berk and Alan C. Monheit, "The Concentration of Health Care Expenditures Revisited," *Health Affairs* 20 (March/April 2001), 9, 12.

children and young adults who see a doctor once or twice a year) averaged only $122 per person in that year.[7] Obviously, however, there is no necessary positive correlation between high incurred health-care costs and wealth. Indeed, one would expect that many of those health-care consumers whose health-care costs are highest—the elderly and those in poor health—would also tend often to be among the less wealthy in our society.[8] In fact, poverty seems to be clearly related to poor health status.[9] Many of those whose health-care costs are highest, therefore, cannot be expected to meet these expenses from current income.

Of course, there is a way to deal with skewed risk distributions: insurance. The costs of automobile accidents and house fires also are very skewed in their distribution, but automobile and home owners routinely purchase insurance. Insurance is a means of pooling risk to make them manageable, to shift risk from the risk-averse individuals to insurers who can pool the risk and thus make it less risky. For much of the past century, therefore, many Americans have carried private health insurance to assist with the costs of health care.

## The Unusual Characteristics of Health Insurance

Health risks are different from other insurable risks, however, and health insurance is different from other forms of insurance. First, other forms of insurance are designed to insure an existing endowment of wealth against loss.

I purchase homeowner's insurance to insure my existing house and personal property, auto insurance to insure my current car, life insurance to provide income replacement for my survivors. Even liability insurance is purchased primarily (where there is a choice) to ensure that my current wealth is not wiped out by a liability judgment.

However, in most lines of insurance (other than health insurance) there is a correlation between cost and ability to pay: it costs more to insure a Bentley than a Kia, a $5 million mansion than a mobile home. But the person who buys the high-end car or the mansion can presumably also afford to insure it. Similarly, those who purchase multimillion-dollar life or liability insurance policies are presumably those who have the most to lose financially to death or lawsuits.

Health insurance, however, does not insure a person's existing wealth but, rather, that person's existing health.[10] In fact, it often covers treatment aimed at improving the current health of the insured. Indeed, a major function of health insurance, public or private, is to ensure access to health care that might never be otherwise affordable—to provide a means of financing extraordinary expensive forms of health care.[11]

Moreover, because casualty, life, and (to a certain extent) liability insurance are intended to insure existing wealth, those without substantial wealth can do without them. In some states, one can own an auto without insurance (if one is able to demonstrate financial responsibility upon having an accident),[12] and, unless a lending institution insists on it, a homeowner can go without homeowner's insurance. If auto or homeowner's insurance is in fact a precondition to auto or home ownership and yet is unaffordable, one can always take public transportation or rent an apartment. But, as noted in the previous chapter, health care can be literally a matter of life and death. Doing without inexpensive health care can in some instances lead to the later need for high-cost care; doing without high-cost care can in some instances cause death or serious disability. Doing without health insurance, therefore, is a very risky proposition, even (or especially) for the poor.[13]

Although the consequences of remaining uninsured constitute the most salient difference between health insurance and other forms of insurance, they are not the only difference. Premiums for other forms of insurance are often set with an eye toward encouraging preventive activities or discouraging risky behavior.[14] Premiums for homeowner's insurance may be reduced in response to the installation of smoke detectors or deadbolt locks, while premiums for auto insurance might be increased (or insurance denied) to reflect a history of traffic violations.

While health insurance premiums vary depending on participation in unhealthy behavior such as smoking, they are also based on factors such as age, gender, health status, claims history, and geographic location—characteristics about which the insured can do little or nothing—or on the presence of pre-existing medical conditions which the insured person has, at least in the present, little control over.[15] Typically, a 60-year-old male pays more than three times the premium paid by a 25-year-old male for the same coverage.[16] Although health insurers do not currently seem to be abusing genetic information for underwriting (and are limited in their ability to do so by the laws of many states), it is quite possible that health insurance premiums eventually could be determined by genetic predispositions totally beyond the control of the insured.

## Problems Presented by Private Health Insurance

### The Problem of Affordability

The greatest barrier that many face in purchasing health insurance, however, is that it simply is not affordable. While auto or homeowner's insurance may cost hundreds of dollars, health insurance can cost thousands. The average cost of group family insurance, purchased through an employer, was over $6,000 in 2001, while mid-range premiums for family insurance in the nongroup market ran to over $7,000.[17] One survey of individual health insurance policies available on the Internet in 10 states in 2000 found that individual health insurance policies cost on average $313 per month for a healthy 55-year-old male.[18] If that person earned the poverty level income for a single individual of $8,860 in 2002, health insurance premiums would consume 43% of his income.[19]

Because health insurance is so expensive, many low-income Americans do without it. This is presumably the case because the costs of food and shelter—or of clothing, transportation, and child care necessary to make employment possible—present a more immediate demand on income than does insurance against health risks that may or may not eventuate. It is also true that persons without health insurance can ultimately, in an emergency, claim the protection of a federal law that requires hospitals with emergency rooms to screen and stabilize patients first and seek compensation later.[20] They also may be able to obtain free or reduced-cost care from safety-net providers. Thus, lower-income Americans might gamble that foregoing health insurance will not result in lack of access to care in an emergency. Moreover, bankruptcy may be an alternative to health insurance for those overwhelmed with health-care costs, although this is only true for those who can first find health-care providers willing to provide care on credit.[21] But filing for bankruptcy may end all hope of continuing relationships with existing sources of medical care.

One reason that it is rational for poor persons to pass up buying health insurance in the individual market is that inexpensive insurance, which might be affordable, has very little value to the poor. There is obviously a great range of cost for most essentials, such as food, housing, or clothing. If one has little money, one can eat food from cans and live in a mobile home. An inexpensive "bare-bones" health insurance policy, however, usually imposes high deductibles and high cost sharing.[22] In fact, it insures primarily against catastrophic costs (and even these may be subject to caps). But the poor are already insured by the bankruptcy laws against catastrophic costs, and what they need is access to primary care, which bare-bones policies often do not provide. Thus, the value of bare-bones policies to the poor is even less than their low cost, and few are sold.

## The Problem of Biased Selection

While affordability is a problem for many Americans, the possibility of being able to afford health insurance varies based on the circumstances and characteristics of the applicant. Here the problem of insurance underwriting comes to the fore. As has already been noted, the price of health insurance, and thus its affordability, varies considerably from applicant to applicant. This is true because, as noted, health-care costs are reasonably predictable from the characteristics of the insured. Elderly people are more likely to need health care than younger persons; persons with chronic conditions will need more than those in good health.

Because the need for health care is, to a large degree, predictable, health insurers are able to vary their premium rates, often dramatically, based on the predicted exposure of potential insureds to health-care costs. In a competitive market for health insurance, insurers must underwrite based on risk if they want to stay in business. No single insurer will choose to offer the same price to all purchasers of insurance (i.e., to "community-rate") voluntarily.[23] Any insurer that tried to do so would obviously have to charge each person it insured a premium that is high enough to cover its total risks (plus administrative expenses and profits) divided by the total number of insured persons. This premium would have to yield enough income to cover the costs anticipated from extraordinarily expensive cases, as well as the cost of a much greater number of more moderately expensive services.

Because of the extraordinarily skewed nature of health-care costs, however, an insurer that decided to charge a community rate would have to charge hefty premiums to many insureds who, in fact, would incur few insured expenses over the course of the year. More important, the insurer would have to convince many persons who did not anticipate any health-care expenses during the year (young, healthy males, for example) to subsidize the health-care costs of those who fully expected high medical costs.

Faced with sizeable premiums and little anticipation of need for insurance, some low-risk insureds will undoubtedly decline insurance coverage, for the reasons already noted.[24] High-risk insureds, in contrast, will find community-rated insurance very attractive.[25] In other words, insurers who charge the same rate to all applicants will be exposed to "adverse selection" (the preferential choice of insurance by high-risk individuals).[26]

If at least one insurer offers insurance at a lower price (as would be expected in competitive markets), however, low-risk individuals will abandon the high-cost insurer and flock to the insurer with lower premiums.[27] But so will high-risk insureds, thus seriously threatening the viability of the lower-cost insurer. To make money with its low rates, the lower-cost insurer will have to try to discourage high-risk insureds by offering a less generous product (for example, a product subject to lower caps or higher cost-sharing, or covering fewer services).[28] Such policies will be of little value to high-risk insureds, who are unlikely to buy them. If the lower-cost insurer succeeds in warding off high-risk insureds, however, the high-risk insureds will remain with the higher-cost, higher-coverage insurer, which will now need to raise its premiums to cover the ever more expensive population it retains.[29] Once the high-cost insurer does this, however, its policies will become even less attractive to those low-risk insureds who had remained loyal to it.

In the end, an insurer that community-rates voluntarily will slip into the insurance "death spiral," as it is left with an ever more unfavorable risk pool and must charge ever higher rates.[30] Similarly, plans with generous benefits that do not risk-underwrite will be driven out of the market by adverse selection.[31] In short, a stable "pooling equilibrium"—in which every insured is in a common pool paying the same amount for insurance—is not possible in competitive health insurance markets.[32]

As soon as at least one insurer risk-underwrites or "experience-rates,"[33] however, offering higher rates for higher-risk applicants and lower rates for lower-risk applicants, the market will sort itself out into a "separation equilibrium."[34] Community-rated plans will be forced to move to risk underwriting or be priced out of the market.

As already noted, however, there is no necessary positive correlation between health-care risk and ability to pay. Thus, high-risk individuals facing high health insurance premiums in a risk-segmented market may not be able to afford them. Even persons with incomes well above the poverty level may find health insurance, however necessary, beyond their means.

Although risk selection on the part of insurers is often referred to in morally-laden terms, such as "cherry picking" or "cream skimming," it is simply economically rational behavior. One can hardly object to a business trying to cover its costs, and any insurer that charges high-risk insureds premiums that are not high enough to cover expected claims cannot expect to stay in business long. Yet risk underwriting presents high-risk individuals with a serious problem. It is, moreover, a bad deal not only for those with health problems but also for almost everyone else because of its high administrative costs.

The High Administrative Costs of Individual Insurance

The need for health insurers to choose risks carefully substantially increases the cost of health insurance, especially in the individual market. Insurers must pay for underwriting, for bearing the increased uncertainty of insuring individuals, for marketing to attract good risks, and for commissions to agents who help them locate potential customers and screen out bad risks before the applicant is even presented to the insurance company (so-called field underwriting).[35] These costs may equal as much as 40% of premiums for individual policies, and as little as 6% of premiums for the large group policies. None of the money spent on these costs, however, goes for health care. Although these expenses add considerably to the cost of health insurance, and thus diminish its affordability, they add little, if any, value for insureds.

## The Solution to the Health Insurance Conundrum—Entitlements

Because the distribution of the risk of incurring health-care costs is so skewed, health insurance is commonly available throughout the world. Because of the problem of affordability of health insurance, all developed countries have recognized some form of public entitlement to health insurance or health-care services.[36] Because of the high administrative costs attending individual insurance, and because biased selection makes individual insurance unaffordable to those who need it most, no country relies on individual health insurance sold in private markets to cover its entire population. Rather, health insurance (or health care) is publicly provided by other countries to all, or most, of their residents. Where health insurance is available in private markets, moreover, it is often provided through group, rather than individual, health insurance policies.[37]

In most countries health-care entitlements have evolved over time. In many countries these entitlements first covered industrial workers, spreading only later to pensioners, agricultural and domestic workers, and others.[38] In a number of European countries they began as quasi-private social insurance programs, evolving later into national health insurance programs.[39] In a few countries they still do not cover the entire population. In Germany, for example, public medical insurance is optional for those whose income exceeds a relatively high level (40,500 euros a year in 2002). In the Netherlands, those whose income exceeds 30,700 euros annually (in 2002) are barred from some parts of the social insurance program; while in Ireland certain forms of public insurance are only accessible to those who are relatively poor.[40] In some countries, public health insurance is administered at the local or regional level, and entitlements may vary somewhat throughout the country. But in virtually all developed nations, a resident is entitled to basic health-care services as a matter of law. In many developing nations, incidentally, health access entitlements also exist as a matter of law, although the reality of access may not.[41]

These entitlement programs are fundamentally based on the notion of social solidarity—on the belief that all of us are vulnerable to disease and accident, and thus all should be insured against these perils:

> [Solidarity] denotes a behavioral orientation of non-indifference, namely, to deliberately put one's own utility maximization, at least temporarily, behind the pursuit of utility of others for the sake of promoting the welfare of the collectivity to which one belongs. Solidarity presupposes recognition of "others" as people like myself and thus as legitimate recipients of immediate advantages; and as trustworthy in that they can be expected to dutifully reciprocate if roles were reversed and [to] . . . abstain from exploitative behavior.[42]

Thus, all insureds contribute—through general taxation for national health services plans or wage-based contributions for social insurance plans—and all are insured.

The three American health-care entitlement programs that are the focus of this book—Medicare, Medicaid, and tax subsidies for employment-related health insurance—also address the three problems of biased selection, affordability, and high administrative costs for individual insurance. They are all based to a greater or lesser extent on a solidarity principle.

This is most obviously true with the Medicaid program. A welfare program, Medicaid entitles indigent persons over 65, the blind, the disabled, children and their families, and pregnant women to a broad array of medical services. Medicaid programs are operated by the states, but at least half the cost of the program is paid for by the federal government, and states must comply with federal program requirements. Medicaid covered about 36.5 million persons at a cost of about $226 billion in 2001.[43]

Medicaid is available without charge except for very low cost sharing. It is available only to the very poor, few of whom could afford individual commercial insurance policies, and in particular to the elderly and disabled, who would otherwise have a very hard time purchasing adequate insurance coverage because of underwriting requirements.

Medicare Part A, a traditional social insurance program, entitles persons over 65, the long-term disabled, and those needing renal dialysis to hospital care, home health care, limited nursing-home care, and hospice care. Medicare Part B, a tax-subsidized insurance program, covers physicians' services, durable medical equipment, home health, the services of a variety of therapies, and a number of other health-care goods and services, but only for those who pay Part B premiums. Medicare covered about 40 million Americans, at a cost of about $247 billion in 2001.[44]

Though Medicare is not free, affordability is rarely an issue. Part A is financed by payroll taxes that are collected from employees and the self-employed. Although its financing is not very progressive, Medicare Part A is at least financed by those who are healthy enough to work. At present, moreover, these taxes amount to a small proportion of income—1.45% taxed to the employee—and, in any event, are mandatory, so the question of affordability does not pose a dilemma to enrollees. Part B premiums, in contrast, are paid by insureds but are so heavily subsidized ($3 of subsidy for every $1 of premium) that few pass up enrollment in Part B. The fact that Part B premiums are taken directly out of Social Security premiums unless there is an objection by the beneficiary also undoubtedly contributes to the high enrollment rate.[45]

The third major program covered in this book is less commonly thought of as an entitlement, although it does create legally enforceable rights to which eligible persons are entitled. This is the federal tax subsidy that excludes from income and payroll taxation money spent on group health insurance for employees.[46] Any employee whose employer offers group health insurance benefits is legally entitled to the benefit of this entitlement. Some 172 million Americans currently benefit from this entitlement, at a cost of $111 billion in federal tax subsidies in 1998.[47]

Because only group, rather than individual, insurance has historically been supported by our tax subsidies, Americans have tended to be insured in employment-related groups. Because the cost of insurance has traditionally been community-rated within groups by custom and is now community-rated by federal law, group insurance has covered older and less healthy people, as well as the younger and healthier.[48] A recent study found that for persons aged 55, individual insurance coverage costs 60% more than group insurance, even though individual plans offer less coverage than group plans.[49] While individual insurance may be less expensive than group insurance for young healthy males, the tax subsidy (and the fact that insureds often believe, falsely, that the cost of employment-related insurance is borne by the employer) tends to make group insurance attractive to the young as well. Because the underwriting and marketing costs are much lower for insuring groups, particularly large groups, employment-related group health insurance would be more affordable than individual policies even without the tax subsidy.[50]

Although we have far more uninsured people in the United States than other developed countries have, our three primary health-care entitlement programs have made health insurance widely available to much of the population. They have extended health coverage to the elderly, the long-term disabled, poor children, pregnant women, and 85% of the working population. There are still significant gaps, including many of the near-elderly, the working poor, and young adults. Also, Medicare coverage excludes important services such as long-term care and prescription drugs, and Medicaid payment rates are so low in most states that the program brings about two-tier medicine. Attempts to move forward to universal coverage seem persistently stalled.

## The Reaction—Disentitlement

More alarmingly, policy proposals in recent years threaten to roll back our current entitlement programs and to bring about disentitlement. In recent years, conservative policy analysts have persistently argued for replacing the solidarity principle with markets.[51] In their ideal system, all would pay their own way (with the assistance of tax credits for the poor), and all would purchase as individuals in health insurance markets.

This approach is based on several related articles of faith. The first is that the most significant problem we face in health-care financing is moral hazard caused by overinsurance. "Moral hazard" is an awkward term used to describe the propensity of those who are insured to inappropriately take advantage of their insurance. Historically, it was used to describe the phenomena of insured ships sinking inexplicably or insured houses mysteriously burning down. In the health insurance context, it refers to the excessive use of health-care services by those who are insured for those services. It is often asserted by conservative health-care analysts that this phenomenon is common enough to be the major cause of escalating health-care costs.[52] The solutions they propose are to create managed competition, where more of the costs of health insurance are passed on to insureds, or to use medical savings accounts coupled with catastrophic coverage to make insureds more sensitive to the cost of medical care.[53]

It is undoubtedly the case that people who are insured use more health-care services than those who are not. The problem, however, is determining whether this reflects inappropriate and opportunistic use of unneeded health-care services by the insured, or inappropriate and potentially dangerous failure to use needed health-care services by those who are not insured. The case for moral hazard in health care is built largely on the Rand Health Care Experiment, conducted in the early 1970s.[54] The Rand experiment did demonstrate that lower cost sharing results in higher health-care use, and that, in general, higher use did not result in better health-care outcomes. It also showed, alternatively, that poorer people with some chronic diseases have worse outcomes if they have higher cost-sharing obligations.[55] The most important point about the Rand experiment, however, is that it was conducted a quarter century ago in a fee-for-service environment and thus has little to tell us about the prevalence or effects of moral hazard in our radically different, managed-care-driven system. All 14 of the plans with cost sharing in the study were fee-for-service plans, though the study also included two groups enrolled in one of the few established HMOs available at that time.[56] Most managed-care plans, and most of the health-care systems of other countries, use supply-side controls, such as budgets, utilization review, or risk (capitation), rather than (or in addition to) cost sharing to control moral hazard. The Rand study tells us nothing about the comparative effectiveness of these strategies. Many of the other studies that find evidence of overinsurance also are badly dated.[57] Nevertheless, these studies continue to form the bedrock of conservative health policy advocacy.

Conservative health advocates put forth other arguments in favor of reliance on markets in which individuals purchase health insurance for insuring the American population. First, they believe simply in the virtues of markets to bring about an efficient allocation and use of resources. There is, of course, ample evidence of markets working this way in other sectors. The ability of markets to serve as the exclusive means of organizing the health-care sector, however, has long been contested.[58] In particular, the problems of biased selection, affordability, and high administrative costs make markets for individual health insurance inefficient.

Conservative health advocates also believe in the virtue of choice regarding health insurance in itself.[59] In individual insurance markets, they argue, individuals can choose the insurance policy that meets their needs. While choice is usually a good thing, in this context it comes at a very high price. In particular, because of the affordability and biased selection problems, markets, although they offer greater choice to some, effectively exclude choice by others. Because of the higher administrative costs of individually purchased policies, moreover, most individuals get a worse deal in individual markets than they get in group markets, regardless of their health status.

Finally, some (though not all) conservative advocates embrace biased selection as a positive good. These advocates reject the vision of health insurance pooling based on solidarity in favor of a belief that everyone should pay his or her own way, that subsidization of the chronically ill and elderly is a bad thing in itself.[60] In turn, this conviction is based on a distorted and erroneous belief that persons who are insured are more likely to engage in unhealthy behaviors[61] and, in extreme cases, on a commitment to a form of natural selection ("let the poor and sick die off, who needs them?").[62] It is a belief that has been rejected by all other major health-care systems in the world.[63]

Later in this book I address the conservative argument in greater detail. First, however, I examine in the next two chapters the nature and history of the entitlements that have arisen in the United States to deal with the problems of affordability, biased selection, and administrative costs.

## Notes

1. Marc L. Berk and Alan C. Monheit, "The Concentration of Health Care Expenditures, Revisited," *Health Affairs* 20 (March/April 2001): 9, 12. Berk and Monheit's study (which followed up on two earlier studies published in 1988 and 1992), was based

on an analysis of the 1996 Medical Expenditure Panel Survey (MEPS). The MEPS is a two-year survey of 10,000 households consisting of 23,000 individuals, conducted by the Agency for Healthcare Research and Quality. Ibid., 17 n. 6.

2. Ibid, 10–11.

3. See Anne A. Scitovsky, "The High Cost of Dying Revisited," *Milbank Quarterly* 72, no. 4 (1994): 561.

4. See, e.g., L. Com-Ruelle, S. Dumesnil, Centre de Recherche d'Etude et de Documentation en Economie de la Santé (CREDES), "Concentration des despenses et grands consommateurs de soins medicaux," 1999, available at http://www.credes.fr/Publications/bulletins/QuestEco/1999.htm#20 (cited Oct. 20, 2002). These disparities lessen, but do not disappear, when expenditures are considered over long periods of time. See Marian Gornick, Alma McMillan, and James Lubitz, "A Longitudinal Perspective on Patterns of Medicare Payments," *Health Affairs* 12 (summer 1993): 140–150.

5. Berk and Monheit, "Concentration of Health Care Expenditures," 13.

6. Benjamin G. Druss et al., "The Most Expensive Medical Conditions in America," *Health Affairs* 21 (July/August 2002): 105–111.

7. Berk and Monheit, "Concentration of Health Care Expenses," 13.

8. Nancy E. Adler and Katherine Newman, "Socioeconomic Disparities in Health: Pathways and Policies," *Health Affairs* 21 (March/April 2002): 60–76.

9. Angus Deaton, "Policy Implications of the Gradient of Health and Wealth," *Health Affairs* 21 (March/April 2002): 13–30; Michael Marmot, "The Influence of Income on Health: Views of an Epidemiologist," *Health Affairs* 21 (March/April 2002): 31–46.

10. My thinking on this point was assisted by a presentation given by Peter J. Hammer at the American Society of Law, Medicine, and Ethics Health Law Teachers' Conference held at Indianapolis, Indiana in Spring 2002.

11. John A. Nyman, "The Value of Health Insurance: The Access Motive," *Journal of Health Economics* 18, no. 2 (1999): 141–152.

12. Robert L. Joost, *Automobile Insurance and No Fault Laws*, 2nd ed. (Deerfield, Ill.: Clark Boardman Callaghan, 1992), 2001 Supp, ¶ 1.8.

13. Institute of Medicine, *Care Without Coverage: Too Little, Too Late* (Washington D.C.: National Institute Press, 2002), 81.

14. See Scott E. Harrington and Gregory R. Niehaus, *Risk Management and Insurance* (Columbus, Oh.: Irwin/McGraw-Hill, 1999), 120–121.

15. See Deborah J. Chollet and Adele M. Kirk, *Understanding Individual Health Insurance Markets: Structure, Practices, and Products in Ten States* (Washington, D.C.: Kaiser Family Foundation, 1998). Both auto and homeowner's insurance depend heavily on geographic location, which might not always be wholly within the control of the insured, while life insurance depends heavily on age and health condition, and auto insurance rates are much higher for young males. But older people can forego life insurance (which often becomes less important once children are raised), and teenagers who get good grades can earn lower auto insurance premiums.

16. Ibid., 43.

17. Iris J. Lav and Joel Friedman, *Tax Credits for Individuals to Buy Health Insurance Won't Help Many Uninsured Adults* (Washington, D.C.: Center on Budget and Policy Priorities, 2001).

18. Jon Gabel et al., "Individual Insurance: How Much Financial Protection Does It Provide?" *Health Affairs Web Exclusive*, available at www.healthaffairs.com (cited April 17, 2002).

19. This is not to say that all persons currently uninsured cannot afford health in-

surance. In a recent paper M. Kate Bundorf and Mark V. Pauly, attempting to define the concept of affordability, contend that (a) half of the uninsured could purchase health insurance without reducing their remaining income below 1.75 times the poverty level (a proposed normative definition of affordability), and that (b) half of the population with an income equal to or less than that of 60% of the uninsured (adjusting for a number of factors that affect affordability) purchase health insurance, thus indicating that health insurance is in fact affordable to at least 60% of the uninsured (a proposed behavioral definition). Though there are methodological problems with their analysis (they do not differentiate between the short term uninsured, who may be gambling on doing without coverage for a brief period of time, and the long-term uninsured, and do not appear to adjust fully for differences in premiums based on health status) their overall point that many uninsured could in fact afford insurance is probably accurate. M. Kate Bundorf and Mark V. Pauly, *Is Health Insurance Affordable for the Uninsured?* (Cambridge, Mass: National Bureau of Economic Research, 2002).

20. The Emergency Medical Treatment and Active Labor Act, 42 U.S.C. § 1395dd.

21. See Hugh F. Daly III, Leslie M. Oblak, Robert W. Seifert, and Kimberly Shellenberger, "Into the Red to Stay in the Pink: The Hidden Cost of Being Uninsured," *Health Matrix* 12, no. 1 (winter 2002): 39–61.

22. Sherry Glied, Cathi Callahan, James Mays, and Jennifer N. Edwards, "Issue Brief," *Bare-Bones Health Plans: Are They Worth the Money?* (New York: Commonwealth Fund, 2002).

23. The classic demonstration of this is found in Michael Rothschild and Joseph Stiglitz, "Equilibrium in Competitive Insurance Markets: An Essay on the Economics of Imperfect Information," *Quarterly Journal of Economics* 90 (1976): 629.

24. John V. Jacobi, "The Ends of Health Insurance," *University of California at Davis Law Review* 30 (1997): 311, 387–388.

25. Mark A. Hall, *Reforming Private Health Insurance* (Washington, D.C.: American Enterprise Institute Press, 1994), 11.

26. See ibid., and Leah Wortham, "The Economics of Insurance Classification: The Sound of One Invisible Hand Clapping," *Ohio State Law Journal* 47 (1986): 836, 844. Adverse selection may occur either when insurers are unable to identify high-risk applicants or, when rate regulation limits their ability to respond, to act on their identification of such applicants. Wynand P.M.M. van de Ven, et al., "Access to Coverage for High Risks in a Competitive Individual Health Insurance Market: Via Premium Rate Restrictions or Risk-Adjusted Premium Subsidies?" *Journal of Health Economics* 19 (2000): 311.

27. Rothschild and Stiglitz, "Equilibrium in Competitive Insurance Markets," 637.

28. Mark V. Pauly, "Is Cream-Skimming a Problem for the Competitive Medical Market?" *Journal of Health Economics* 3 (1984): 92.

29. Jacobi, "The Ends of Health Insurance," 388–389.

30. Deborah Chollet, "Consumers, Insurers, and Market Behavior," *Journal of Health Politics, Policy and Law* 25 (2000): 27, 37; Jacobi, "The Ends of Health Insurance," 389.

31. See M. Susan Marquis, "Adverse Selection with a Multiple Choice among Health Insurance Plans: A Simulation Analysis," *Journal of Health Economy* 11 (1992): 129. Marquis demonstrates this elimination through a simulation based on the Rand Health Insurance experiment.

32. Rothschild and Stiglitz, "Equilibrium in Competitive Insurance Markets," 634.

33. That is, it offers rates to groups or to individuals based on experience with health-care costs.

34. See Pauly, "Is Cream-Skimming a Problem?" 90.

35. Hall, *Reforming Private Health Insurance*, 21 (citing U.S. Congressional Research Service, Private Health Insurance, Options for Reform, 1990). See also Wortham, "The Economics of Insurance Classification," 863–869 (discussing insurance transaction costs).

36. See World Health Organization, *World Health Report 2000: Improving Performance* (Geneva: World Health Organization, 2000).

37. Timothy S. Jost, "Private or Public Approaches to Insuring the Uninsured: Lessons from International Experience with Private Insurance," *New York University Law Review* 76 (2001): 471.

38. This was the case in Germany, as described in Chapter 10.

39. This was the case in Great Britain, as described in Chapter 9.

40. See, describing these systems, Elias Mossialos and Julian Le Grand, eds., *Health Care and Cost Containment in the European Union* (Burlington, Eng.: Ashgate, 1999).

41. See, e.g., Pan American Health Organization, *The Right to Health in the Americas* (Washington, D.C.: Pan American Health Organization, 1989).

42. Karl Hinrichs, *Health Care Policy in the German Social Insurance State: From Solidarity to Privatization?* (Bremen: Center for Social Policy Research, 1999), 6.

43. Center for Medicare Services, *National Summary of Medicaid Managed Care Programs, and Enrollment* (Washington, D.C.: CMS, 2001); Health Care Financing Administration, "National Health Care Expenditures Projections Tables," available at http://www.hcfa.gov/stats/NHE-Proj/proj2001/tables (cited July 2, 2002).

44. Kaiser Family Foundation, "Medicare Quick Facts," available at http://www.kff.org/docs/sections/medicare/quickfacts.html (cited October 23, 2002).

45. Boards of Trustees, Federal Hospital Insurance, and Federal Supplementary Medical Insurance Trust Funds, *2002 Annual Report of the Boards of Trustees of the Federal Hospital Insurance and Federal Supplementary Medical Insurance Trust Funds* (Washington, D.C.: Federal Hospital Insurance and Federal Supplementary Medical Insurance Trust Funds, 2002), 4.

46. Other provisions allow tax exclusions or deductions for (*a*) health insurance premiums paid by the self-insured, (*b*) long-term care insurance premiums and medical savings accounts under certain circumstances, and (*c*) money contributed to employees for cafeteria accounts. See Chapter 8 for a detailed discussion of these benefits.

47. William S. Custer and Pat Ketsche, *Employment-Based Health Insurance* (Washington, D.C.: Health Insurance Association of America, 2000), 9; John Sheils and Paul Hogan, "Cost of Tax-Exempt Health Benefits in 1998," *Health Affairs* 18 (2001): 176–181.

48. 29 U.S.C. § 1182. This provision of the Health Insurance Portability and Accountability Act of 1996 prohibits discrimination in premiums in group health plans based on health status.

49. Jon Gabel et al., "Individual Insurance: How Much Financial Protection Does It Provide?" *Health Affairs Web Exclusive* available at http://healthaffairs.org/WebExclusives/2103Gabel.pdf (cited April 12, 2002).

50. Administrative expenses consume 25%–40% of each premium dollar for individual policies, compared to 10% for large groups and 15%–25% for small groups. Mark A. Hall, "The Geography of Health Insurance Regulation," *Health Affairs* 19 (March/April 2000): 173–184.

51. Although the views described in this section are widely held by conservative health economists, the group that has been primarily responsible for bringing them to the na-

tional political agenda has been the Heritage Foundation. For over a decade, the Heritage Foundation has maintained a persistent and effective campaign to publicize and popularize these proposals. See Trudy Lieberman, *Slanting the Story: The Forces That Shape the News* (New York: New Press, 2000), 117–148.

52. See, e.g., Michael Tanner, "What's Wrong with the Present System?" in *Empowering Health Care Consumers through Tax Reform*, edited by Grace-Marie Arnett (Ann Arbor: University of Michigan Press, 1999), 27–34.

53. See, e.g., Robert Emmet Moffit, "High Anxiety: Working Families Need Market-Based Health Care Reform," in *Empowering Health Care Consumers through Tax Reform*, edited by Grace-Marie Arnett (Ann Arbor: University of Michigan Press, 1999), 35–53.

54. Joseph P. Newhouse, *Free for All? Lessons from the Rand Health Insurance Experiment* (Cambridge, Mass.: Harvard University Press, 1993).

55. Ibid., 243, 255.

56. Ibid., 8–9.

57. See Peter Zweifel and Willard G. Manning, "Moral Hazard and Consumer Incentives in Health Care," in *Handbook of Health Economics*, edited by A. J. Culyer and J. P. Newhouse (Amsterdam: Elsevier, 2000), 429–444.

58. The classic article on this was Kenneth J. Arrow, "Uncertainty and the Welfare Economics of Medical Care," *American Economic Review* 53 (1963): 851–883.

59. See, e.g., Moffit, "High Anxiety," 35–53.

60. See, e.g., Richard A. Epstein, *Mortal Peril: Our Inalienable Right to Health Care?* (Reading, Mass.: Addison-Wesley, 1997). See also, describing this vision of the role of health insurance, Deborah A. Stone, "The Struggle for the Soul of Health Insurance," *Journal of Health Politics, Policy, and Law* 18 (1993): 287–317.

61. In fact, the absence of insurance may lead to diminished use of preventive care, and thus to a greater need for medical services later. Peter Zweiffel and Williard G. Manning, "Moral Hazard and Consumer Incentives in Health Care" in A. J. Culyer and J. P. Newhouse, eds., *Handbook of Health Economics* (Amsterdam: Elsevier, 2000), 418–420.

62. See Epstein, *Mortal Peril*, 114–115 (suggesting this approach).

63. See, e.g., stating the opinion of many European health law and policy scholars: The United States "stands apart from every other industrialized nation in its misguided belief in the applicability of the market to health care." Elias Mossialos et al., *The Influence of EU Law on the Social Characteristics of Health Care Systems in the European Market* (London: European Observatory, 1991).

# 3

# The Nature of
# American Health-Care
# Entitlements

W HAT exactly is a health-care "entitlement"? More specifically, what are the legal ramifications of entitlement status? Yet more specifically, how does the concept of entitlement apply to the three programs with which this book is primarily concerned—Medicare, Medicaid, and the tax exclusions that are available for subsidizing employment-related health insurance?

The dictionary defines the verb *entitle* as "to furnish with a right or claim to something."[1] The noun *entitlement,* therefore, is a claim or right that has been furnished. In the context of Medicare and Medicaid, the claim or right is obviously that of the beneficiary or recipient to health-care goods and services.[2] By extension, providers may also have a claim or right to be paid for goods or services that they provide to recipients. Employers and employees have a legal claim to tax exclusions and deductions for employment-related health insurance. Employees have legal rights against the programs employers adopt because of these subsidies. What is the nature of these claims or rights, however? And by what means are they "furnished"?

In this chapter I consider the nature of American health-care entitlements from a variety of, primarily legal, perspectives. I begin by asking whether Americans (or, perhaps, some Americans) have a fundamental, constitutional, right to health care. Concluding that no such right exists (but that the Constitution does have relevance for health-care entitlements), I next examine the nature of statutory entitlements to health care under the three programs considered in this book. Third, I turn from rights to remedies, recognizing that rights are of little value unless remedies are available to protect them. Indeed, federal entitlements arguably exist legally to the extent that they are protected by the federal courts. Fourth, I explore the functional meaning of entitlement for program beneficiaries and for providers: what concrete difference does it make that each of the programs examined here is an entitlement for those who depend on that program? Fifth, entitlement as a budgetary concept is explored. Here we see that in our American system, entitlement means an open-ended budgetary commitment, and entitlements are often discussed in terms of this commitment. Finally, I turn to the notion of entitlement as a political concept: What difference does it make politically that a program is an entitlement?

## Do Americans Have a Constitutional Entitlement to Health?

The most powerful legal claim that one can make in our constitutional system is that a right is guaranteed by the U.S. Constitution. The practical effect of such a claim is that the right is not wholly under the control of the explicitly political branches of government—Congress and the executive branch. Under our constitutional system, the courts—and, more specifically, the Supreme Court—have the ultimate responsibility for protecting constitutional rights. When the political branches of the federal government (or the state governments) interfere with constitutional rights, the courts have the obligation to intervene at the instance of the person whose rights have been violated.

If Medicare and Medicaid or tax subsidies for health insurance were constitutionally protected entitlements, therefore, the courts could order either Congress or the federal government agency responsible for these programs (currently the Center for Medicare and Medicaid Services (CMS) within the Department of Health and Human Services (HHS) for Medicare and Medicaid, and the Internal Revenue Service (IRS) for tax subsidies)—or the states (who administer Medicaid)—to honor these entitlements.

The strongest constitutional health-care entitlement would be a constitutional right to public health insurance or public provision of health-care services. Although the U.S. Constitution does not guarantee such a right, such a fundamental human right to health care is widely recognized throughout the world, both in international human rights law and in the constitutions of many nations. Article 25 of the 1948 Universal Declaration of Human Rights states:

> Everyone has the right to a standard of living adequate for the health and well-being of himself and of his family, including food, clothing, housing and medical

care and necessary social services, an the right to security in the event of . . . sickness, [and] disability.

The International Covenant on Economic, Social, and Cultural Rights (ICESCR) provides more explicitly at Article 12:

The States Parties . . . recognize the right to everyone to the enjoyment of the highest attainable standard of physical and mental health.

The Universal Declaration of Human Rights is not self-executing in American courts,[3] however, and the United States has not signed the ICESCR,[4] which in any event is more aspirational than proscriptive in nature.[5]

Many national constitutions of recent vintage also recognize a right to health, health provision, or health security.[6] Litigation enforcing these provisions is rare, however, and even more rarely successful.[7] In most nations these provisions have served primarily a hortatory function and have not been specifically enforced.[8]

The U.S. Constitution is the product of the late eighteenth century, not of the late twentieth century. It reflects a time when the primary concern of nation builders was to protect citizens from arbitrary and oppressive government.[9] The framers of the Constitution did not see the federal government as a benevolent means for extending health and welfare benefits to the populace but, rather, as a necessary evil to be contained.[10] Many of the framers were also more concerned with protecting property than with protecting those who lacked it (most of whom, including slaves and women—but also propertyless men—were excluded from voting and thus lacked a political voice).[11] Health and welfare protection were at the time local concerns.[12] The framers did not contemplate shifting responsibility for them to the national government.[13] The focus of the Constitution, therefore, is on negative, not positive, rights.[14]

Given this historical context, it is not surprising that nowhere in the Constitution is there a hint of a right to health care.[15] Although the federal, state, and local governments have long funded health-care programs, there is no credible argument that the federal Constitution obligates them to do so.[16]

But a constitutional entitlement to a universal public program for health insurance or provision is not necessarily the only form that a constitutional right to health care might take. A less comprehensive claim could be that, even if Congress has no general obligation to provide universal health insurance, at least indigents, who cannot otherwise afford private health insurance, have a right to some form of public health coverage. This right would not be focused specifically on health care but, rather, on the right of all Americans to have their basic needs met, including the need for health care.

The claim that the Constitution provides some form of protection for welfare rights has retained remarkable resiliency in the academic commentary over the years, even though it has enjoyed little success in the courts. For several decades, distinguished academicians have attempted to find "welfare rights," described variously as "rights to a livelihood" or rights to a "minimum protection from economic hazard" in the Thirteenth or Fourteenth Amendment or elsewhere in the Constitution.[17]

For a time in the 1960s and 1970s it seemed possible that the Supreme Court would recognize some version of such a right.[18] In particular, the argument was pressed that the right to welfare was a "fundamental right" or that the poor were a "suspect class," and that the courts should therefore subject welfare legislation to the heightened scrutiny appropriate for reviewing legislation that affects fundamental rights or suspect classes under the Equal Protection Clause of the Fourteenth Amendment.[19]

In a series of cases involving the joint federal and state Aid to Families with Dependent Children (AFDC) program in the early 1970s, the Supreme Court and the lower federal courts read the federal statutes governing these programs expansively to protect the rights of indigents against arbitrary and oppressive conditions imposed by state administrators.[20] The Court also suggested—in cases invalidating the Virginia poll tax[21] and protecting the rights of indigent criminal defendants[22]—that indigents as a class might be entitled to special constitutional protection. When pushed to go further, however, and recognize some form of heightened scrutiny of welfare cases under the Fourteenth Amendment Equal Protection Clause, the Court in 1970 demurred, finding that welfare programs constituted economic and social legislation, subject to a minimal "reasonableness" standard of equal protection review.[23] Three years later, the Supreme Court definitively rejected the claim that indigents belonged to a "suspect class," which, if accepted, would have given indigents heightened protections from disadvantageous state actions.[24]

Moreover, in subsequent cases, the Court held that indigents have no particular right to public funding of health care. The issue arose in the context of abortion rights. In *Roe v. Wade* in 1973 the Supreme Court had held that states could not prohibit a woman from choosing to have an abortion, at least not in the early months of pregnancy.[25] Three years later, however, when the Court addressed the question of whether states had an obligation to fund Medicaid abortions for indigent women who would not otherwise be able to afford them, the Court stated: "The Constitution imposes no obligation on the States to pay for pregnancy-related medical expenses of indigent women, or indeed to pay any of the medical expenses of indigents."[26] In other words, even when a person has a recognized constitutional right to choose to undergo a health-care procedure, the government has no obligation to fund that service.

During the 1960s and 1970s, welfare rights advocates argued as an alternative position that even if the government has no constitutional obligation to establish any particular form of welfare or public health insurance program as such, once it does so, the rights of beneficiaries or recipients become in some sense vested property or contract rights and cannot be revoked or substantially altered without just compensation, or at least without due process.[27]

Insofar as the Constitution was clearly intended to protect property from confiscation by the government, recasting a right to welfare as a property right seemed for a time to be a promising strategy for those who sought justice for the poor. In a very influential article published in 1964, Charles Reich, then a professor at Yale Law School, argued that public licenses and benefits, including welfare benefits, had become a new form of property, equally worthy of constitutional protection as traditional property.[28]

Even before the "new property" theory entered the realm of public debate, however, a similar argument based on vested rights had been pressed with respect to American social insurance. The history of the development of the Medicare entitlement will be more fully explored in the next chapter. For the moment, however, suffice it to say that Medicare was established through an amendment to the Social Security Act, and it built on the model of the Social Security program as it was established in the 1930s.[29]

The Social Security program is funded through "contributions" or payroll taxes, assessed against workers who actively participate in the labor market. As the program was originally established, these contributions were to be paid into a trust fund that would be invested, with the invested capital eventually used to fund the retirement pension.[30] Beginning with the 1939 amendments to the Social Security Act, the program began to depend on the payroll tax to fund current obligations of the program, with the expectation that future contributions would pay for the retirement of current contributors.[31]

From the outset, however, supporters of the program encouraged contributors in the belief that they were paying now for their future retirement.[32] There was reason to believe this: Social Security contributions were accounted for in a Social Security trust fund, and only persons who had contributed to the program were eligible for benefits (indeed, no benefits were payable under the original act until 1942 to allow accumulation of individual contributions before disbursement). In addition, payments were proportionately related to income, and thus to contributions. The program was widely understood to be based on a contract between the government and contributors.[33]

In 1960, however, the Secretary of Health, Education and Welfare revoked the Social Security benefits of Ephram Nestor, an alien who for a time in the 1930s had been a member of the Communist Party. When Nestor challenged this action, claiming an "accrued property right" in Social Security benefits, the Supreme Court rejected his claim.[34] The Court recognized at the outset that

> the "right" to Social Security benefits is in one sense "earned," for the entire scheme rests on the legislative judgment that those who in their productive years were functioning members of the economy may justly call upon that economy, in their later years, for protection from "the rigors of the poor house as well as from the haunting fear that such a lot awaits them when journey's end is near."[35]

The Court proceeded to hold that "to engraft upon the Social Security system a concept of 'accrued property rights' would deprive it of the flexibility and boldness in adjustment to ever changing conditions which it demands."[36]

Thus, at the time Congress established the Medicare program six years later, the law was clear. A person who contributed to the Part A trust fund through Medicare payroll taxes could hope some day to receive Part A benefits, but any legal rights that a beneficiary had against the program were based on a statute that Congress was free to amend, even to repeal, and not on vested contract or property rights.

*Flemming v. Nestor* did not totally reject constitutional protection of social insurance entitlements, however. Having rejected the strong claim to vested entitlements, the Court observed:

> This is not to say, however, that Congress may exercise its power to modify the statutory scheme free of all constitutional restraint. The interest of a covered employee under the Act is of sufficient substance to fall within the protection from arbitrary governmental action afforded by the Due Process clause.[37]

Ten years later, in *Goldberg v. Kelly*,[38] the Court went further, recognizing that the due process clause also required that welfare recipients must be afforded an evidentiary hearing before their benefits could be terminated.[39] Although the defendant welfare department had in that case conceded that due process rights attended the termination of welfare benefits, Justice Brennan's majority opinion acknowledged Reich's "new property" thesis in a footnote[40] and went on to discuss the vital importance of welfare—not only to the recipient who depends on it "for the very means by which to live" but also for society, which benefits when the poor enjoy the opportunity to "participate meaningfully in the life of the community," as well as from the protection welfare affords from "the societal malaise that may flow from a widespread sense of unjustified frustration and insecurity."[41]

Although *Goldberg v. Kelly* aroused great hope among the advocates of broader constitutional rights in public benefits, it proved to be the high-water mark of judicial recognition of welfare rights.[42] A decade beyond *Goldberg v. Kelly*, a new majority in the Supreme Court opined the following in *Harris v.*

*McRae* (one of the abortion funding cases): "Although the liberty protected by the Due Process Clause affords protection against unwarranted government interference . . . it does not confer an entitlement to such [governmental aid] as may be necessary to realize all the advantages of that freedom."[43] Yet a decade further on, an ever more conservative Court noted, "Our cases have recognized that the Due Process Clauses generally confer no affirmative right to governmental aid, even when such aid may be necessary to secure life, liberty, or property interests of which the government may not deprive the individual."[44]

Although the Court never went beyond *Goldberg* in recognizing welfare rights—and has, in fact, since abandoned the rhetoric and reasoning on which *Goldberg* was based—the core holding of Goldberg remains intact. Ever since *Goldberg v. Kelly*, the Supreme Court has continued to accept the argument (conceded by the defendants in that case) that programs based on the Social Security Act create interests that are protected against precipitous termination by the due process clause. A recipient of Medicare or Medicaid enjoys an interest in the benefits of those programs that can only be terminated by an appropriate notice and hearing.[45] This constitutional "entitlement," however, is built on a property interest created by statute, not by the Constitution itself.

Two years after *Goldberg*, the Supreme Court decided in *Board of Regents of State Colleges v. Roth* that whether the due process clause attached to a particular claim against the government depends on the nature of the interest at issue, as defined by the relevant substantive law.[46] Literally read, the due process clause only provides due process when there is a threatened deprivation of "life, liberty, or property." The Supreme Court has basically settled on a positivist definition of property rights: property exists when it is recognized by law.[47] This creates a paradoxical situation in that neither the state nor the federal government can deprive a person of property without due process, but due process only protects property rights that are otherwise recognized by the state or federal government.[48]

In the area of public benefits, this understanding of property rights has made the character of statutory entitlements all the more important. Once Congress creates statutory entitlements the Constitution gives them real substance. Recipients of entitlements do not simply receive charity, subject to the whim of program administrators, but they have legal rights, much like those enjoyed by owners of traditional property. Before we move on to examine statutory entitlements, a few final comments on constitutional health-care entitlements are in order.

First, it should be noted (and has, in fact, frequently been noted by academic commentators), that the quest to establish constitutional welfare entitlements, including entitlements to health care, has always been a bit quixotic. Public health insurance programs are very costly and terribly complex. They are subject to the conflicting political claims of a variety of powerful provider (and consumer) groups. Although the courts can play, and have played, a useful role in constraining illegal or irrational actions of state and federal administrative agencies in their management of our public health-care programs, it is difficult to conceive of a court mandating the establishment of a public health insurance program or of playing a significant role in the expansion of such a program.[49]

Moreover, there are practical problems with relying on the judicial branch to define and effectuate an entitlement to health care. Persons in need of public health insurance are generally not in a position to pay lawyers to argue their cause. If they had money to pay lawyers, they could pay doctors. Public legal service programs, however, have very limited resources and have been under almost continuous attack since the 1970s.[50] Restrictions imposed on the federal legal services program in recent years have left it very limited in its ability to bring law reform litigation. A high proportion of the judges currently sitting on the federal bench, moreover, are appointees of conservative presidents and are thus unlikely to support judicial activism toward the end of expanding federal health-care programs.[51] Indeed, some conservative judges are more likely to pursue an activist role to limit these programs.[52]

These factors also are considerations in other countries with constitutional rights to health care. As noted at the outset of this chapter, constitutional provisions in other nations are usually quite vague and rarely result in litigation, much less in enforceable orders.[53] But they do express national aspirations, and they do become relevant in litigation that interprets the scope of entitlements. Thus, as discussed more fully later in Chapter 10, the German constitutional provision that expresses Germany's identity as a "social state," however vague, is a touchstone for the identity of Germany and for defining the character of its social health insurance system. Equally important, the absence of such a provision in the U.S. Constitution evidences the lack of such a national aspiration in our foundational documents, resulting in the lack of a fundamental commitment to a public health-care entitlement on our part. Thus, although the absence of a constitutional entitlement to health-care coverage in the United States has not ultimately blocked the development of legal health-care entitlements, it has rendered those entitlements more vulnerable to the proposed changes I discuss in later chapters.

## Medicare, Medicaid, and Federal Tax Subsidies as Statutory Entitlements

Just because we lack constitutional guarantees to health care, however, does not mean that we lack legal health-care entitlements. If mere repetition of the word *entitlement* in a government benefit statute created entitlements,

Medicare and Medicaid clearly qualify. The language of entitlement is deeply embedded in the Medicare and Medicaid statutes. For example, 42 U.S.C. § 426, which establishes the basic eligibility requirements for Medicare Part A (hospital) benefits, begins:

> (a) Every individual who—
>     (1) has attained age 65, and
>     [meets other program requirements]
> shall be entitled to hospital insurance benefits under part A of subchapter XVIII of this chapter . . .

Section 426 further states that persons who have been entitled to disability benefits for 24 months are also entitled to Part A hospital insurance.[54]

The language of entitlement is also found throughout Title XVIII of the Social Security Act (the Medicare statute) itself. 42 U.S.C. § 1395c, which describes the Medicare program:

> The insurance program for which entitlement is established by §§ 426 and 426-1 of this title provides basic protection against the costs of hospital, related post-hospital, home health services, and hospice care . . . [to persons entitled by virtue of meeting program requirements].

Also, 42 U.S.C. § 1395d describes the benefits available under Part A, the Hospital Insurance program, stating:

> The benefits provided to an individual by the insurance program under this part shall consist of entitlement to have payment made on his behalf [for Part A services].

The benefits provided under Part B of the Medicare program, the Supplementary Medical Insurance Program, are also described by 42 U.S.C. § 1395k as consisting of "entitlement to have payment made for him or on his behalf" for listed services.

Throughout Title XVIII, Medicare beneficiaries are referred to as "persons entitled to benefits" under Title XVIII or one of its subparts, a phrase that appears over 100 times in Title XVIII. The statute also occasionally refers to beneficiaries as "entitled" to specific services or payment for specific services.[55] In a few instances, Title XVIII also describes providers as "entitled" to payments for services.[56] Finally, the Medicare statute also uses the word *entitled* to describe the rights of beneficiaries of providers to fair hearings or other remedies.[57]

The words *entitled* and *entitlement* are also found throughout Title XIX of the Social Security Act, which created the Medicaid program, although Medicaid is not quite as forthright as Medicare in announcing itself to be an entitlement program. Medicaid is a joint federal and state program, and the decisions as to who will be eligible for services, what benefits they receive, and how providers will be paid for providing those services are to a considerable degree in the control of the states. Thus, 42 U.S.C. § 1396 describes the program as follows:

> For the purpose of enabling each State, as far as practicable under the conditions in such State, to furnish (1) medical assistance on behalf of families with dependent children and of aged, blind, or disabled individuals, whose income and resources are insufficient to meet the costs of necessary medical services, and (2) rehabilitation and other services to help such families and individuals attain or retain capability for independence or self-care, there is hereby authorized to be appropriated for each fiscal year a sum sufficient to carry out the purposes of this subchapter. The[se] sums . . . shall be used for making payments to States which have submitted, and had approved by the Secretary State plans for medical assistance.

The following section, 1396a,[58] describes the required contents of the state plan, and section 1396b provides for a state "entitlement" to funding for services under the state plan.[59]

Title XIX of the Social Security Act, like Title XVIII (though not nearly so often), identifies Medicaid recipients as "persons entitled to medical assistance" under Title XIX[60] or under a state plan approved under Title XIX.[61] This phrase is used most persistently in § 1396r—which governs program participation by nursing homes—where some variant of it is used eight times. Several sections of the Medicare statute also refer to persons entitled to medical assistance under Title XIX.[62] Title XIX, like Title XVIII, also occasionally refers to persons "entitled" to specific Medicaid services.[63] And it refers to recipients whose entitlement is limited to a particular service[64] or for a particular period of time[65] and to the entitlement of providers to Medicaid payments.[66] Finally, with respect to one particular Medicaid benefit—coverage on a first-come, first-served basis of Medicare cost sharing for a limited number of low-income individuals not otherwise eligible for Medicaid—Title XIX explicitly provides that "nothing in this subchapter shall be construed as establishing any entitlement" of these individuals to covered services.[67]

Even though Medicaid is a cooperative federal/state program, the federal statute takes precedence over the state law in specifying program requirements.[68] Although states are not required to participate in the Medicaid program, if they do so, they must conform to federal requirements.[69] The federal Medicaid statute thus creates an important federal entitlement against the states.

The sections of the Internal Revenue code that create income tax exclusions and deductions for amounts paid for and by employment-related group health-benefit plans do not use the word *entitlement*. Nonetheless, they create legally enforceable rights—our working definition of entitlements. Section 105(b) of the Internal Revenue Code, for example, states that "gross income does not include amounts [received through health insurance attributable to contributions of the employer] . . . if such amounts are paid, directly or indirectly, to the taxpayer to reimburse the taxpayer for expenses incurred by him for the medical care . . . of the taxpayer, his spouse, and his dependents." Section 106(a) provides that the "gross income of an employee does not include employer-provided coverage under an accident or health plan."[70] Section 3121(a)(2) also authorizes an employer to exclude the cost of employer-provided health insurance from payroll taxes. These provisions give employer and employees a legally enforceable right to exclude from their income amounts covered by these provisions.

The entitlement to exclusions and deductions for employment-related health insurance payments is structured in such a way that disputes rarely arise. The amount paid for health insurance and by insurers is not reported to the IRS by or with respect to any particular employee. Rather, employers report to the Internal Revenue Service (IRS) the amount they pay in total for employee benefits on the employer's tax return. Only where an audit brings the legitimacy of these deductions into question (as where a self-insured plan discriminates impermissibly in favor of "highly-compensated" employees), might the IRS question a deduction or exclusion under these provisions.[71] In the rare and unlikely event that the IRS questioned a deduction or exclusion for employer-financed employee health insurance, an administrative appeal would be available through the IRS Appeals Division, followed by an appeal to the tax court. Alternatively, the taxpayer could pay the tax and sue in the federal district court or the court of federal claims for a refund.[72]

In reality, however, a bigger issue is the nature of the entitlement that employees have to health-care services under their employee benefit plans. Historically, employee benefit plans were regarded as contracts, enforceable under contract law in state court. Traditionally, these contracts were regarded as adhesion contracts and interpreted very favorably to insureds. This was all changed by the Employee Retirement Income Security Act of 1974, ERISA.

ERISA was adopted to address abuses in employee retirement plans, but it also governs employee benefit plans, including employment-related health insurance. Section 514 of ERISA preempts state laws that "relate to" employee benefit plans. Although § 514(b)(2)(A) permits the states to regulate insurers that insure ERISA plans, § 514(b)(2)(B) prohibits the states from regulating ERISA plans themselves, which includes self-insured ERISA plans. Many employers currently self-insure, thus freeing themselves completely from state regulation. Until recently, the courts also interpreted the savings clause quite narrowly, freeing ERISA plan administrators, for example, from liability for bad faith denial of insurance benefits.[73] The Supreme Court's most recent pronouncement on the savings clause, however, signals a willingness to allow the states more leeway in regulating insured ERISA plans, even to the extent of strengthening the remedial rights of ERISA beneficiaries.[74] Moreover, ERISA does provide for federal remedies for plan members who have been denied benefits. These will be described further in subsequent sections of this chapter. Suffice it to say here that its overall thrust has been to provide only a limited entitlement of employees to insurance coverage.

To summarize, then, the Medicare and Medicaid statutes create statutory entitlements in their beneficiaries and recipients. Also, the Internal Revenue Code provisions dealing with tax deductions and exclusions for employment-related health-care benefits create an entitlement to a tax subsidy, but not to health insurance itself. ERISA, however, limits the rights of employees to health benefits even when their employer chooses to offer health benefits, although it also provides some protection for these rights.

Legal rights are hollow, however, unless they are protected by legal remedies, the topic to which we now turn.

## Entitlement to Federal Court Jurisdiction

Medicare, Medicaid, and federal health insurance tax subsidy entitlements are protected not only by federal law but also by the federal courts. A fuller history of the development of federal court jurisdiction in the Medicare and Medicaid programs is presented in Chapter 4. Because of the importance of this topic to a full understanding of the nature of the federal health-care entitlements, however, this subject is introduced here.

From the outset, the Medicare statute provided for judicial review of entitlement decisions and of Part A benefit decisions where the value of the claim was $1,000 or more.[75] In fact, the Medicare statute simply piggy-backed on earlier provisions found in the Social Security Act. When the Provider Reimbursement Review Board (PRRB) was established in 1972, judicial review was recognized for PRRB claims that exceed $10,000.[76] The statute was further amended in 1984 to provide for judicial review of Part B benefit determinations worth $1,000 or more.[77]

In fact, judicial review of Medicare decisions is subject to a number of limitations. First, in most instances, judicial review is available only after the exhaustion of lengthy administrative processes that involve multiple levels of review.[78] Second, judicial review of certain technical and methodological issues is specifically precluded by the Medicare statute.[79] Third, judicial review is not available as a matter of law, or as a practical matter, with respect to some other categories of cases—for example, there is no judicial review available for Part

A and B claims involving less than $1,000. Further, if a provider refuses to deliver services that the Centers for Medicare and Medicaid Services (CMS) has specified are not covered by Medicare, thereby making it impossible for the beneficiary to file a claim for the service and exhaust administrative remedies, the exhaustion requirement simply precludes the beneficiary from attacking the policy.[80] Finally, remedies available to courts reviewing certain decisions are limited by statute. For example, national coverage determinations, which decide whether a particular class of items or services is covered under Medicare, cannot be held unlawful or set aside for lack of compliance with the Administrative Procedure Act (APA) rule-making provisions.[81]

Attempts to obtain judicial review when it is not available by statute and precluded by 42 U.S.C. 405(h) have generally been rejected by the Supreme Court, despite repeated attempts by the lower courts to find some jurisdictional toehold. Successive Supreme Court cases have rejected arguments for review under general federal question jurisdiction,[82] through the Administrative Procedures Act,[83] or in the Court of Claims.[84]

In sum, Medicare beneficiaries and providers are entitled to appeal adverse individual or group claims that involve significant sums of money to the federal courts. Although policy issues involving payment or coverage can often be raised through individual claims, review of other policy decisions is limited or strictly forbidden. But although a very small percentage of Medicare cases get to court, decisions in these cases help guide the decisions of administrative law judges (ALJs) in administrative appeals. The ALJs can consider federal judicial opinions as precedent binding on the agency, and thus court decisions involving Medicare have a greater effect on the program than their number would indicate.

Unlike the Medicare statute, the Medicaid statute does not explicitly provide for federal judicial review of Medicaid eligibility or claims decisions. Nevertheless, almost from the outset, the federal courts have allowed Medicaid beneficiaries to challenge state Medicaid decisions under 42 U.S.C. § 1983, a Reconstruction-era civil-rights law that states:

> Every person who, under color of any statute, . . . of any State . . . subjects, or causes to be subjected, any citizen of the United States or other person within the jurisdiction thereof to the deprivation of any rights, privileges, or immunities secured by the Constitution and laws, shall be liable to the party injured in an action at law, suit in equity, or other proper proceeding for redress.

In 1990 the Supreme Court went further, explicitly recognizing the right of providers to bring § 1983 suits as well.[85] Federal courts generally do not require exhaustion of state administrative or judicial remedies prior to the initiation of a § 1983 action,[86] although they may abstain to permit resolution of an issue of state law.[87] As federal administrative remedies are not generally available for review of state Medicaid policies, exhaustion of federal administrative remedies is not an issue.[88] Therefore, it is much easier to get into federal court with a Medicaid claim than with a Medicare claim.[89]

Once a Medicaid claimant gets into federal court, however, the remedies available are much more limited than those available in a Medicare case. The Eleventh Amendment does not permit a suit to be brought against a state without the state's consent, and a state does not consent to suit simply by participating in Medicaid.[90] Suit may be brought against officials who administer a state Medicaid program, but only for prospective relief.[91] Retroactive relief that affects the state treasury is prohibited.

Despite these jurisdictional limitations, however, the federal courts seem somewhat more willing to consider challenges to Medicaid than to Medicare policies. In recent years the federal courts have been remarkably deferential to the Department of Health and Human Services (HSS) in its administration of Medicare, and the level of deference becomes greater the higher the court. The secretary of HSS won each of the six Supreme Court Medicare cases litigated in the 1990s.[92] During two recent years surveyed in a study by the author,[93] DHHS prevailed in 88% of the Medicare cases it litigated at the court of appeals level and 70% of the cases it litigated at the district court level.[94] In Medicare cases, the courts have rigorously applied the doctrine of *Chevron v. Natural Resources Defense Council*, under which they must defer to an administrative agency in its interpretation of a statute that it administers if the interpretation is not clearly contrary to the plain meaning of a statute and is reasonable.[95] The courts also defer to HHS in its interpretations of its own rules, which, under *Thomas Jefferson v. Shalala*,[96] the courts may not ignore unless the agency's interpretation is "plainly erroneous or inconsistent with the regulation."[97] The courts show little interest in taking control of the complex and technical Medicare program from HHS, and they rarely intervene except where HHS seems clearly to be overreaching.

Plaintiffs seem to be somewhat more successful in reported cases challenging Medicaid program decisions or requirements in federal court; although again, the level of deference varies by level of court. During 1999, recipients and providers prevailed in 53% of the reported cases that they brought against Medicaid programs, while in 2000 they prevailed in 48% of these cases.[98] In the courts of appeals, however, Medicaid agencies prevailed 83% of the time in 1999 and 81% of the time in the year 2000. Success rates varied dramatically between providers and recipients, moreover. Recipients prevailed 61% of the time in suits against Medicaid agencies in both 1999 and 2000, while providers prevailed only 35% of the time in 1999 and 38% of the time in 2000.

Federal courts commonly assert that they accord substantial deference to the states in administering their Medicaid programs.[99] Judges claim that they will only invalidate state Medicaid regulations or decisions shown to be arbitrary and capricious or in violation of federal law.[100] Federal courts, however, are not reluctant to make this finding if a state is sufficiently unreasonable, particularly if the rights of an indigent recipient are at issue.[101] Federal administrative approval of a state plan, moreover, is commonly provided little deference by the courts, which recognize the cursory nature of federal review.[102] The Supreme Court's recent decision in *Wisconsin Department of Social Services v. Blumer*, is typical of these cases.[103] While the Supreme Court ultimately upheld Wisconsin's approach to determining eligibility in that case, ostensibly deferring to the state and to the HHS which had authorized the methodology used by the state, the Court also engaged in a searching analysis of the statute and statutory scheme, and three justices dissented, claiming the state and HHS had misinterpreted the statute.

Litigants have been only slightly less successful in state than in federal court in Medicaid cases. During 2000, state Medicaid agencies prevailed in 59% of reported cases against recipients and providers, while in 1999, they prevailed in 54%.[104] Recipients were substantially less successful in state than in federal court, however. In 2000 they won only 41% of state court reported cases (compared to 61% in federal court), while in 1999 recipients won 50% of reported state court cases (compared to 61% in federal court.

The nature of federal Medicaid litigation is very different, however, from litigation brought in state court. In the year 2000, three-quarters of reported cases challenging Medicaid agency policies or decisions in federal court were brought as class actions or had multiple or organizational plaintiffs, and only one-quarter were brought by individuals. In reported state court cases, the statistics were almost precisely the reverse: three-quarters of the cases involved individuals, and only one-quarter class actions, associations, or multiple plaintiffs. Nearly three-quarters of the cases, moreover, were cases appealing administrative decisions rather than original cases brought to challenge agency policies.

These statistics illustrate why federal court jurisdiction has long been thought to be important for challenging state Medicaid policies.[105] State court judges, appointed by the state governor or elected in periodic elections, are understandably reluctant to order the state to adopt policies that might significantly increase state expenditures.[106] Moreover, state court cases tend to involve individual appeals and to have far less influence on state Medicaid policy than does corresponding federal litigation involving class actions. In addition, state courts might come up with inconsistent interpretations of federal law, thus undermining the national scope of the Medicaid program. Also, suits against state Medicaid programs in federal court provide leverage for state Medicaid directors to argue for state budget allocations for their programs.[107] Finally, it makes sense for the federal courts to take responsibility for hearing disputes involving such a massive federal program.

Federal jurisdiction is even more readily available in federal court over disputes that involve tax subsidies for employment-related group insurance. Depending on the procedures followed, adverse IRS decisions involving these exclusions can be challenged in the tax courts, the federal district courts, or the Court of Federal Claims, and internal IRS appeals procedures need not even be fully exhausted before judicial review is sought. In fact, however, there are few reported cases involving these exclusions, indicating that they rarely figure in disputes. Disputes only arise under these provisions if the IRS challenges a claim for tax exclusion or deduction, and the grounds under which these exclusions can be challenged are relatively few. Although federal jurisdiction is readily available under these provisions, therefore, it is rarely invoked.

More important to employees insured under employee benefit plans is the federal jurisdiction available under ERISA for disputes concerning the coverage of those plans. Section 502 of ERISA provides federal court jurisdiction over the decisions of ERISA plan administrators.[108] Indeed, the Supreme Court has interpreted ERISA to preempt state court jurisdiction over ERISA benefit claims in favor of federal jurisdiction, even though ERISA itself provides for concurrent jurisdiction.[109]

As noted in the preceding section, the lack of a constitutional right to health care means that the courts cannot generally call into question the decisions that the legislature makes with respect to health care. American courts, however, do take responsibility for interpreting legislation and thus will hear challenges against the acts of administrative agencies in applying entitlement law. The federal courts also exercise authority over the states when questions of federal rights arise, even rejecting state constitutional provisions when they come into conflict with federal entitlement program requirements.[110] The involvement of the American courts, however, is far from consistent. The next section presents a more nuanced overview of their role.

## Functional Meanings of Entitlements for Providers and Beneficiaries

Entitlement claims arise primarily in four different types of disputes. First, and most basic, are disputes involving recipient eligibility for programs. Second are disputes that arise when persons who are eligible for programs are denied coverage for particular services. Third are disputes involving providers for whom program participation is denied or revoked. Fourth are payment amount disputes, which will normally involve providers, but may involve beneficiaries if they receive services for which they must pay and seek indemnification.

## Eligibility

Eligibility disputes under both Parts A and B of Medicare are subject to administrative and judicial review. Anyone eligible for Social Security old age assistance or Railroad Retirement (and since 1972, who has been receiving Social Security disability for two or more years) is eligible for Part A.[111] Any citizen of the United States or person legally resident in the United States for five or more years who is over 65 or disabled and enrolls in Part B is entitled to Part B services.[112] Decisions regarding the entitlement of beneficiaries for Part A or Part B benefits are made by the Social Security Administration, subject to reconsideration, review by a Social Security administrative law judge, the Appeals Council, and, ultimately judicial review.[113] Disputes as to Medicare's straightforward eligibility requirements should be relatively uncommon, however.

Eligibility for Medicaid is much more contentious. First, Medicaid eligibility is based on membership in a "worthy poor" category, which, when the program was established, meant the aged, the blind, the permanently and totally disabled, and the families of dependent children. Covered categories have expanded over time to include, for example, pregnant women or children whose family incomes are below the federal poverty level, and there are currently about 60 categories of Medicaid eligibles.[114] Medicaid recipients must also be financially eligible for services—that is, their income and assets must be low enough to qualify under federal or state limits.

Medicaid eligibility requirements offer many opportunities for disputes to arise. Although these disputes can involve whole classes of individuals, they more often turn on the facts of individual cases. A recurrent cause of disputes, for example, is the application of prohibitions against transfers of assets to create eligibility.[115]

Eligibility for tax subsidies for employment-related group insurance, in contrast, rarely results in disputes. Self-insured plans must not discriminate in favor of highly-compensated employees.[116] Yet the paucity of reported cases involving §§ 105 and 106 indicates that eligibility seldom comes up as an issue. Cafeteria plans must meet more requirements, and result in more disputes, but legislation and regulations promulgated in the past two decades have resolved many of the more contentious issues regarding these programs.[117]

## Benefit Coverage

Benefit coverage disputes have proved more contentious, under both the Medicare and Medicaid programs. Medicare is not a comprehensive program, but it does cover about 55 different types of goods and services. Many of the categories, however, such as physician or hospital services, are quite broad. The

Medicare statute provides that "payment cannot be made for any services determined to be not reasonable and necessary for the diagnosis or treatment of illness or injury, to improve the functioning of a malformed body member."[118] Thus decisions must be made regarding coverage of specific goods or services.

Most coverage decisions are made initially by Medicare carriers or intermediaries. A beneficiary dissatisfied with an initial decision regarding coverage of Medicare goods or services may request a redetermination by the carrier or intermediary.[119] If the beneficiary remains dissatisfied, he or she may, under a new procedure effective 1 October 2002, receive an independent medical review by one of 12 qualified independent contractors that contracts with Medicare for this purpose, and which is directed to consider "clinical experience and medical, technical, and scientific evidence."[120] A beneficiary who loses at the reconsideration stage may request a hearing before an ALJ if the amount in controversy is $100 or more.[121] The ALJ decision may be appealed to the Departmental Appeals Board (DAB).[122] Final decisions may be reviewed by the federal courts if $1,000 or more is at issue.[123] The Benefits Improvement and Protection Act (BIPA) of 2000 has imposed time frames for each step of this process (including expedited time frames for decisions to discharge an individual from a provider institution or where a physician certifies that delay could pose a significant risk to the beneficiary's health).[124]

Medicare disputes have focused in particular on coverage of new technologies or new applications of existing technologies.[125] Historically, most coverage decisions have been made by intermediaries and carriers at the local level, but HHS has always made national coverage decisions in some circumstances— such as where there are conflicting local policies, a new service represents a significant medical advance or has provoked considerable controversy as to effectiveness, a service is currently covered but considered obsolete, or a service raises particular program integrity issues.[126] HCFA published proposed rules for making such decisions in late 1989, but the proposals faced strong opposition and were never implemented.[127] Much of the controversy concerned the position taken by the proposed rules that the cost of a new technology should be considered in coverage decisions. Unable to overcome this controversy, HCFA proceeded informally, publishing its coverage decisions in its *Coverage Issues Manual*.[128]

In late 1998 HCFA created a Medicare Coverage Advisory Committee (MCAC), consisting of 120 health-care experts to assist it in developing Medicare coverage policy.[129] In May 1999, HCFA published a notice describing the procedures it intended to use for making national coverage decisions using the MCAC.[130] In 2000, BIPA established procedures for reviewing national coverage decisions.[131]

A beneficiary in need of a noncovered item or service may request a national coverage determination, and the secretary of HHS must act on the request within 90 days (even though one of the actions the secretary may take is to state that the review will take longer than 90 days, and explain why).[132] HCFA makes coverage decisions using the MCAC, together with review by its own staff and independent research and extramural assessment, to develop coverage policy. A beneficiary adversely affected by a coverage decision may seek review by the Departmental Appeals Board, subject to judicial review.[133]

Medicare coverage decisions have proved very contentious over the years. Coverage decisions most commonly concern drugs and devices and bring well-funded pharmaceutical companies and medical equipment manufacturers, who are not themselves Medicare providers, into conflict with the governing agency, now the Center for Medicare and Medicaid Services (CMS). The agency takes the position that new technologies should not be approved unless they in fact demonstrate medical benefit and offer "added value" to the program, either in terms of lower cost or in terms of benefits not available through existing covered technologies. Nevertheless, technology manufacturers (and sometimes beneficiaries and their physicians) have complained that Medicare should approve all technologies that are not demonstrably unnecessary or ineffective and should not itself make decisions that are properly medical decisions. They also argue that Medicare's coverage determination process deprives beneficiaries of beneficial technologies that are available to privately insured patients.[134]

Medicaid benefit coverage is established by each state, subject to very broad federal guidelines. States must cover a limited range of essential services but may cover a long and exhaustive list of additional services. A state's Medicaid plan must specify the amount, duration, and scope of each service that it provides for the categorically needy and each group of the medically needy.[135] According to the regulations, "Each service must be of sufficient amount, duration, and scope to reasonably achieve its purpose."[136] State restrictions on benefits may be challenged in state or federal court.

While a Medicaid recipient is in theory entitled by virtue of eligibility to receive covered services, states retain a great deal of discretion in determining coverage. A state Medicaid regulation limiting reimbursable physician visits to three per month, except in emergencies, was upheld, for example, against a challenge under the "amount, duration, and scope" regulation,[137] but an excessively restrictive drug formulary was not.[138] The Medicaid agency is prohibited from arbitrarily denying or reducing the "amount, duration, or scope of a required service . . . solely because of the diagnosis, type of illness, or condition."[139] Thus a state provision covering eyeglasses for individuals suffering from eye disease, but not for individuals with refractive error, was invalidated,[140] as was a $50,000 cap on payment for hospital services that precluded coverage of $200,000 liver transplants. A state may place appropriate limits on a service based on medical necessity or utilization control criteria, however.[141] On the whole, the Medicaid program presents more opportunities for benefit coverage disputes than does the Medicare program, but because recipients often lack access to legal representation, few disputes actually end up in court, and when they do, courts usually afford the state a fair amount of discretion to state administrators in determining coverage.

The laws that create tax subsidies for employment-related insurance do not specify any benefits that must be covered by such insurance.[142] ERISA, moreover, gives employers completely unbridled discretion to determine the benefits that may be covered or not covered under ERISA plans.[143] ERISA also, as noted, preempts state laws that mandate coverage of specific benefits, even though such laws may be saved as laws regulating insurance, except insofar as they attempt to cover self-insured plans.

ERISA only provides a federal remedy if plans fail to comply with contractual requirements or breach their fiduciary obligations. The remedies available to beneficiaries denied services by an ERISA plan, therefore, are quite limited. In *Firestone Tire Co. v. Bruch*, the Supreme Court interpreted ERISA to require the courts to engage in de novo review of plan benefit decisions.[144] *Firestone*, however, recognized an exception that swallowed the rule: plans could reserve discretion in themselves to make plans decisions and thereby only expose themselves to "abuse of discretion" review. Because ERISA plans now routinely do this, ERISA benefit claims cases have effectively become administrative review cases, in which the federal courts review plan decisions for arbitrariness and capriciousness.[145] Only where the court can be convinced that the plan faced a conflict of interest in its decision making (and the courts vary widely in their willingness to find conflicts)[146] will a court engage in a more searching review of plan decisions. The upshot is that courts are rarely willing to second-guess plan decision makers.

## Provider Participation

Providers who meet program certification requirements are entitled to participate in both the Medicare and Medicaid programs. In an effort to appease providers who were either hostile to or suspicious of these programs at their founding, Medicare and Medicaid imposed minimal participation requirements on providers.[147] Both programs initially guaranteed recipients free choice of providers. Hospitals could participate in Medicare if they met either Joint Commission on Accreditation of Hospitals or Medicare certification requirements. Physicians needed merely to be licensed. Nursing homes had to be certified by the states as meeting minimal requirements.

Over time, as scandal after scandal broke in the nursing-home industry, Medicare and Medicaid tightened up program participation requirements. For a very brief period in the late 1980s, moreover, Medicare Peer Review Organizations (PROs) attempted to exclude from program participation a few physicians who were grossly incompetent.[148] More providers were excluded from program participation under program fraud provisions as fraud and abuse enforcement was stepped up in the 1990s. Finally, the move to managed care contracting, discussed in Chapter 5, augmented by Medicaid amendments in 1997 that allowed limitation of recipient freedom of choice, has led to exclusive contracting by some state Medicaid plans.

The initial decision as to whether a provider or supplier qualifies to participate in the Medicare program is made by the CMS.[149] Prospective providers and suppliers dissatisfied with this determination may request a reconsideration.[150] Providers and suppliers dissatisfied with a reconsidered determination—as well as terminated or suspended providers, suppliers, or practitioners—may appeal to an ALJ and then to the Departmental Appeals Board.[151] Medicare+Choice (M+C) organizations that are denied contracts, are terminated, or are not renewed may appeal to an ALJ, and M+C organizations that are terminated or not renewed may further appeal to the administrator.[152]

While both Medicare and Medicaid have historically attempted to encourage maximum program participation by providers, on the relatively rare occasions that program participation has been denied or revoked, the courts have been ambivalent about recognizing a provider entitlement in participation. The issue has commonly come up in situations where providers have lost participation status and have sought equitable relief to bar their exclusion before an administrative hearing is conducted. In these cases, the courts have repeatedly refused to require pretermination hearings. Although the reason given most commonly is that a posttermination hearing (generally provided by statute) is adequate,[153] some courts have gone further to deny the applicability of due process requirements at all. Some of these cases have denied the existence of a property right in providers to program participation, and some have recognized that providers denied program participation might suffer deprivation of a liberty interest by virtues of damage to reputation.[154]

Providers have no rights to participation in employment-related group insurance programs under the federal tax laws. Also, ERISA provides no guarantees for provider participation. In fact, in recent years, private health-care plans have increasingly limited coverage to "in-network" providers. A few states have adopted "any willing provider" laws, protecting the rights of providers to participate in health plans, while other states offer due process review rights to providers terminated from health plans, but ERISA preempts these laws with respect to self-insured health plans.[155]

## Provider Payment

Providers who care for Medicare beneficiaries and Medicaid recipients are entitled to payment, but both Medicare and Medicaid generally set payment rates administratively and offer them on a take it or leave it basis. The Medicare statute provides for a special forum, the PRRB, for hearing appeals involving payment of hospitals and other institutional providers, PRRB if the amount in controversy is $10,000 or more.[156] Decisions of the PRRB are reviewable by the administrator of the CMS at his or her discretion.[157] The provider may then seek judicial review of the PRRB or administrator's decision. Finally, the Medicare statute also provides special provisions for Medicare+Choice appeals.[158]

Initially, Medicare paid for most Part A services on a cost basis and Part B services on a charge basis. These methods generated endless disputes, and, beginning with diagnosis-related-group prospective hospital payment in 1983, Medicare has moved to prospective payment for almost all services.[159] Each of the statutes creating prospective payment programs has removed more and more issues from judicial review. At this point, therefore, providers are only able to raise a narrow range of issues in Medicare payment disputes. In sum, providers are entitled to payment for Medicare services, but only to payment at the level Medicare determines appropriate.

The Supreme Court's 1990 decision in *Wilder v. Virginia Hospital Association*[160] established the right of Medicaid providers to go directly into federal court to contest payment rates. Medicaid payment cases have historically been brought primarily by hospitals and nursing homes, which usually have little choice but to participate in Medicaid, but which suffer greatly under low payment rates. Attempts by the states to limit hospital and nursing-home payments during the 1970s, 1980s, and early 1990s provoked numerous lawsuits under the 1976 "Boren Amendment," which required the states to pay for hospital, skilled nursing facility, and intermediate-care facilities on a "reasonable cost related basis, as determined in accordance with methods and standards . . . developed . . . on the basis of cost-finding methods approved and verified" by HHS.[161]

Boren Amendment litigation was always a risky enterprise for providers, at best resulting in a temporary reprieve from budget cuts while the state reconstructed its rates following proper procedures. Such litigation, however, was a major source of annoyance to the states. In the 1997 BBA, therefore, Congress abolished the Boren Amendment, putting in its place much less burdensome procedural requirements, which a subsequent court decision has held to preclude future litigation in federal court involving state provider-rate setting.[162]

The 1997 Balanced Budget Act did not end litigation over Medicaid rates, however. Federal Medicaid law also requires payment rates to be "consistent with efficiency, economy, and quality of care and . . . sufficient to enlist enough providers so that care and services are available under the plan at least to the extent that such care and services are available to the general population in the geographic area."[163] Several courts have held that this statute gives providers enforceable rights,[164] but others have rejected this position,[165] while still others have held that the provision does not compel the state to follow any particular methodology in setting rates.[166]

In sum, while, in theory, Medicaid entitles providers to payment for services that they provide to Medicaid recipients, the discretion that the states exercise over payment levels is considerable, and only rarely and in egregious situations have providers been successful in compelling states to increase payment rates through litigation.

Providers have no rights to payment under the federal tax laws that subsidize employment-related health insurance. ERISA also does not explicitly afford a remedy to providers, but neither does it explicitly preempt provider remedial rights. Some courts have permitted providers to recover on the basis of an assignment from a beneficiary or on estoppel theories, if the plan had made representations that a service would be covered.[167] Many states have also adopted laws requiring insurers to pay providers promptly, which have increasingly been enforced against insured plans.

## Conclusion

The functional role of legal institutions in the operation of our health-care entitlement programs is complex and inconsistent. The Medicare statute creates the clearest statutory entitlement and explicitly provides for judicial review. In reality, however, the rights of Medicare beneficiaries and providers exist primarily in the context of a multilayered system of administrative review, which must be exhausted before access to the courts becomes possible. Once the aggrieved beneficiary or provider reaches the courts, moreover, the courts usually defer to the decisions of the administrators that preceded their review. This system is not a bad one: it concentrates decision-making authority in those who have the expertise in the pertinent area, conserves judicial resources, and affords more control over expenditures. But it also weakens accountability and can prove frustrating to providers and confusing to beneficiaries.

The Medicaid program is vaguer in the rights and remedies that it affords, but the courts have filled in many of the gaps left by Congress. In fact, the federal courts are more immediately accessible to Medicaid recipients than to Medicare beneficiaries, since they do not impose exhaustion requirements. In addition, federal courts have proved somewhat more amenable to hearing recipient and, occasionally, provider complaints. Because Medicaid recipients, the poorest of the poor, lack the political clout of Medicare beneficiaries and often suffer from a "brutal need"[168] for health-care services, it is appropriate that the courts afford special solicitude to their rights. Nevertheless, the frailty of the statutory protections afforded Medicaid recipients is a real cause for concern. The courts of today are much less sympathetic to the needs of the poor than were the courts of a generation ago, and today's courts cannot always be depended on to protect the poor.

Finally, on its face it seems ironic that employees, the wealthiest and least-dependent beneficiaries of health-care entitlements, seem to enjoy the most limited entitlement claims in our system. Even though their rights to tax subsidies are clear and readily enforceable, these tax subsidies are only of value if they are successful in stimulating employers to offer group insurance coverage. If employers decide to offer coverage, moreover, plan members have only limited rights to benefits under ERISA.

The logic of this situation is discernable, however. If employees depend on the grace of their employers for insurance coverage, then a system that imposes minimal legal risks and obligations on employers who do offer coverage is likely to result in broader coverage than one that imposes greater obligations. Employees with the most bargaining power (who will also probably have the most political clout), moreover, are likely to secure benefit packages that are satisfactory for themselves. Unfortunately, however, this system fails many employees who receive no coverage whatsoever, and it frustrates others who find that their rights are very limited when they need to claim the protection of the insurance they have.

This review of the constitutional, statutory, and remedial aspects of our health-care entitlements does not exhaust our consideration of their implications in our health-care system because entitlements also exist as budgetary and political concepts. To these final meanings of entitlements I now turn.

## Entitlement as a Budget Function

When politicians fret about entitlements, they are usually not thinking about constitutional or statutory entitlements, or about federal court jurisdiction to defend them, but rather about the budget. Both Medicare and Medicaid are classified as entitlement programs for the purposes of the federal budget process. The Congressional Research Service (CRS) defines entitlement in this sense as follows:

> Entitlements are statutory requirements that government payments be made to any individual or unit of government that meets eligibility criteria established in the law. Entitlements are a binding obligation on the government, and eligible recipients have legal recourse if the obligation is not met.[169]

As so defined, federal entitlements have existed since 1776, when the Continental Congress established a pension system for disabled veterans.[170] Pension entitlements became a major federal budget expense following the Civil

War, a story told in the next chapter. By 1910, 28.5% of all American men aged 65 and over were recipients of Civil War pension entitlements.[171] But the modern period of American entitlements dates from 1935, when the Social Security Old Age Pension program was established as an entitlement. When Medicare and Medicaid were created in 1965, they were created as entitlements as well, following the Social Security model.

Entitlements are grouped together with other categories of expenditures, such as interest payments on the national debt or salaries for the federal judiciary, into a budget category called "mandatory" or "direct" expenditures.[172] Mandatory expenditures are contrasted with "discretionary" expenditures. Discretionary expenditures are controlled by the annual congressional appropriations process and are thus subject to the will of Congress.[173] While some mandatory expenditures (such as Medicare) have permanent appropriations, others (including Medicaid) require annual appropriations,[174] but in either case Congress must fund mandatory expenditures as needed to meet program obligations. Mandatory expenditures currently cover about two-thirds of federal government spending.

Under the current federal budgetary process,[175] which is based on the 1974 Congressional Budget and Impoundment Control Act,[176] as modified by the 1985 Balanced Budget and Emergency Deficit Control Act (Gramm–Rudman–Hollings, or GRH) Act,[177] and the Budget Enforcement Act (BEA) of 1990,[178] (with lesser amendments in 1993, and 1997),[179] Congress adopts a budget resolution every spring in response to the president's budget.[180] This resolution establishes budget authority and outlay levels for the next five fiscal years.[181] It also distributes federal spending among 20 functional categories and among the House and Senate committees with jurisdiction over spending, principally the appropriations committees. The appropriations committees further divide their allocations among their 13 subcommittees, which are responsible for the 13 regular appropriations bills that provide discretionary funding for the government.[182]

The appropriations bills submitted by the appropriations committees are usually considered first by the House and then by the Senate.[183] Budget ceilings imposed on these discretionary appropriations measures are enforced through two different processes. First a member can block (a) appropriation bills that exceed committee or subcommittee allocations; (b) amendments that would cause an appropriations bill to exceed allocated authority or program authorization, or to violate the special rules under which a bill is debated (or that are not germane to the bill); or (c) bills or amendments that would cause appropriations in total to exceed total annual discretionary budget limits—by raising a point of order.[184] Second, discretionary appropriations that exceed spending limits are subject to sequestration. If Congress enacts discretionary appropriations that exceed spending limits it has established, the president is required to impose automatic across-the-board reductions to eliminate the excess in the particular category.[185]

Mandatory spending, including entitlement spending, is treated very differently. Although some entitlement programs require annual appropriations, actual outlays are determined by eligibility, benefit, and payment rules, which are established by the legislation that authorizes the programs. That is, mandatory spending is not subject to annual budget limits.

The 1990 BEA established a new procedure that focused on limiting legislated increases in mandatory programs. Under the 1990 Pay-As-You-Go, or PAYGO, procedures, new direct spending and revenue legislation must be revenue neutral.[186] Under these rules, any direct spending or revenue reductions (tax cuts or new tax expenditures) must be offset in an equivalent amount by direct spending reductions or revenue increases, or both.[187] Spending in excess of PAYGO limitations is subject to sequestration. Sequestration is triggered automatically when the Office of Management and Budget (OMB) determines that the net effect of new direct spending or revenue legislation enacted in the current or the immediately prior sessions of Congress increases the deficit or reduces the surplus.[188] Social Security benefits, federal deposit insurance guarantee commitments, tax expenditures, and direct spending or revenue legislation designated as emergency legislation are free from the PAYGO sequestration, while Medicare sequestration is limited to a 4% reduction.[189] PAYGO limits are also enforced by procedural rules in the Senate, where a point of order can be raised challenging legislation violating PAYGO limits, which can only be waived by a three-fifths vote.[190] PAYGO rules and enforcement procedures, however, only apply to legislated changes in entitlement programs and have no application when program expenditures increase due to increases in the number of persons eligible for the program or in the cost of benefits as determined by established payment rules.

Changes in entitlement programs are not enacted through the regular appropriations bills that fund discretionary programs, but rather though omnibus budget reconciliation acts (OBRAs). Although the reconciliation process was originally conceived in the 1974 budget legislation as a wrap-up process for bringing the total budget into balance, it has become the means by which congressional leadership (often through negotiations with the president) changes mandatory spending and revenue programs both to enforce PAYGO requirements and to fulfill their legislative agendas.[191]

Under the reconciliation process, the budget committees adopt reconciliation instructions directing substantive committees to make changes in mandatory spending or revenue programs to meet specific targets.[192] The budget committees collate recommendations from the substantive committees "without any substantive revision," adding their own recommendations when a substantive committee fails to report.[193] The resulting omnibus bills are usually enormous and very complex. Debate and amendments are governed by rules that allow congressional leadership to strictly limit them.[194] In particular, under the 1974 legislation, no amendment can be considered to an OBRA that would increase the deficit or decrease the surplus, and no amendment can be offered that is not germane to the legislation.[195]

While OBRAs have been used to enact significant changes in the Medicare and Medicaid programs over the past two decades, the potential for change through OBRAs is not unlimited. The Byrd Rule in the Senate permits any senator to challenge a provision of an OBRA as "extraneous," which generally means that it is not directed at changing outlays or revenues.[196] A three-fifths vote is required to waive the Byrd Rule, which has been used quite frequently in recent years to block attempts to make substantive changes in entitlement programs through the reconciliation process.

Tax expenditures are not considered to be entitlements for the budget process. Indeed, they are not even considered to be expenditures, and therefore are not subject to the appropriations process. New tax expenditures, however, are subject to the PAYGO procedures, under which they are treated as revenue reductions and must be offset by reductions in direct spending or tax increases.[197] Adjustments in tax expenditures, moreover, are normally handled through OBRAs, where they are included alongside entitlement expansions or reductions. Tax deductions and exclusions (or credits) to subsidize health insurance, therefore, are the budgetary equivalent of entitlement spending.

Much has been made of the contrast between discretionary spending, which is tightly controlled through the budget process, and mandatory spending, which is controlled only by program eligibility and payment limits, and has grown from 40% of total federal spending in 1975 to two-thirds today.[198] Proposals to impose caps on entitlements in general, or on Medicare and Medicaid in particular, were seriously debated in the mid-1990s.[199]

However, mandatory spending seems to be a necessary concomitant of the establishment of entitlements by federal law, enforceable by beneficiaries and providers in the federal courts. Congress can, and frequently does, change program eligibility, benefit, or payment provisions, but unless and until it does, it cannot simply refuse to meet program obligations for budgetary reasons without radically changing what it means to be a legal entitlement. Tax subsidies are even more carefully shielded from budget control, as they are not even considered expenditures.

The open-ended budgetary nature of American health-care entitlements is unusual in the international context. As noted in later chapters in this volume, the health-care systems of other countries operate within a more or less fixed budget and allocate resources within the constraints of that budget. Entitlements, then, do not translate into mandated expenditures on the part of the government. The open-ended nature of American entitlements contributes significantly to their expense and to the uncontrolled nature of American entitlement spending, a theme to which this book returns later. Before concluding this consideration of the nature of health-care entitlements, however, it must be acknowledged that entitlement claims are not just legal and budgetary; they are also political in nature.

## Political Entitlements

Budgetary entitlements and tax expenditures enjoy a special political status in our system. Their exclusion from the annual appropriations process is emblematic of this special political status.

The obvious advantage of a constitutional as opposed to a statutory entitlement is that it would not be subject to the legislative will. It is very difficult to amend the Constitution, and convincing the Supreme Court to change its mind once it has recognized a constitutional right is also a formidable task. In contrast, a legislature may change its mind from session to session.

Certain characteristics of the Medicare and Medicaid programs and of employment-related health insurance tax subsidies, however, make legislative change difficult. The federal tax subsidies for employment-related insurance, for example, constitute our second most expensive tax expenditure (after employer contributions for pensions), and benefit 172 million Americans.[200] Any attempt to eliminate these subsidies would be perceived as a tax increase and would be very unpopular politically.

The financing of Medicare is also structured to provide significant political protection. The entitlement language used in the Medicare program was used intentionally to encourage the belief that the program was, in fact, an insurance program in which contributors had vested rights. Section 1395c uses the term "insurance" in describing the program. The word "insurance" is also used in the titles of Part A and Part B (the "Hospital Insurance" and "Supplementary Medical Insurance" programs). These terms, of course, evoke the notion of contractual rights inherent in private insurance programs.

The funding of the program through payroll tax contributions was also intended to ensure its political sanctity. President Franklin Roosevelt is quoted as having said of Social Security, "We put those payroll contributions in there so as to give the contributors a legal, moral, and political right to collect their pension and their unemployment benefits. With those taxes in there, no damn politician can ever scrap my social security program," and the same psychology carries through into Medicare.[201]

Medicare's "trust fund" financing also contributes to the program's political security. Protecting the Medicare program from future political attack was one factor motivating the trust fund financing of the program.[202] Even though the impending "bankruptcy" of the Medicare Part A trust fund from time to time has been used as an argument for cutting back the program, trust fund funding of the program has both contributed to the sense of ownership that beneficiaries have in the program and to the reliance that Americans place in its continued existence.[203]

Medicaid, of course, is funded through general revenue funds and by state and federal taxes. It is generally thought of as a welfare rather than a social insurance program. One would expect it to be more vulnerable than Medicare—and, in fact, it is. Yet its vulnerability can be overestimated, as it was by the Republican Congress in 1995, when President Bill Clinton's veto of their budget bill, which would have eliminated Medicaid as a federal entitlement, played a part in positioning the then-weak president for reelection a year later. A particular political advantage of the Medicaid program, moreover, is that it funnels money into the states, which can be counted on to support its continued existence, however much they may chafe under the federal control that comes with the federal dollars.[204]

Both Medicare and Medicaid establish what have been referred to by R. Shep Melnick as "programmatic rights":

> Programmatic rights are a hybrid in several senses. Although they are not constitutional in the strict sense of the word, they are more than simply statutory. They are the product of both congressional enactment and extensive judicial interpretation—interpretation usually informed by constitutional precedents and values. . . . Unlike the rights of free speech, religion, property, and privacy, which set limits on the power of government officials, programmatic rights require extensive public programs rather than private autonomy, a welfare state rather than limited government.[205]

Three and a half decades of legislative action, administrative implementation, beneficiary and provider reliance, and judicial interpretation have woven Medicare and Medicaid rights deeply into the fabric of the American state.[206] Similarly, employment-related health insurance tax subsidies have become a fixed landmark in the American political landscape that will not be easily moved. Public opinion polls consistently show that a solid majority of Americans favor the continued existence of—and, indeed, the expansion of—public health-care programs.[207] Ultimately, it is not the Constitution, not even the courts, but the polls that offer the most solid protection to our health-care entitlements.

In the end, our federal entitlement programs are not immutable, however. Although they are not likely to be abolished soon, they are far more vulnerable to "reform" than to abolition. The major threat to entitlements currently is from proposals to improve, reform, or even to "save" them. It is to these challenges that this book turns, but first I examine how our entitlements came to be and look more closely at the character of each of the three programs that has emerged from this historical process.

## Notes

1. *American Heritage Dictionary of the English Language*, 3rd ed. (second meaning).

2. The Social Security Act routinely refers to individuals who receive Medicare as "beneficiaries" and individuals who receive Medicaid as "recipients" or as "recipients of medical assistance." The term *beneficiary* is obviously drawn from the world of private insurance, while *recipient* implies the gratuitous nature of welfare benefits.

3. See *Fuji v. State*, 242 P. 2d 617 (Cal. 1952). See also Randal S. Jeffrey, "Equal Protection in State Courts: The New Economic Equality Right," *Law and Inequality Journal* 17 (1999): 239, 347.

4. Jeffrey. "Equal Protection in State Courts," 347–348.

5. Steven D. Jamar, "The International Right to Health," *Southern University Law Review* 22 (1994): 23–27.

6. Ibid., 50; Art Hendriks, "The Right to Health in National and International Jurisprudence," *European Journal of Health Law* 5 (1998): 389.

7. Timothy Stoltzfus Jost, *Comparative Health Law and Bioethics* (Charlotte, N.C.: Carolina Academic Press, 2001), 15–18.

8. Hendriks, "The Right to Health in National and International Jurisprudence."

9. Frank B. Cross, "The Error of Positive Rights," *U.C.L.A. Law Review* 48 (2001): 857, 872.

10. David P. Currie, "Positive and Negative Constitutional Rights," *University of Chicago Law Review* 53 (1986): 864, 865–866.

11. See Frank E. L. Deale, "The Unhappy History of Economic Rights in the United States and Prospects for Their Creation and Renewal," *Howard Law Journal* 43 (2000): 281, 298–302; David Abraham, "Liberty without Equality: The Property-Rights Connection in a 'Negative Citizenship' Regime," *Law and Society Inquiry* 21 (1966): 1, 4–5. The classic statement of this, not entirely uncontroversial, assertion is Charles Beard, *An Economic Interpretation of the Constitution of the United States* (New York: MacMillan, 1913).

12. Wendy Parmet, "Health Care and the Constitution: Public Health and the Role of the State in the Framing Era," *Hastings Constitutional Law Quarterly* 20 (1992): 267, 293.

13. Parmet, "Health Care and the Constitution," 319–325.

14. *Jackson v. City of Joliet*, 715 F. 2d 1200, 1203 (7th Cir. 1983) (Posner, J.).

15. See Kenneth R. Wing, "The Right to Health Care in the United States," *Annual Health Law* 2 (1993): 161–162. But see also Parmet, "Health Care and the Constitution."

16. There are limited exceptions to this non-duty. Prisoners and others held in institutions by the state have a right to minimal provision of health care. Wing "The Right to Health Care in the United States," 163; *O'Connor v. Donaldson*, 422 U.S. 563 (1975). Also, it should be noted that the constitutions of a number of states recognize a state obligation to provide welfare benefits in general or health-care benefits in particular. Several state supreme courts have held that pregnant women have a state constitutional right to public funding for abortions, although these decisions rely more on the fundamental protected status of the decision to have an abortion than on general constitutional rights to health-care benefits. See *Committee to Defend Reproductive Rights v. Myers*, 625 P. 2d 779 (Cal. 1981); *Doe v. Maher*, 515 A. 2d 134 (Conn. Supr. Ct. 1986); *Moe v. Secretary of Administration and Finance*, 417 N.E. 2d 387 (Mass. 1981); *Women's Health Ctr., Inc. v. Panepinto*, 446 S.E. 2d 658 (W.Va. 1993); *Right to Choose*

*v. Byrne,* 450 A. 2d 925 (N.J. 1982); *Planned Parenthood Ass'n v. Dept. of Human Resources,* 663 P. 2d 1247 (Or. Ct. App. 1983). See Randal S. Jeffrey, "Equal Protection in State Courts," 281–287, 298–299; See also, Helen Hershkoff, "Welfare Devolution and State Constitutions," *Fordham Law Review* 67 (1999): 1403.

17. Among the classic sources in this tradition, see Frank I. Michelman, "The Supreme Court, 1968 Term–Forward: On Protecting the Poor through the Fourteenth Amendment," *Harvard Law Review* 83 (1969): 7 (arguing for a right to "minimum protection against economic hazard" where economic interests were involved); Akil Reed Amar, "Forty Acres and a Mule: A Republican Theory of Minimal Entitlements," *Harvard Journal of Law and Public Policy* 13 (1990): 37 (based in the Thirteenth Amendment); Charles L. Black Jr., "Further Reflections on the Constitutional Justice of Livelihood," *Columbia Law Review* 86 (1986); 1103 (finding a right to "freedom from gnawing hunger and from preventable sickness," in the Ninth Amendment, interpreted in light of the Declaration of Independence and the Preamble of the Constitution); and Peter B. Edelman, "The Next Century of Our Constitution: Rethinking Our Duty to the Poor," *Hastings Law Journal* 39 (1987): 1, 32 ("The framework and structure of our Constitution implicitly create affirmative obligations for government in a democratic society, among them an obligation to provide basic food and shelter"). For a reasonably recent and complete catalogue of academic discussions of welfare rights, see Helen Hershkoff, "Positive Rights and State Constitutions: The Limits of Federal Rationality Review," *Harvard Law Review* 112 (1999): 1131, 1133–1135.

18. See, recounting the welfare rights movement during this period, Elizabeth Bussiere, *(Dis)Entitling the Poor: The Warren Court, Welfare Rights, and the American Political Tradition* (University Park: Pennsylvania State University Press, 1997); Martha F. Davis, *Brutal Need: Lawyers and the Welfare Rights Movement, 1960–1973* (New Haven, Conn.: Yale University Press, 1993); Susan E. Lawrence, *The Poor in Court: The Legal Services Program and Supreme Court Decision Making* (Princeton, N.J.: Princeton University Press, 1990); and William E. Forbath, "Constitutional Welfare Rights: A History, Critique, and Reconstruction," *Fordham Law Review* 69 (2001): 1821.

19. See, Bussiere, *(Dis)Entitling the Poor,* 85–98; Davis, *Brutal Need,* 38. See also Edward Sparer, "The Right to Welfare," in *The Rights of Americans: What They Are—What They Should Be,* edited by Norman Dorsen (New York: Pantheon, 1971), 63 (a contemporaneous description of the welfare rights litigation by the leading theoretician of the movement).

20. See *Carleson v. Remillard,* 406 U.S. 598 (1972); *Townsend v. Swank,* 404 U.S. 282 (1971); *King v. Smith,* 392 U.S. 309 (1968). See R. Shep Melnick, *Between the Lines: Interpreting Welfare Rights* (Washington, D.C.: Brookings Institute, 1993); R. Shep Melnick, "Federalism and the New Rights," *Yale Journal on Regulation* 14 (1996): 332–337.

21. *Harper v. Va. State Bd. of Elections,* 383 U.S. 663 (1966).

22. *Griffin v. Ill.,* 351 U.S. 12 (1956) (right of indigent appellants to trial transcript); *Douglas v. Cal.,* 372 U.S. 353 (1963)(right of indigent to appointed counsel on appeal); and *Gideon v. Wainwright,* 372 U.S. 335 (1963) (right of indigent to appointed counsel at trial).

23. *Dandridge v. Williams,* 397 U.S. 471, 484 (1970). See Bussiere, *(Dis)Entitling the Poor,* 107–111.

24. *Rodriguez v. San Antonio Indep. Sch. Dist.,* 411 U.S. 1, 28–29 (1973).

25. *Roe v. Wade,* 410 U.S. 113 (1973); *Doe v. Bolton,* 410 U.S. 179 (1973).

26. *Maher v. Roe,* 432 U.S. 464, 469 (1976). Four years later in *Harris v. McRae,* 448

U.S. 297, 316–318 (1980), the Court extended the holding of *Maher*, which had involved therapeutic abortions, to uphold a statute prohibiting funding of medically necessary, therapeutic, abortions.

27. See William H. Simon, "The Invention and Reinvention of Welfare Rights," *Maryland Law Review* 44 (1985): 1, 23–28; William H. Simon, "Rights and Redistribution in the Welfare System," *Stanford Law Review* 30 (1986): 1431, 1486–1504.

28. See Charles Reich, "The New Property," *Yale Law Journal* 73 (1964): 733.

29. Robert Cover, "Social Security and Constitutional Entitlement," in *Social Security: Beyond the Rhetoric of Crisis*, edited by Theodore R. Marmor and Jerry L. Mashaw (Princeton, N.J.: Princeton University Press, 1988): 69.

30. William H. Simon, "Rights and Redistributions in the Welfare System," *Stanford Law Review* 38 (1986): 1431, 1450; (citing Ewin E. Witte, *The Development of the Social Security Act: A Memorandum on the History of the Committee on Economic Security and Drafting and Legislative History of the Social Security Act* [Madison: University of Wisconsin Press, 1962], 147–152). See also Cover, "Social Security and Constitutional Entitlement."

31. Simon, "Rights and Redistributions," 1455–1456.

32. See ibid., 1451 (citing Eveline Burns, *Toward Social Security: An Explanation of the Social Security Act and a Survey of the Larger Issues* [New York: McGraw-Hill, 1936], 26–27); Robert Ball, "The American System of Social Security," *Journal of Commerce* 15 (June 1964): 17.

33. Simon, "Rights and Redistributions," 1452–1453. But see Cover, "Social Security and Constitutional Entitlement," 75–76 (discussing why Social Security is not contractual). Cover proceeds to argue that Social Security benefits should be recognized as a form of property. Ibid., 84–87.

34. *Flemming v. Nestor*, 363 U.S. 603, 608 (1960).

35. Ibid., 610 (quoting *Helvering v. Davis*, 301 U.S. 619, 641 [1937], which had originally upheld the constitutionality of the Social Security program).

36. *Flemming v. Nestor*, 610. The Court's decision relied in part on a clause in the Social Security Act that retains in Congress "the right to alter, amend, or repeal any provision" of the act. Ibid., 611, quoting 42 USC § 1304.

37. *Flemming v. Nestor*, 611.

38. *Goldberg v. Kelly*, 397 U.S. 254 (1970).

39. Ibid.

40. Ibid., 262.

41. Ibid., 265.

42. It was followed rapidly by *Dandridge v. Williams*, 397 U.S. 471 (1970); *Wyman v. James*, 400 U.S. 309 (1971); and *Jefferson v. Hackney*, 406 U.S. 535 (1972), all rejecting equal fundamental right and invidious discrimination challenges to welfare practices, and by the collapse of the welfare rights movement. Davis, *Brutal Need*, 119–145.

43. *Harris v. McRae*, 317–318.

44. *Deshaney v. Winnebago County Dept. of Social Serv's*, 489 U.S. 189, 196 (1989).

45. See recent cases applying Goldberg in public benefits cases: *Grijalva v. Shalala*, 152 F. 3d 1115 (9th Cir. 1998), vacated on other grounds in *Shalala v. Grijalva*, 526 U.S. 1096 (1999); *Hart v. Westchester Co. Dept. Soc. Serv's*, 160 F. Supp. 2d 570 (S.D.N.Y. 2001); *Ford v. Shalala*, 87 F. Supp. 2d 163 (E.D.N.Y. 1999); and *Richardson v. Kelaher*, 1998 WL 812042 (S.D.N.Y. 1998). See also *American Manufacturer's Mutual Insurance Company v. Sullivan*, 526 U.S. 40, 60 (1999)(distinguishing but not overruling *Goldberg*).

46. *Board of Regents of State Colleges v. Roth*, 408 U.S. 564 (1972). Specifically, the court held that a university professor teaching under a 1-year contract and without tenure did not have a "legitimate claim of entitlement" in continued employment, protected by the due process clause. Ibid., 578.

47. "Property interest[s], of course, are not created by the Constitution. Rather they are created and their dimensions are defined by existing rules or understandings that stem from an independent source such as state law." Ibid., 577.

48. Taken to its limits, this would mean that the procedures due a person threatened with deprivation of an interest would depend on the dimensions of that interest as defined by nonconstitutional law, including the procedures specified by that law to protect that interest. See *Arnett v. Kennedy*, 416 U.S. 134, 151–154 (Rehnquist, J. [1974]. This situation was described by Professor Jerry Mashaw and by subsequent commentators as "the positivist trap." Mashaw, "Administrative Due Process: The Quest for a Dignitary Theory," *Boston University Law Review* 61 (1981): 885, 888. The Supreme Court subsequently rejected this extreme position in *Cleveland Bd. of Ed. v. Loudermill*, 470 U.S. 532 (1985), but the question of whether entitlements are protected by the due process clause continues to be defined by substantive, nonconstitutional law. For recent survey and analysis of this area, see Thomas W. Merrill, "The Landscape of Constitutional Property," *Virginia Law Review* 86 (2000): 885..

49. See Frank B. Cross, "The Error of Positive Rights," *U.C.L.A. Law Review* 48 (2001): 857, 879–901; Wing, "The Right to Health Care in the United States," 184–186.

50. See Alan W. Houseman, "Civil Legal Assistance for Low-Income Persons: Looking Back and Looking Forward," *Fordham Urban Law Journal* 29 (2002): 1213.

51. Ibid., 905–913.

52. A striking example of this is the opinion of an activist conservative judge in *Westside Mothers v. Haveman*, 133 F. Supp. 2d 549 (E.D. Mich. 2001), who overruled decades of Supreme Court precedent to effectively abolish Medicaid as a federal entitlement. The decision was reversed on appeal, in 289 F. 3d 852 (6th Cir. 2002).

53. Because some of the countries in which they exist also lack the tradition of judical supremacy that we have in the United States, resort to the courts might not be possible.

54. The next section, 426-1, contains similar language in creating an entitlement for persons with end-stage renal disease. 42 U.S.C. § 426-2(a).

55. See e.g., 42 U.S.C. §§ 1395e(a)(1)(B) (each day of hospital services for which beneficiary is entitled to have payment made), 1395(h)(1) (person entitled to hospital benefits), 1395w-22(g) (health services to which beneficiary entitled from Medicare+Choice organizations), and 1395cc(a)(1)(A)(i) (items and services for which an individual is entitled to have payment made).

56. See, e.g., 42 U.S.C. §§ 1395mm(a)(6) (health maintenance organizations), 1395ww(j)(3)(A) (rehabilitation facility), and 1395bbb(f)(2)(A)(ii) (home health agencies).

57. See, e.g., 42 U.S.C. §§ 1320c-5(a)(4) (practitioner entitled to notice and hearing of Peer Review Organization determination).

58. 42 U.S.C. § 1396a. Subsection (a) of this section, describing the content of state plans, is written as a single sentence. At over 10,800 words, it is probably the longest sentence in the English language.

59. 42 U.S.C. § 1396b(d).

60. See, e.g., 42 U.S.C. §§ 1396b(k) and 1396e(a)(1).

61. 42 U.S.C. §§ 1396b(m)(2)(A)(vii), 1396r-4(d)(1), and 1396r-4(g)(2)(B).

62. See, e.g. 42 U.S.C. §§ 1320(b)(1)(A), 1395i–e(c)(1)(A), 1395ss(d)(3)(B)(iii)(III), 1395ss(q)(5)(A), and 1395eee(c)(1)(B).

63. See, e.g., 42 U.S.C. §§ 1396a(a)(10(D) (individuals entitled to payment for nursing facility services), 1396n(c)(2)(B)(i) (individuals entitled to inpatient hospital services, nursing facility services, and intermediate-care facility for the mentally retarded), and 1396n(d)(2)(B)(i) (individuals 65 years of age and older entitled to medical assistance for nursing facility services).

64. 42 U.S.C. § 1396a(a)(10) (Medicare beneficiaries entitled only to payments for Medicare cost-sharing obligations).

65. 42 U.S.C. §§ 1396a and 1396u-3(b)(4).

66. 42 U.S.C. §§ 1396m(d) and 1396m(f).

67. 42 U.S.C. § 1396u-3(e).

68. *Addis v. Whitburn*, 153 F. 3d 836 (7th Cir. 1998); *Elizabeth Blackwell Health Center for Women v. Knoll*, 61 F. 3d 170 (3rd. Cir. 1995).

69. *Harris v. McRae*, 448 U.S. 297, 301 (1980).

70. Further provisions of § 106 also exclude from employee income employer contributions to Archer Medical Savings Accounts.

71. See e.g. *Larkin v. C.I.R.*, 394 F. 2d 494 (1st Cir. 1968) (medical reimbursement payments for stockholder-officer-employees not "plan for employees" under § 105).

72. See Willam A. Raabe et al., *West's Federal Tax Research*, 6th ed. (Mason, Oh.: Thompson Learning, 2003), 118–119, 121–122, 130–132, 382–385.

73. *Pilot Life Ins. Co. v. Dadeaux*, 481 U.S. 41 (1987). See generally on ERISA preemption, Barry R. Furrow et al., *Health Law*, 2d ed. (St. Paul: Westgroup, 2000), § 8-3.

74. *Rush Prudential HMO, Inc. v. Moran*, 122 S.Ct. 2151 (2002).

75. 42 U.S.C. § 1395ff(b)(E)(i).

76. 42 U.S.C. § 1395oo(a) and (f).

77. 42 U.S.C. § 1395ff(b)(E)(i).

78. 42 U.S.C. §§ 405(h) and 1395ii. See *Heckler v. Ringer*, 466 U.S. 602 (1984).

79. 42 U.S.C. § 1395ww(d)(7) and 42 U.S.C. § 1395w–4(i)(1). Certain technical and methodological issues under other prospective payment systems established by the 1997 Balanced Budget Act are also not subject to review; see 42 U.S.C. §§ 1395ww(j)(7) (rehabilitation services), 42 U.S.C. § 1395yy(e)(8) (skilled nursing facility services), 42 U.S.C. § 1395l(t)(9) (outpatient hospital services), and 42 U.S.C. § 1395fff(d) (home health benefits).

80. *Heckler v. Ringer*, 466 U.S. 602.

81. 42 U.S.C. § 1395ff(b)(3)(B). See also *Friedrich v. Secretary of HHS*, 894 F. 2d 829 (6th Cir. 1990), cert. denied 498 U.S. 817 (1990) (holding national coverage determinations to be interpretive rules not subject to APA rule-making requirements).

82. *Illinois Council for Long Term Care v. Shalala*, 529 U.S. 1 (2000); *Weinberger v. Salfi*, 422 U.S. 74 (1975).

83. *Califano v. Sanders*, 430 U.S. 99 (1977).

84. *United States v. Erika, Inc.*, 456 U.S. 201 (1982). See also, *St. Vincent's Medical Center v. United States*, 32 F. 3d 548 (Fed. Cir. 1994); *Bloomington Hosp. v. United States*, 29 Fed. Cl. 286 (Ct. of Claims, 1993) (recent cases denying Court of Claims jurisdiction over Medicare disputes).

85. *Wilder v. Virginia Hosp. Ass'n*, 496 U.S. 498 (1990). A provider, however, has no right to be a Medicaid provider if the state chooses to limit its provider contracts. *Macombs Pharmacy v. Wing*, 1998 WL 696008 (S.D.N.Y. Oct. 5, 1998).

86. See *Wilder v. Virginia Hosp. Ass'n*, 496 U.S. 498, 523–525; *Skubel v. Fuoroli*, 113 F. 3d 330 (2d Cir. 1997); *Alacare, Inc.–North v. Baggiano*, 785 F. 2d 963, 965–970 (11th Cir. 1986), cert. denied 479 U.S. 829 (1986).

87. *Heartland Hosp. v. Stangler*, 792 F. Supp. 670 (W.D. Mo. 1992) (abstention ap-

propriate where state administrative remedy and federal intervention would disrupt state efforts to establish a coherent policy); *St. Michael Hosp. v. Thompson*, 725 F. Supp. 1038, 1045 (W.D. Wis. 1989) (issues under review predominantly local issues appropriate to resolution in state appeal); *St. Joseph Hosp. v. Electronic Data Systems Corp.*, 573 F. Supp. 443, 451–452 (S.D. Tex. 1983) (abstention appropriate where complex state administrative framework is available to address important state issues).

88. But see *Greenery Rehab. Group v. Sabol*, 841 F. Supp. 58 (N.D.N.Y. 1993) (exhaustion of federal remedies not required where state sues federal government in third-party claim).

89. This situation may be changing. In a series of cases in recent years, the Supreme Court has been cutting back on the reach of § 1983. In its most recent consideration of the issue, the Court held that nothing "short of an unambiguously conferred right [will] support a cause of action brought under § 1983" and stated that Congress must create rights enforceable under § 1983 in "clear and unambiguous terms." *Gonzaga University v. Doe*, 122 S.Ct. 2268, 2275, 2279 (2002). However, the Court expressly did not overrule *Wilder*, which it said met these criteria.

90. *Florida Dept. of Health and Rehab. Servs. v. Florida Nursing Home Ass'n*, 450 U.S. 147 (1981).

91. See *Edelman v. Jordan*, 415 U.S. 651, 662–664 (1974); *Doe v. Chiles*, 136 F. 3d 709 (11th Cir. 1998); *Amisub (PSL), Inc. v. Colorado Dep't of Social Services*, 879 F. 2d 789, 792–793, n. 7 (10th Cir. 1989), cert. denied 496 U.S. 935 (1990).

92. *Illinois Council for Long Term Care v. Shalala*, 529 U.S. 1 (2000); In *Your Home Visiting Nurse Servs., Inc. v. Shalala*, 525 U.S. 449 (1998); *Regions Hospital v. Shalala*, 522 U.S. 548 (1998); *Shalala v. Guernsey Mem. Hosp.*, 514 U.S. 87 (1995); *Thomas Jefferson Univ. v. Shalala*, 512 U.S. 504 (1994); and *Good Samaritan Hosp. v. Shalala*, 508 U.S. 402 (1993).

93. The two years were 1995 and the second half of 1997 and the first half of 1998.

94. Timothy Stoltzfus Jost, "Governing Medicare," *Administrative Law Review* 51 (1999): 39, 56.

95. *Chevron v. Natural Resources Defense Council, Inc.*, 467 U.S. 837, 842 (1984). See, applying Chevron, *Good Samaritan Hosp. v. Shalala*, 508 U.S. 402 (1993), and *Regions Hospital v. Shalala*, 522 U.S. 548 (1998).

96. *Thomas Jefferson Univ. v. Shalala*, 512 U.S. 504 (1994).

97. 512 U.S. at 512. These cases were decided before the Supreme Court's recent decision in *United States v. Mead Corp*, 533 U.S. 218 (2001), in which the Court seems to back off of the extreme deference that it has shown to administrative agencies in recent years toward a more nuanced standard of deference. However, the first Medicare case to apply *Mead* distinguished it in favor of a more traditional deference standard. *Robert Wood Johnson Hosp. v. Thompson*, 297 F. 3d 273 (3rd Cir. 2002).

98. Reported cases were identified using a Westlaw search of the ALLFEDS database for 1999 and 2000 cases, including a citation to a provision of 42 U.S.C. 1396, and the word *Medicaid*. Only cases in which a Medicaid agency was the defendant were included. Fraud and abuse and qui tam cases were excluded, as were cases challenging or seeking a share of tobacco tort litigation settlements. Cases involving purely procedural issues such as class certification or attorneys' fees awards were also excluded. Cases were coded as either wins for the plaintiff or for the Medicaid agency. Cases in which both parties won on some issues were coded for computing win/loss statistics as favoring each party half and half.

99. See, e.g., *Unicare Health Facilities v. Miller*, 481 F. Supp. 496, 498 (N.D. Ill. 1979).

100. *Colorado Health Care Ass'n v. Colorado Dep't of Social Services*, 842 F. 2d 1158,

1164 (10th Cir. 1988); *Mississippi Hosp. Ass'n v. Heckler*, 701 F. 2d 511, 516 (5th Cir. 1983).

101. See, e.g., *Temple Univ. v. White*, 729 F. Supp. 1093 (E.D. Pa. 1990), affirmed 941 F. 2d 201 (3d Cir. 1991).

102. *Ala. Hosp. Ass'n v. Beasley*, 702 F. 2d 955, 961–962 (11th Cir. 1983).

103. *Wisconsin Department of Social Services v. Blumer*, 534 U.S. 473 (2002).

104. These statistics are based on a Westlaw search of the Allstates database of 1999 and 2000 cases using the search described in note 98. Again, only cases in which a Medicaid agency was the defendant or respondent were considered. Again, fraud and abuse cases were excluded. Cases involving Medicaid as secondary payer liens on tort settlements and judgments or private insurance claims were also excluded. Cases brought by recipients' estates or by survivors who were challenging liens imposed on recipient's assets at death were included, however, as these are cases challenging state program requirements or their application. Obviously, this search would capture only a tiny fraction of state cases involving Medicaid claims, as most would be unreported. There is no obvious reason, however, to believe that these statistics would not be representative of win–loss statistics in general.

105. Note "Federal Judicial Review of State Welfare Practices," *Columbia Law Review* 67 (1967): 84.

106. I still remember the shock and surprise expressed by a state court judge once the judge finally comprehended the fact that a suit I filed (when I was a legal services lawyer) was asking the judge to order the state to increase grants to welfare recipients to comply with state law.

107. See Carol S. Weissert and William G. Weissert, *Governing Health* (Baltimore: Johns Hopkins University Press, 1996), 175.

108. 29 U.S.C. § 1132(a)(1).

109. *Pilot Life v. Dedeaux*, 481 U.S. 41, 52–53 (1987).

110. See *Little Rock Family Planning Services v. Dalton*, 60 F. 3d 497 (8th Cir. 1995), reversed in part on other grounds in *Dalton v. Little Rock Family Planning Services*, 516 U.S. 474 (1996) (Arkansas constitutional amendment prohibiting funding of abortions except to save mother's life invalid insofar as it limits Medicaid funding for abortions in cases of rape and incest).

111. 42 U.S.C. §§ 426 and 1395c.

112. 42 U.S.C. § 1395o.

113. 42 U.S.C. § 1395ff(a) and (b); 20 C.F.R. §§ 404.900–404.999(d).

114. 42 U.S.C. § 1396a(10). See Jane Perkins, "Medicaid: Past Successes and Future Challenges," *Health Matrix* 12 (2002): 7, 11.

115. See Furrow et al., *Health Law*, § 12–14.

116. 26 U.S.C. § 105(h).

117. See Cafeteria Plans, BNA Tax Management Portfolio, 397-3rd (2000).

118. 42 U.S.C. § 1395y(a)(1)(A).

119. 42 U.S.C. § 1395ff(a)(3).

120. 42 U.S.C. § 1395ff(b)(1).

121. 42 U.S.C. §§ 1395ff(b)(1)(A), (E), and (d)(1).

122. 42 U.S.C. § 1395ff(d)(2).

123. 42 U.S.C. § 1395ff(b)(1)(E).

124. 42 U.S.C. § 1395ff(b)(1)(F), (c)(3)(C), and (d).

125. See David M. Frankford, "Food Allergy and the Health Care Financing Administration: A Story of Rage," *Widener Law Symposium Journal* 1 (1996): 160; Gordon B. Schatz, "Medical Technology Coverage and Coding," in *Health Law Handbook*, edited by Alice G. Gosfield (New York: Clark Boardman, 1990), 413; Louis B. Hays,

"Medicare Coverage," *Journal of the American Medical Association* 262 (1989): 2794 (describing the coverage determination process); Eleanor Kinney, "Setting Limits: A Realistic Assignment for the Medicare Program," *St. Louis Law Journal* 33 (1989): 631; Kinney, "National Coverage Policy under the Medicare Program: Problems and Proposals for Change," *St. Louis Law Journal* 32 (1988): 869.

126. "Procedures for Making National Coverage Decisions," *Federal Register* 64 (April 27, 1999): 22,619.

127. "Proposed Rule: Criteria and Procedures for Making Medical Services Courage Decisions that Relate to Health Care Technology," *Federal Register* 54 (January 30, 1989): 4,302.

128. "Notice, Medicare Program National Coverage Decisions," *Federal Register* 54 (August 21, 1989), 34,555.

129. "Notice, Medicare Program, Establishment of the Medicare Coverage Advisory Committee," *Federal Register* 63 (December 14, 1998): 68,780.

130. "Notice Medicare Program, Procedures for Making National Coverage Determination," *Federal Register* 64 (April 27, 1999): 22,619.

131. 42 U.S.C. § 1395ff(f).

132. 42 U.S.C. § 1395ff(f)(4).

133. 42 U.S.C. § 1395ff(f)(1).

134. See Eleanor Kinney, ed., *Guide to Medicare Coverage Decision Making and Appeals* (Chicago: American Bar Association, 2002).

135. 42 C.F.R. § 440.230(a).

136. 42 C.F.R. § 440.230(b).

137. *Curtis v. Taylor*, 625 F. 2d 645 (5th Cir. 1980), rehearing denied, opinion modified 648 F. 2d 946 (1980).

138. *Dodson v. Parham*, 427 F. Supp. 97 (N.D. Ga. 1977).

139. 42 C.F.R. § 440.230(c).

140. *White v. Beal*, 555 F. 2d 1146 (3d Cir. 1977).

141. 42 C.F.R. § 440.230(d). See, e.g., *Medical Soc'y of N.Y. v. Toia*, 560 F. 2d 535 (2d Cir. 1977); *Cowan v. Myers*, 232 Cal. Rptr. 299 (Cal. App. 1986), cert. denied 484 U.S. 846 (1987).

142. However, the law does describe in some detail long-term care policies and medical savings account policies eligible for the health insurance exclusion. 42 U.S.C. §§ 106(b), 220, and 7702-B.

143. See *Shaw v. Delta Airlines*, 463 U.S. 85 (1983) and *Nazay v. Miller*, 949 F. 2d 1323 (3rd Cir. 1991). In fact, a few federal statutes adopted in recent years impose specific limitations on ERISA plans, prohibiting, for example, "drive-through deliveries" or requiring coverage for breast reconstruction for plans that cover mastectomies.

144. *Firestone Tire Co. v. Bruch*, 489 U.S. 101 (1989).

145. See Furrow, *Health Law*, § 8-6 describing relevant authorities.

146. See Judith C. Brostron, "The Conflict of Interest Standard in ERISA case: Can it be Avoided in the Denial of High Dose Chemotherapy Treatment for Breast Cancer," *DePaul Journal of Health Care Law* 3 (1999): 1; "Haavi Morreim, Benefits Decisions in ERISA Plans: Diminishing Deference to Fiduciaries and an Emerging Problem for Provider Sponsored Organizations," *Tennessee Law Journal,* 65 (1998): 511.

147. See Jost, "Governing Medicare," 84–86.

148. See Timothy Stoltzfus Jost, "Administrative Law Issues Involving the Medicare Utilization and Quality Control Peer Review Organization (PRO) Program: Analysis and Recommendations," *Ohio State Law Journal* 50 (1989): 1–71.

149. 42 C.F.R. § 498.3(b).

150. 42 C.F.R. § 498.5(a).

151. 42 C.F.R. § 498.5(b).

152. 42 C.F.R. §§ 422.641–422.698.

153. See *Erickson v. United States Dep't of Health & Human Servs.*, 67 F. 3d 858 (9th Cir. 1994) and *Ram v. Heckler*, 792 F. 2d 444 (4th Cir. 1986).

154. See *Erickson v. United States Dep't of Health & Human Servs.*, 67 F.3d 858, 862–863 (liberty interest in loss of provider status, no property interest in continued Medicare participation where mandatory exclusion was imposed based on conviction still on appeal); but see *Doe v. Bowen*, 682 F. Supp. 637 (D. Mass. 1987) (finding both liberty and property interest) and *Gellman v. Sullivan*, 758 F. Supp. 830 (E.D.N.Y. 1991) (no property interest in continued participation in Medicare, liberty issue not presented). See also *Kahn v. Inspector General*, 848 F. Supp. 432, 438 (S.D.N.Y. 1994) (holding that exclusion cannot violate the takings clause because there is no property right in continued participation in Medicare).

155. See Furrow, *Health Law*, § 9-8.

156. 42 U.S.C. § 1395oo. See Phyllis E. Bernard, "Empowering the Provider: A Better Way to Resolve Medicare Hospital Payment Disputes," *Administrative Law Review* 49 (1997): 269; and Phyllis E. Bernard, "Social Security and Medicare Adjudications at HHS: Two Approaches to Administration of Justice in an Ever-Expanding Bureaucracy," *Health Matrix* 3 (1993): 339.

157. 42 U.S.C. § 1395oo(f)(1); 42 C.F.R. § 405.1875.

158. 42 U.S.C. § 1395w-22(g)(4) and (5); 42 C.F.R. §§ 422.592–.616. See, e.g., *Rogers v. Shalala*, 1998 WL 325248 (N.D. Ill. 1998); *Kelly v. Bowen*, 1987 WL 120016 (W.D. Wash. 1997) (reviewing HMO coverage determination).

159. See Furrow, *Health Law*, § 11-16.

160. *Wilder v. Virginia Hospital Association*, 496 U.S. 498(1990).

161. Former 42 U.S.C. § 1396a(a)(13)(E). See Michael MacDonald et al., *Treatise on Health Care Law*, § 8.26 (New York: Mathew Bender, 1991); Joel M. Hamme, "Medicaid Reimbursement Litigation by Hospitals and Nursing Homes," in *1991 Health Law Handbook*, (New York: Clark Boardman, 1991), 301; Joel Hamme, "Long–Term Care Reimbursement," in *1990 Health Law Handbook*, (New York: Clark Boardman, 1990) 345; and Robert A. Ringer, "Boren Amendment Litigation: An Analysis," *Journal of Health and Hospital Law*, (March 1994): 65. Academic consideration of Boren Amendment litigation is found in Gerard F. Anderson and Mark A. Hall, "The Adequacy of Hospital Reimbursement under Medicaid's Boren Amendment," *Journal of Legal Medicine* 13 (1992): 205. See also Rand E. Rosenblatt, "Statutory Interpretation and Distributive Justice: Medicaid Hospital Reimbursement and the Debate over Public Choice," *St. Louis Uuniversity Law Journal* 35 (1991): 793.

162. 42 U.S.C. § 1396a(a)(13)(A). *HCMF Corp. v. Gilmore*, 26 F. Supp. 2d 873 (W.D. Va. 1998). Because repeal of the Boren Amendment was not retroactive, pre-1997 Boren Amendment litigation continued after its adoption. See *Exeter Memorial Hospital Assn v. Belshe*, 145 F. 3d 1106 (9th Cir. 1998).

163. 42 U.S.C. § 1396a(a)(30).

164. *Orthopaedic Hospital v. Belshe*, 103 F. 3d 1491 (9th Cir. 1997); *Arkansas Medical Soc'y v. Reynolds*, 6 F. 3d 519 (8th Cir. 1993); *Visiting Nurse Ass'n of N. Shore, Inc. v. Bullen*, 93 F. 3d 997 (1st Cir. 1996). But see *Evergreen Presbyterian Ministries v. Hood*, 235 F. 3d 908 (5th Cir. 2000) (beneficiaries have right to sue under equal access provision, but not providers).

165. *Florida Pharmacy Ass'n v. Cook*, 17 F. Supp. 2d 1293 (N.D. Fla. 1998).

166. *Minnesota Home Care Ass'n, Inc. v. Gomez,* 108 F. 3d 917 (8th Cir. 1997), and *Rite Aid of Pennsylvania v. Houston,* 171 F. 3d 842 (3rd. Cir. 1999).

167. See, e.g., *Transitional Hospitals Corp. v. Blue Cross and Blue Shield of Texas,* 164 F. 2d 952 (5th Cir. 1999); Furrow, *Health Law,* § 8-6.

168. *Goldberg v. Kelly,* 397 U.S. at 261.

169. Sandy Streeter for the Congressional Research Service, *The Congressional Appropriation Process: An Introduction* (Washington, D.C.: The Library of Congress, 1999), 14 n. 33.

170. Charles Tiefer, "Budgetized Health Entitlements and Fiscal Constitution in Congress's 1995–1996 Budget Battle," *Harvard Journal on Legislation* 33 (1996): 411, 416 n. 12.

171. Theda Skocpol, *Protecting Soldiers and Mothers,* (Cambridge: Harvard University Press, 1992), 132.

172. See Streeter, *Congressional Appropriations Process,* 13–14; General Accounting Office, *Budget Policy Issues in Capping Mandatory Spending* (Washington, D.C.: GAO/AIMD94-155 (Washington, D.C.: GAO, 1994); Elizabeth Garrett, "Rethinking the Structures of Decisionmaking in the Federal Budget Process," *Harvard Journal on Legislation* 35 (1998): 387, 388, 400; Tiefer, "Budgetized Health Entitlements."

173. See Streeter, *Congressional Appropriations Process,* explaining this process.

174. This allows Congress to impose restrictions on funding through the appropriations process, the most well known of which is the Hyde amendment banning Medicaid funding for abortions.

175. 2 U.S.C. §§ 601–688.

176. Congressional Budget and Impoundment Control Act, Pub. L. 93-344, 88 Stat. 297 (1974).

177. Balanced Budget and Emergency Deficit Control Act (Gramm–Rudman–Hollings), Pub. L. 99-177, 99 Stat. 1037 (1985).

178. Budget Enforcement Act, Pub. L. 101-508, 104 Stat 1388-573–1388-630 (1990).

179. The balanced budget and Emergency Deficit Control Reaffirmation Act of 1987 (Pub. L. 100-119 (101 Stat. 754); the Omnibus Budget Reconciliation Act of 1993, Pub. L. 103-66 (107 Stat. 312), and the Budget Enforcement Act of 1997, Pub. L. 105-33 (111 Stat. 251.)

180. See Streeter, *Congressional Appropriations Process,* CRS-3–CRS-4.

181. Ibid.

182. Ibid., CRS-11. In some years, these bills are packaged together, resulting in fewer than 13 appropriation acts. Ibid., CRS-12 and CRS-13. Also, in some years, Congress funds certain functions on a short-term or long-term basis through continuing resolutions if it is unable to enact an appropriations bill. Ibid., CRS-15–CRS-16.

183. Ibid., CRS-6.

184. Ibid., CRS-7–CRS-8, CRS-24–CRS-25. The House may waive or suspend points of order by majority vote, the Senate by a three-fifths vote. Congress and the president may also (and often do) designate legislation as "emergency-designated discretionary spending," freeing it from the constraints of the budget act.

185. Ibid., CRS-26–CRS-28. The categories are very broad, such as defense and non-defense spending, but a few special categories—currently, highway, mass transit, and violent crime reduction—are excluded from these categories. Ibid.

186. Congressional Research Service (CRS), *Pay-As-You-Go Rules in the Federal Budget Process* (Washington, D.C.: The Library of Congress, 2001).

187. Ibid. See, exploring justifications for this approach, Garrett, "Rethinking the Structures of Decisionmaking," 387, 401–405.

188. CRS, *PAYGO Rules*, 2.

189. Garrett, "Rethinking the Structures of Decisionmaking," 400 n. 43.

190. CRS, *PAYGO Rules*, 2.

191. See Elizabeth Garrett, "The Congressional Budget Process: Strengthening the Party-in-Power," *Columbia Law Review* 100 (2000): 702, 718–723; Anita S. Krishnakumar, "Reconciliation and the Fiscal Constitution: The Anatomy of the 1995–96 Budget 'Train Wreck,'" *Harvard Journal on Legislation* 35 (1998): 589, 591–600.

192. Garrett, "The Congressional Budget Process," 719–720.

193. Ibid., 720; Bill Heniff Jr., *Budget Reconciliation Legislation: Development and Consideration*: CRS Report to Congress (Washington, D.C.: The Library of Congress, 1998). Under the 1974 budget legislation, reconciliation legislation cannot recommend changes to the Social Security program.

194. Garrett, "The Congressional Budget Process," 720–722.

195. Pub.L. 93-344 § 310(d) 88 Stat. 310 (1974).

196. Robert Keith, *The Senate's Byrd Rule against Extraneous Matter in Reconciliation Measures* (Washington, D.C.: The Library of Congress: Congressional Research Service, 1998).

197. See Elisabeth Garrett, "Harnessing Politics: The Dynamics of Offset Requirements in the Tax Legislative Process," *University of Chicago Law Review* 65 (1998): 501–569 (exploring the ramifications of PAYGO for tax expenditures).

198. See General Accounting Office (GAO), *Budget Policy Issues in Capping Mandatory Spending* (Washington, D.C.: GAO, 1994).

199. See ibid., and Tiefer, "Budgetized Requirements."

200. See Office of Management and Budget (OMB), *Budget of the United States Government*, Table 22-4, Tax Expenditures by Function, 2002, available at http://www.whitehouse.gov/omb/budget/fy2002/bud22_4.html (cited October 21, 2002).

201. Arthur M. Schlesinger Jr., The Age of Roosevelt: The Coming of the New Deal (Boston: Houghton Mifflin, 1959), 308–309.

202. See Eric M. Patashnik, *Putting Trust in the U.S. Budget* (Cambridge: Cambridge University Press, 2000), 96. Patashnik contends that the primary driving force in establishing the Medicare trust funds was Wilbur Mills, the head of the House Ways and Means Committee, who is generally credited with creating the Medicare program. Patashnik argues that Mills insisted on separate Medicare trust funds to preserve the fiscal integrity of Social Security. Ibid., 97–100. See also Eric M. Patashnik and Julian Zelizer, "Paying for Medicare: Benefits, Budgets, and Wilbur Mills' Policy Legacy," *Journal of Health Politics Policy and Law* 26 (2001): 7.

203. Patashnik and Zelizer, "Paying for Medicare," 196–201.

204. See Aaron Wildavsky, "The Politics of the Entitlement Process," in Marc K. Landy and Martin A. Levin, *The New Politics of Public Policy*, (Baltimore: Johns Hopkins University Press, 1995), 143, 151–157.

205. R. Shep Melnick, "Federalism and the New Rights," *Yale Journal on Regulation* 14 (1996): 325, 327.

206. See Wing, "The Right to Health Care in the United States," 189–193.

207. According to a recent survey, 71% of Americans favor increased public spending for health care and 70% for Medicare. See *Public Agenda Online*, available at http://www.publicagenda.org/issues/major_proposals_detail.cfm?issue_type=Medicare&list=1 (cited July 9, 2002).

# 4

# The Historical
# Foundations of
# American Health-Care
# Entitlements

THE two primary public health insurance entitlement programs of the United States, Medicare and Medicaid, were created by the Social Security Amendments of 1965 and became effective on July 1, 1966. Although these programs were the product of a vigorous, decades-long debate to which many contributed, they were most immediately the creation of Wilbur Mills, the then-powerful chairman of the powerful House Ways and Means Committee. Mills combined three proposals—President Lyndon B. Johnson's administration's Medicare proposal then before Congress as the King–Anderson bill; the American Medical Association's "Eldercare" proposal; and a Republican alternative sponsored by Representative John W. Byrnes, sometimes referred to as "Bettercare"—to form the "three-layer cake," that became Medicare and Medicaid.[1] The Johnson administration's Medicare proposal, a traditional social insurance program, became the Part A hospital insurance program; the AMA's Eldercare, a limited, means-tested approach to insuring the elderly, became Medicaid; and Byrnes's proposal for subsidizing private insurance became Part B of Medicare.

Each of these three approaches to providing government funding for health-care service—social insurance, means-tested welfare programs, and tax-subsidized private insurance—has a venerable history in the United States. The earliest government approach to providing health-care services to the poor in the

United States were local means-tested programs that, in turn, had their origins in the English poor laws. This tradition formed the basis of the New Deal public assistance programs for the elderly, the blind, and dependent children, which, in turn, laid the foundation for the 1960 Kerr–Mills legislation, and, in the end, for Medicaid. Medicare Part A, in contrast, was grounded in the tradition of the New Deal social insurance programs of the 1930s, which trace their roots to the European social insurance programs of the late nineteenth and early twentieth centuries, but which also resemble in many respects the American Civil War pension system of the nineteenth century. The Republican subsidized private insurance proposal was of more recent origin, but by the 1960s, medical expenses had already been tax deductible for a half century, while the use of tax subsidies to fund the purchase of private health insurance had grounded our private, employment-related, health insurance programs for two decades, and the idea of using explicit cash subsidies to encourage the purchase of private health insurance had been on the table for at least half a decade.

All three of these approaches to health-care entitlements remain very much alive in the public debate. The social insurance strategy of health-care financing, represented by Medicare Part A, is still relied on in many other countries throughout the world, retains great political support in the United States, and is likely to continue to form the basis of our health-care entitlements for some time. At times, however, when the affordability of social insurance programs becomes questionable, proposals for downsizing our health-care entitlements and focusing them on the poor through means-testing return to the fore. Finally, the idea of public subsidies for private insurance lies at the basis of the Medicare Part C, Medicare+Choice program, created by the 1997 Balanced Budget Act, and is being pushed aggressively as the basis for "Medicare reform" based on vouchers or premium support. There is also considerable interest in expanding the use of tax credits as a primary strategy for making health insurance available to the general population.

Each of these three approaches is based on a distinct vision of entitlement. The foundations of social insurance entitlements are clear: one who meets statutory eligibility criteria is legally entitled to receive the social insurance benefits specified by law. Social insurance statutes afford applicants who are denied coverage or beneficiaries who are refused benefits the opportunity for both administrative appeal and judicial review. Undergirding these statutory rights, however, is a deeper understanding of entitlement as exchange. Social insurance program participants make regular "contributions" to social insurance trust funds during their working lives, which in the United States take the form of payroll taxes. When participants subsequently become eligible for social insurance (by retiring, by reaching a specified age, or by becoming unemployed or disabled), they are entitled to receive social insurance benefits in return.

Although, in fact, the relationship between contributions made and pensions withdrawn from social insurance funds is quite tenuous, supporters of social insurance have long promoted a belief that social insurance payments are earned, that they are the result of a quasi-contractual, quid pro quo kind of exchange relationship.[2] This has created a psychology of entitlement that transcends actual legal rights.

Paradoxically, although the absence of a real equivalence between payments and benefits means that at any one time the funds withdrawn from the program by any particular beneficiary are based by and large on current contributions from current contributors rather than on earlier contributions by the specific beneficiary, the conceptualization of the program as self-funded frees it from the constraints of annual congressional appropriations that confine the expenditures of nonentitlement programs. The belief that beneficiaries are entitled to recover their previous investments in the program make cutting program benefits very difficult. Alternatively, the correlative argument that new or expanded benefits must be funded by new or expanded payroll taxes makes contributory social insurance programs attractive to fiscal conservatives.[3] Social insurance benefits must bear some relationship to contributions, making social insurance programs more fiscally acceptable than welfare programs, which provoke anxious fears of bottomless pits.[4]

The quasi-contractual philosophy of entitlement that grounds social insurance has also long allowed these programs to escape the stigma that has always attended "welfare" programs in the United States. Americans have always put a high value on self-reliant individualism. Dependence on the community or state, it is widely believed, is shameful; an admission of personal and moral failure. American welfare administrators, moreover, have often further humiliated welfare applicants by investigating the intimate details of their lives, imposing financial obligations on their adult children, or forcing them to give up their homes to receive assistance.[5] Social insurance, because it is thought of as "earned," is free from taint. It is consistent with self-support, self-respect, and self-confidence—words often used by early advocates of the American Social Security program.[6] In contrast, ideological conservatives have long favored means-tested public health insurance programs because they are inherently marginalized. In the words of Senator Robert Taft, an early proponent of the approach later taken by Medicaid:

> It has always been assumed in this country that those able to pay for medical care would buy their own medical service, just as under any system, except a socialistic system, they buy their own food, their own housing, their own clothing, and their own automobiles. . . . Undoubtedly, in that system there are gaps . . . and we have a very definite interest in trying to fill up those gaps.[7]

Because of their "unearned" and gratuitous nature, entitlements to welfare-type benefits have historically been more vulnerable politically. In nineteenth-century America, welfare payments were clearly considered to be gratuities, available at the discretion of local authorities. The state may have a moral, even a legal obligation to help the less fortunate, but no individual was entitled to support.[8] While the 1935 Social Security Act created statutory rights to welfare, the states still exercised considerable discretion over these benefits. Indeed, the leadership of the Social Security Board, which implemented the 1935 public assistance statute, at first equivocated on whether public assistance was granted as a right, even though they were clear from the outset that Social Security insurance was.[9] The 1965 Medicaid legislation lacked any provision for judicial review of Medicaid eligibility, benefit, or payment determinations, although it did provide for eligibility appeals to the state Medicaid agency.

During the following decade, however, the Supreme Court came to recognize a property-like entitlement in public assistance benefits (discussed in the previous chapter) which continues to benefit Medicaid recipients and providers to this day. Philosophically and psychologically, however, the entitlement nature of welfare programs has always been less well grounded than that of social insurance programs. Benefits under these programs continue to be much more subject to the whims of policymakers, as was evidenced by the abolition of Aid to Families with Dependent Children (AFDC) in 1996 and the creation of an explicitly nonentitlement state Children's Health Insurance Program (SCHIP) in 1997. Indeed, the existence of a federal cause of action to enforce program entitlements, firmly established for three decades, has recently been called into question by an activist conservative judge.[10]

Finally, the character of entitlements under subsidized insurance programs remains even less certain. Legal rights can be specified in a subsidy (or voucher or premium contribution) as the actual benefit of a public insurance program. As noted in Chapter 3 in this volume, legal claims to our current employment-based insurance tax subsidies are clear and enforceable. Rights to and within private programs purchased through the use of such subsidies, however, are much less definite, at least at the constitutional level. For example, employers are currently clearly under no obligation to offer subsidized employment-related group health insurance. Moreover, there is no guarantee that proposed tax credit programs would be sufficient to actually purchase insurance; indeed, there is every likelihood that they would be insufficient for most Americans.

In this chapter I examine the background of these three visions of entitlement by recounting the history of the origins of health-care entitlement programs in the United States. I begin by tracing the emergence of welfare and social insurance programs up through the New Deal and discuss federal health-care programs that preceded the Medicare and Medicaid programs, including tax subsidies for employment-based health insurance. I examine the debate surrounding the Social Security amendments of 1965 that created these programs, focusing in particular on their entitlement characteristics. Finally, I consider the development of Medicare and Medicaid as entitlement programs in the decades following their creation, as well as the evolution of claims to employment-related insurance benefits under ERISA. This chapter lays the groundwork for the following four chapters, in which I explore recent and proposed changes that would restrict the entitlements whose creation and growth is described in this chapter.

## The Origins of Entitlements

The poor have always been with us. At least since the emergence of the modern state in the sixteenth century, some public provision has been made for their support.[11] The Elizabethan poor laws of 1597 to 1601 were the culmination of a series of laws dating back to the fourteenth century directed at dealing with the problem of the poor.[12] Like earlier laws, they imposed harsh penalties on "rogues, vagabonds, and sturdy beggars," who were to be stripped and whipped, or worse.[13] But they also imposed on local parishes the responsibility for the "impotent poor" who were not able to support themselves.[14] The fact that welfare was a local responsibility made the issue of "settlement," or place of residence, a key issue in the handling of the poor, as indigents who had recently entered a parish would be "removed" to their place of origin, which would then be responsible for their upkeep.[15] The tradition of local responsibility for the poor has continued to have a major role in American welfare policy.

The Elizabethan poor laws provided the basis of relief for the poor in Britain until the reforms of 1834, and they influenced American developments even longer.[16] Although better opportunities to find work and to obtain land existed in the American colonies than in England, some provision still remained necessary for the sick, the disabled, and the elderly. As in England, paupers who were capable of working received no sympathy and were subjected to whippings, jail, and removal if possible, and compulsory labor if not; poor, orphaned, or illegitimate children were apprenticed.[17] Nevertheless, communities seem to have taken seriously their responsibility to care for the elderly, widows, and those too disabled to work, at least for residents who were Caucasian.[18] Over time, responsibility for relief increasingly was formalized in the township or county, although eventually the states began to take some responsibility, particularly for the blind, deaf, mentally ill, and others with special needs.[19]

During the nineteenth century, two primary trends became apparent in the treatment of the poor. First, the poor were increasingly regarded with resentment and distrust. Americans seem to have had a growing belief that there was no excuse for poverty in the United States, given the great bounty of its resources. Americans were encouraged in their distaste for poor relief by the writings of economists like Adam Smith and Thomas Malthus, as well as by the Protestant work ethic, which found new life in the Second Great Awakening.[20] Poverty became a moral issue: the poor were not only unfortunate, they were personally responsible for their condition. Moreover, as the poor increasingly consisted of impoverished German and Irish Catholics, who came to the United States in great numbers in the mid-nineteenth century, charity wore thinner among the predominantly English Protestant population that had come before them.[21] Finally, growing concern about alcohol abuse, which was certainly very prevalent at the time, led to a growing apprehension that relief might be used to support alcohol dependency. In combination, all of these factors led to an increasing emphasis on the distinction between the worthy and unworthy poor, an increasing insistence that the unworthy poor should be refused assistance, and an increasing reluctance to help the worthy poor lest the unworthy inadvertently receive help as well.[22]

Yet poverty did not go away just because it was regarded less charitably. Indeed, it got worse as increasing industrialization and urbanization led to population dislocations and to an ever greater incidence of industrial accidents; as seasonal employment became more common; as immigrants flooded the country, often destitute and in ill health; and as Americans continued to fall ill, to grow old, or to die leaving dependents.[23]

The programmatic response to this poverty represents the second major change in the treatment of the poor in the nineteenth century: the emergence of the poorhouse. Throughout the first half of the nineteenth century, counties attempted to cut back on outdoor relief, increasingly confining indigents in poorhouses. In 1824, Massachusetts had 83 almshouses; by 1860, it had 219.[24] The poorhouse was based, as was relief through much of the nineteenth century, on the principle of "less eligibility." This principle, as described in the 1834 Chadwick Report, which provided the philosophical underpinnings of the British poor law reforms, meant that the situation of the individual receiving relief "shall not be made really or apparently so eligible [satisfactory] as the situation of the independent labourer of the lowest class."[25] In other words, the conditions of the poor should be kept so miserable that no one would prefer relief to work. This principle continues to be a lodestar of welfare policy in the United States.

County poorhouses were indeed miserable places. The mentally ill and physically ill, men and women, the elderly and hardened criminals, were thrown together in common residence; fed and clothed poorly (in ill-fitting poorhouse uniforms); and cared for by overseers who were often cruel and corrupt.[26] Although the poorhouse never completely displaced outdoor relief, the opponents of outdoor relief became increasingly vocal and successful as the century wore on. In particular, the Scientific Charity movement of the latter half of the nineteenth century opposed public outdoor relief, which they believed should be replaced, where necessary, by private charity, coordinated in an efficient manner.[27] If poverty was grounded in depravity, as they believed, the appropriate response was spiritual, not material.[28] Only at the end of the nineteenth century did reformers begin to understand that, in fact, poverty was in most cases attributable to technological, cyclical, or other involuntary unemployment or to sickness and disability, and only rarely to laziness or intemperance.[29]

Even though various forms of aid were offered to the poor throughout this period, assistance was offered as a gratuity, not an entitlement. Relief was distributed at the discretion of the local officials; no individual had a legal claim to it.[30] Indeed, in some cities, relief was awarded by local politicians to influence voters, if not votes.[31] As recently as 1935 the governor of Ohio raised old age assistance by 10% right before Christmas and then sent a letter to all recipients requesting that they ask their friends and relatives to vote for him.[32] As the century wore on, this discretion was increasingly used also to exclude the able-bodied from almshouses, as these institutions began to take on the character of infirmaries or hospitals.[33] Tax financing of entitlements was also anathema to reformers of the time. Josephine Shaw Lowell, reflecting the beliefs of the Scientific Charity movement of which she was a leader, stated, "It is not right to tax one part of the community for the benefit of another part; it is not right to take money by law from one man and give it to another, unless for the benefit of both."[34]

This belief that welfare was a gratuity, not an entitlement, continued well into the twentieth century. A description of the Ohio state old age pension program as it existed in 1935 noted that applications were made to the county board, which personally considered each application because the board members, in the words of a contemporary, "know pretty nearly everybody in the county and they can either refuse to approve [a welfare grant], hold it up, [or] make their own personal investigation."[35] Persons granted a pension could lose it if they misspent or wasted it. According to the state director at the time, recipients of the pension had no "recourse to the law at all . . . no right in court. It is purely a gratuity, in other words."[36] Even though the concept of welfare as a pure discretionary gratuity came later to be rejected by the courts with respect to federal public assistance programs, it remains an important theme in American welfare policy.

## The Rise of Entitlements

The fact that welfare grants to the poor were not entitlements in the nineteenth century does not mean that the entitlement concept did not exist at that time. One need only look elsewhere for it.

Over two million men served in the Union army and navy during the Civil War.[37] By the close of the war, 364,511 of these men had lost their lives (most to disease), while 281,881 returned home wounded.[38] Even before the war was half over, Congress had created a pension program for veterans and their widows. The 1862 law provided benefits for those disabled as a "direct consequence of . . . military duty," as well as benefits for the dependents of soldiers whose death was directly traceable to military service.[39] As the century wore on, moreover, repeated amendments made the program ever more generous. In particular, the 1879 Arrears of Pension Act allowed veterans with newly discovered injuries to apply for pensions and receive back payments equivalent to what they would have received had they been continuously receiving benefits since the war, leading to the discovery of many old war injuries as veterans showed up to collect substantial sums of money.[40] The 1890 Dependent Pension Act finally dispensed with the war injury requirement, allowing any veteran who had honorably served 90 days in the Union military to draw a pension if he subsequently became disabled for manual labor, regardless of whether he had served in combat or had sustained a war injury. This change effectively made the veterans' pension program into an old age pension; indeed, in 1906 the law was amended to recognize old age explicitly as grounds for drawing a pension. By 1910, 28.5% of American men aged 65 and over were recipients of Civil War pensions.[41] At its peak in 1893, the program consumed 42.5% of the federal government's income.[42]

In many respects, the Civil War pension program resembled a modern social insurance program. Eligibility requirements were fixed in law. Eligibility was determined by a federal bureaucracy, the Pension Bureau.[43] All eligible persons were entitled to assistance, and Congress simply appropriated the money needed to fund the program for those eligible.[44] Persons denied assistance could appeal to the secretary of the Interior, who received nearly 3,000 appeals in 1886.[45] There was no shame in receiving benefits; indeed, recipient status was honorable. Unlike later social insurance programs, the Civil War pension program was not based on prior financial contributions. It was based on prior military service, however, which served effectively as a functional quid pro quo. That is, benefits were considered to be earned.

The program stood in stark contrast to contemporary relief programs. While aid to the poor in the United States was granted begrudgingly, stingily, and with resentment and condescension, Civil War pensions were generous and provided without recrimination. This was true even though (and perhaps because) they often went to persons who were reasonably well-off members of the working or middle class.[46] Pension recipients were overwhelmingly native-born, white, rural, non-Catholic men from the North, and excluded many of those who in the late nineteenth century were most in need of assistance.[47] Far more was spent on this population, however, than on those more truly in need. In 1915, the state of Massachusetts spent $801,000 on indoor and outdoor relief for the elderly poor.[48] During that same year, Massachusetts awarded $1.8 million, over twice as much, for military aid and local soldier's relief to the elderly.[49] But federal civil war pensions in Massachusetts, amounted to $6.4 million, making the total available to elderly veterans and their dependants $8.2 million, over 10 times that spent on poor relief for seniors. In short, the program not only established a precedent for later entitlement programs but also initiated a pattern that continues to this day in American entitlement programs: generous provision for those who are "worthy" regardless of need, but parsimonious funding for programs for the needy, regardless of worthiness.

## The Emergence of Social Insurance in Europe

While the Civil War pension program may have been America's first modern entitlement program, Medicare and our other modern social insurance programs also find their roots to social insurance programs that emerged in late-nineteenth- and early-twentieth-century Europe. Modern social insurance is usually traced back to the sickness and industrial accident insurance programs created in Bismarck's Germany in the 1880s.[50] Later chapters will consider more closely the nature of European health-care entitlements; we will only touch here briefly on their origins.

Bismarck's 1883 sickness insurance legislation is a central event in the history of social insurance. Bismarck's motivation in urging the Reichstag to adopt this legislation is clear. A growing socialist movement in Germany was viewed as a threat by the conservative leadership of the recently united Germany.[51] Bismarck pushed legislation through the Reichstag in 1878 to ban the Socialist Labor Party, but he understood that repression alone would not protect the state—it was also necessary to win the allegiance of the working class.[52] His social insurance legislation was directed toward this end.

Although social insurance legislation may have been motivated primarily by a desire to co-opt the working classes, it was also consistent with the philosophy of Germany's conservative monarchy. Continental European conservatives never adopted the extreme emphasis on individualism that characterized the United States in the late nineteenth century. Instead, the organic—indeed, paternalistic—view of society that characterized nineteenth-century European conservatism supported the government's obligation to care for those who were, for whatever reason, unable to support themselves.[53] In nineteenth century Europe, as in America, sickness was one of the primary causes of economic insecurity, and social sickness insurance was a natural response to it. The notion of social solidarity as a basis for public health insurance has always enjoyed a much firmer foundation in Europe than in the United States, across political boundaries.

The sickness insurance program enacted by the Reichstag in 1886 built on the preexisting German mutual insurance system. Workers employed in certain designated industries whose incomes were less than 2000 Marks a year were required to contribute to sickness insurance funds at rates that varied by fund between 1.5% and 6% of income.[54] Employers paid one-third of the contributions; the insured paid two-thirds. The sickness funds were governed by a board and general assembly in which employers and employees were represented according to their contributions. At first, the most important benefit provided by the sickness funds was replacement pay for those who were too sick to work.[55] From the outset, however, the funds also paid for medical care, a feature that became increasingly important as time went on.[56] Eligibility and benefit coverage criteria were governed by statute, and decisions were made by the supervisory board of the fund. Legal proceedings could be brought to dispute these decisions. The Imperial Insurance Office oversaw the administration of the funds, and in the early twentieth century became the highest forum for deciding sickness insurance matters.[57] The program formed the pattern for, and in many respects closely resembled, modern social insurance entitlement programs.

## The American Response

Social health insurance spread slowly throughout Europe following its introduction in Germany. Austria adopted social health insurance in 1888, and Hungary in 1891, followed by Norway in 1909, Serbia in 1910, and Britain, Russia, and Italy in 1911.[58]

At first, however, European developments received little attention in the United States.[59] The Progressive Movement's reaction to the extreme laissez faire approach of late-nineteenth-century American individualism began, however, to bear fruit in social insurance experiments at the end of the nineteenth century. The devastating effects of the depression of 1893 seemed to give lie to the belief that poverty was based solely on individual depravity.[60] Social progressives came to believe that some sort of societal response to poverty was appropriate.

Early social insurance initiatives took place at the state level. The first wave of state legislation established mother's pensions (which were adopted by 40 states between 1910 and 1920) and workers' compensation programs, 43 of which were established between 1909 and 1920.[61] Widows and orphans had long been treated more charitably than other indigents, and the women's movement early in the twentieth century was successful in convincing most of the states to establish welfare programs for their support.[62] Workers' compensation proposals had strong support from labor. As the protection from liability that employers had long enjoyed in the courts began to fray in the late nineteenth century, employers began to see the wisdom of state administrative programs to establish, but also to limit, employer liability for worker's injuries.[63] Also at this time, states began more slowly to adopt old age assistance programs, 10 of which were in place by 1930.[64]

In the late 1910s, the time finally seemed ripe to push for a national sickness insurance program as well. The success of movements to establish widow's pensions and workers' compensation programs encouraged progressives, led by the American Association for Labor Legislation (AALL), to believe that sickness insurance might also find support.[65] They argued that health insurance would relieve poverty by protecting against the devastating and indiscriminate costs of illness, while at the same time reducing the total cost of illness by encouraging prevention.[66] German experience with social health insurance seemed to support arguments for reform.[67] The AALL marshaled a coalition of progressive academics and enlightened business people, who pushed for reform based largely on the German model.[68] Even, for a brief moment, medical leaders seemed to be in support.[69] By 1917 initiatives were being pressed at the national level, and a standard health insurance bill had been introduced in 15 state legislatures.[70]

Then everything fell apart. Labor leaders, especially Samuel Gompers of the American Federation of Labor, opposed the government taking over the provision of welfare benefits to workers, a role that they coveted for themselves.[71] Employers also consolidated their opposition to the legislation.[72] After a brief initial period of openness to change, organized medicine came around rather rapidly to a stance of obdurate, and highly effective, opposition, which it assumed toward public health insurance for decades thereafter.[73] Insurance companies, who as of then sold little health insurance but who did make a great deal of money from "industrial life insurance" policies (policies that were paid for with very small monthly premiums and that offered burial payments at death), opposed the proposal, which would have offered burial policies as part of the sickness benefit.[74] The program was also opposed by the Pharmaceutical Manufacturer's Association. Finally, as America was drawn into World War I, enthusiasm for things German quickly waned.[75] By 1918, social health insurance was no longer on the table.

While the failure of social health insurance in the early twentieth century was primarily due to political factors, there was also a serious underlying concern as to whether federal sponsorship of social insurance would be permitted under the U.S. Constitution. In response to the persistent importuning of Dorothea Dix, Congress had in 1854 adopted legislation to appropriate 10 million acres of land to the states to help pay for the construction and maintenance of mental hospitals.[76] President Franklin Pierce vetoed the legislation, stating, "If Congress has the power to make provision for the indigent insane

. . . it has the same power for the indigent who are not insane."[77] "I cannot find any authority in the Constitution for making the Federal Government the great almoner of public charity throughout the United States," Pierce contended. A federal welfare program, he argued, "would be contrary to the letter and spirit of the Constitution, and subversive of the whole theory upon which the union of these states is founded."[78]

In the late nineteenth and early twentieth century, the U.S. Supreme Court and many of the state courts also took a hostile stance to social legislation. Time and again during this period, the courts struck down progressive labor legislation as violating private freedom of contract and private property rights.[79] This hostility continued right up to the New Deal, and whether or not the Court would accept the constitutionality of the 1935 Social Security Act remained an open question until the Court decided *Helvering v. Davis* in 1937.[80] The problem of industrial accidents was addressed at the state rather than the federal level in part because of a concern that federal legislation would face constitutional obstacles.[81] While social codes were used as a positive force to create entitlements in Europe, conservative interpretations of the U.S. and state constitutions retarded the growth of social entitlements in the United States.

## Entitlements under the New Deal

The Social Security Act of 1935 was the seminal event in the creation of entitlements in the United States. The severe economic dislocation of the Great Depression quickly overwhelmed state, local, and private relief efforts.[82] President Herbert Hoover initially rejected the possibility of a federal relief effort to address the problem.[83] Federal policy changed dramatically, however, with the election of Franklin Roosevelt, who initiated a massive federal relief and jobs program.

President Franklin D. Roosevelt and many of his conservative supporters, however, felt very uncomfortable with these federal relief efforts and job programs.[84] The largest of the programs, the Civilian Work Administration (CWA) and Federal Emergency Relief Administration (FERA) were of short duration, while funding for others was cut as the Depression wore on.[85] Roosevelt preferred to put the problem of support for the poor on the more secure foundation of social insurance.

By 1935, the president and Congress had begun to focus their attention to the problem of the elderly. A primary motivating factor was the increasing militance of labor and of the elderly.[86] Francis Townsend's plan for a flat federal pension of $200 a month to be paid to persons over 60 who stopped working and agreed to spend the entire pension every month, galvanized the elderly, who flooded Congress with mail.[87] The Democratic landslide of 1934, moreover, brought to Washington a Congress eager to move forward with social insurance.[88]

Roosevelt favored contributory social insurance rather than a noncontributory welfare program for the elderly. His Retirement Annuity Program was to be constructed on fiscally conservative social insurance principles. Eligibility was to be based on status rather than need and therefore no means test would be applied. The program would be funded through social insurance "contributions" rather than general taxes. The program's benefits were to be based on earlier earnings and would not strive for equality.[89] In the words of one of the program's architects: "Only to a very minor degree does it modify the distribution of wealth and it does not alter at all the fundamentals of our capitalistic and individualistic economy. Nor does it relieve the individual of primary responsibility for his own support and that of his dependents."[90]

Because the program was to be funded through contributions, regular pension payments were deferred until after 1942 when persons would begin to retire who had paid into the fund for a sufficient period of time.[91] To provide assistance in the interim, Congress also created an old age assistance program through which the states would provide federally subsidized welfare payments for those in need.[92] In addition, this program provided federal matching funds for state welfare programs for dependent children and for the blind.[93] Participation in the program was at the option of the states, and state responses varied widely: for a considerable time after 1935, many more people received old age assistance than received social security insurance, and in some states assistance payments were considerably higher than social insurance payments.[94]

The Social Security Act was significantly amended in 1939 to advance the date of payments to 1940, increase payments for married couples, extend coverage to survivors, change the method through which benefits were computed, and (to a significant extent) delink payments from contributions.[95] Nevertheless, the principles found in the 1935 act continue to define social insurance entitlements in the United States.

These defining characteristics are as follows: eligibility requirements for social security insurance beneficiaries are established by federal law. A person meeting these eligibility requirements is entitled to benefits.[96] Eligibility is determined by a federal bureaucracy. Administrative review is available to those adversely affected by bureaucratic decisions.[97] Entitlement is linked to contributions. This linkage became even more explicit after the Supreme Court's decision in *Helvering v. Davis* cleared the way for federal operation of a contributory social insurance system.[98] Early advocates of Social Security attempted, in fact, to create the impression that Social Security had created an essentially contractual obligation—that the contributions were the quid pro quo for a government pension that would be paid upon retirement.[99] Finally, Social Security payments do not depend on federal appropriations. Eligible persons have the right to benefits, regardless of the actions taken by Congress in any particular year.[100]

The federal public assistance programs created under the Social Security Act also laid the groundwork for future welfare programs, including Medicaid. Many of the key provisions of the current Title XIX of the Social Security Act (the Medicaid statute) are found for the first time in this statute.[101] These include requirements that the assistance be provided under a state plan that operates statewide and is approved by the federal government; that there be a single state agency to administer the program, staffed through a civil service system; that all be afforded an opportunity to apply for assistance; that aid be provided with reasonable promptness; and that the confidentiality of information concerning applicants and recipients be maintained. The statute also required that the states provide for fair hearings for aggrieved public assistance applicants and recipients, an early recognition that assistance was in some sense a right, not merely a gratuity.[102]

## Public Health Insurance in the United States

While President Franklin D. Roosevelt was successful in securing adoption of both a social insurance and a public assistance program for the elderly in 1935, his program did not include a federal health insurance program. While there was considerable support for a federal social insurance program that would provide health benefits, and adoption of such programs had generally preceded the adoption of old age pension programs in Europe, fervent opposition to national health insurance, led by the American Medical Association, threatened to bring down the entire social insurance program if health insurance was a part of it.[103] Edwin Witte, the chair of Roosevelt's Committee on Economic Security, which drafted the 1935 Social Security legislation, reported that there had been one line in the original bill requiring the Social Security Board to study the problem of health insurance and report back to Congress, but that this provision provoked so many telegrams to Congress that it was unanimously stricken from the bill by the House Ways and Means Committee in order to save the legislation.[104] The only health-care provisions found in the 1935 Social Security Act were block grant provisions, which provided $3.8 million in federal grants to the states for maternal and child health services and $2.85 million for crippled children services.[105]

By 1935, however, government provision of health care in the United States was well established. Medical services were among the many goods and services furnished in kind to paupers by traditional local outdoor relief programs.[106] During the nineteenth century, poor people routinely received primary care from "dispensaries," which were usually provided through private charities and staffed by volunteer part-time physicians and their students.[107] These were complemented by public and voluntary hospitals. By the mid-nineteenth century, some poorhouses had begun to evolve into hospitals or nursing homes.[108] In some parts of the country, counties or municipalities additionally founded their own hospitals, which, although they offered services to all residents, often served the poor in particular.[109] Municipal hospitals and clinics were well established by the 1930s (New York had 23 by 1935), and by the early 1930s some cities and counties were paying for indigent care in private hospitals.[110] States, on the other hand, began to open hospitals to treat the mentally ill or persons with tuberculosis.[111] Of course, much health care was still provided through private charity: doctors still provided a great deal of free care, and families were expected to take care of their poorer relations.[112]

The federal government was also not entirely absent from the payment and provision of health care. As early as 1798, the government created a program to provide medical care to merchant seamen based on contributions by ship owners of 20 cents per month for each sailor in their employ.[113] During wars the federal government provided medical care to its troops; after wars it cared for its veterans. The War Risk Insurance Act of 1917 required the government to supply "medical, surgical, and hospital services" to injured veterans.[114] Services to veterans were expanded through the 1920s, and in 1930 Congress created the Veterans Administration (VA) to take charge of these activities.[115] By World War II, the VAs 91 institutions comprised the largest health-care system in the United States, and between 1945 and 1955 the number of VA facilities nearly doubled again.[116] For the brief period of reconstruction following the Civil War, the Freedman's Bureau in the South operated a system of hospitals for former slaves.[117] For an even briefer period immediately before World War I, the Sheppard–Towner Act provided federal funding for preventative health services for mothers and infants.[118]

## The Birth of Tax-Subsidized Employment-Related Health Insurance

While a few government programs began to address the need for health care in the United States in the first half of the twentieth century, the United States did not initially follow the path of European (and Latin American) nations towards developing social health insurance programs. Instead, between 1930 and 1960, private insurance coverage, mostly employment-related expanded rapidly, within a generation becoming the dominant means of financing health care in the country. The rapid rise of health insurance was encouraged, but not initially driven, by government policy. By the end of the 1950s, however, the federal tax entitlements discussed in the last chapter had become a major force in consolidating our employment-related health insurance system.

Private health insurance in the United States dates back to the late nineteenth and early twentieth century, when a number of employers and unions had offered some job-related health benefits, although the focus of benefits was often more on income replacement than on medical cost coverage.[119] Health insurance (initially primarily hospital insurance) first really came into its own during the 1930s, when Blue Cross plans began to appear. The first hospital service plan was started in 1929, and Blue Cross membership grew quickly, reaching six million by 1940, 19 million by 1945 and 79 million by 1958.[120] Commercial insurers noticed the success of the Blue Cross hospital insurance plans (and after 1939, of the Blue Shield medical benefit plans), and aggressively entered the health insurance market. By the early 1950s, commercial insurers covered more insured lives than Blue Cross plans.[121]

Early Blue Cross, Blue Shield, and commercial plans were predominantly group policies, and most were employment-related.[122] The insurers quickly realized that selling individual policies was a risky business, exposing the insurer to adverse selection, and the insured to high marketing and underwriting costs.[123] Early group policies, however, were paid for almost exclusively by employees. Though employers permitted the sale of group policies to their employees, and often deducted the premiums from pay checks through a payroll deduction system, they rarely contributed to the premiums during the 1940s.[124] By the end of the war, only 7.6% of Blue Cross enrollees were participants in employer contribution groups.[125]

After 1940, federal government policy began to encourage the spread of health insurance. In 1942 the War Labor Board had imposed wage and price controls to stanch wartime inflation, but in 1943 the Board ruled that contribution to insurance and pension funds did not constitute wages.[126] Some employers responded by offering health insurance as a fringe benefit to attract scarce workers. Contributions for health insurance also were recognized as deductible by employers for purposes of the wartime excess profits tax.[127] The National Labor Relations Board recognized fringe benefits as a proper subject for collective bargaining in 1948 (a position upheld by the courts), and and over half the strikes in 1949 and the first half of 1950 concerned health and welfare issues.[128] During the Korean war, health insurance benefits were again exempted from a general wage-price freeze, making them again an attractive means of competing for labor.[129]

Tax policy also contributed to the spread of health insurance. Contributions by employers for fringe benefits, including health insurance, had always been compensation and thus business expenses, excludable by employers in calculating their income for tax purposes. The greater issue, however, was whether employees would be taxed on these benefits. The original 1919 Internal Revenue Code excluded from income "Amounts received, through accident or health insurance . . . as compensation for personal injuries or sickness."[130] The 1939

Code was amended in 1942 to allow a deduction for medical expenses not covered by insurance.[131] While it was clear that the insurance exclusion covered payments from commercial insurance policies, it was less clear whether it covered benefits received directly from employers or unions.[132] It was also unclear whether employer contributions to employee health insurance policies were income or not.[133] In 1943 the Internal Revenue Service (IRS) ruled that employer payments for group medical and hospital insurance policies were not taxable as income to employees,[134] creating an additional incentive for employers to contribute to health insurance benefits. But the importance of the tax code to the phenomenal growth of health insurance during the 1940s has probably been overrated. In fact most employees purchased health insurance, including employment-related group policies, out of their own after-tax compensation.

All this changed in the 1950s. The 1954 Internal Revenue Code finally and conclusively established the deductibility of employment-related health insurance benefit through sections 105 and 106 discussed in Chapter 3. Once it became clear that neither the employer nor the employee had to pay taxes on health insurance, employers rapidly began to take responsibility for premiums. Whereas in 1953, 77% of insured households paid their own insurance premiums, and only 17% had their premiums partially covered by their employer and 7% entirely covered, by 1958, only 58% paid the full premium, 25% had partial employer contributions, and 18% had full employer contributions.[135] As employers began to cover an increasing share of premiums, insurance coverage expanded even more rapidly. By 1958, 74% of Americans had private health insurance coverage, and 67% had access to group insurance.[136]

Subsequent amendments to the code have broadened tax subsidies for health insurance. First, § 125, adopted in 1978 and amended several times since, authorizes employers to establish "cafeteria plans" and to cover otherwise nondeductible medical expenses. It permits employees to deposit contributions into flexible savings accounts and to withdraw funds from them to cover health insurance premiums and medical expenses free from taxation.[137] About half of American employees work in firms that offer flexible benefit plans.[138] Second, § 162(l) of the code permits self-employed persons to deduct from their income a portion of the cost of health insurance premiums (100% as of 2003 and afterward).[139] Third, recently adopted amendments to the tax code permit small employers and the self-employed to make tax-free contributions to medical savings accounts and allow employees to obtain benefits under these programs free from taxation if certain requirements are met.[140] Other recent code amendments extend to long-term care insurance the same tax treatment afforded health insurance if certain requirements are met.[141] Finally, a revenue ruling issued in 2002 permits employer funding of Health Reimbursement Accounts (HRAs) to cover employee medical expenses in coordination with high-deductible health insurance policies.[142]

Employment-related coverage expanded rapidly during the 1950s, 1960s, and 1970s, when productivity was high and health insurance costs were relatively low. By 1977 over 70% of the American population under age 65 had employment-related coverage.[143] During the 1980s, as, simultaneously, health insurance costs shot up, wage growth leveled off, tax rates declined, and public insurance spread, the growth of employment-related insurance flattened. During the 1990s, as health insurance cost growth moderated and the economy prospered, employer offers of insurance again increased, but employee take-up, and with it overall levels of employment-related coverage, fell.[144] Only at the very end of the 1990s, as a strong economy drove unemployment down and compensation up, did employment-related coverage again expand, even though it did not rise again to the levels of coverage seen in the early 1980s.

At the outset of the twenty-first century, health insurance costs are again on the increase, and the number of those insured through their place of employment is again dropping.[145] But employment-related health insurance remains our primary source of insurance coverage.

## The Birth of Public Assistance Health-Care Programs

While America made dramatic progress in expanding health insurance for the middle class during the first half of the twentieth century, explicit public health programs for the poor developed more slowly. The first inkling of provision of health-care entitlements within the framework of the Social Security Act is found in the Social Security Act Amendments of 1950.[146] These provisions for the first time committed the federal government to match, to a very limited extent, state expenditures for in-kind medical services ("vendor payments") through the matching fund provisions of the federal/state public assistance programs for the elderly, blind, and disabled and for families with dependent children. Federal payments were minimal (three-quarters of total state expenditures for cash assistance and vendor payments up to $20, and half of the next $30, for any particular elderly individual), and only 20 states submitted federally approved plans for making vendor payments during the first six years of the program.[147] In 1957 the federal matching formula was changed to permit federal payments of up to one-half of the sum of $6 per adult and $3 per child for money spent by a state on average for medical vendor payments; a year later federal matching funds were made generally available for medical vendor payments and cash assistance based on a statewide average rather than on an individual recipient basis.[148] By 1960, 40 states had federally approved vendor payment plans, and $514 million was being spent on medical care by public assistance programs.[149]

Federal assistance for state indigent health-care plans was dramatically expanded by the Social Security Act Amendments of 1960, which created the Kerr–Mills program.[150] Kerr–Mills (sponsored by Senator Robert Kerr and Congressman Wilbur Mills) expanded federal matching funds for medical services for the elderly receiving old age assistance, while also creating a new program to pay for services for what would come to be known as the "medically needy" elderly—those who were "not recipients of old-age assistance but whose income and resources [were] insufficient to meet the costs of necessary medical services."[151] Kerr–Mills authorized federal matching funds for state programs for up to an average of $12 per recipient.

Many requirements found in the later 1965 Medicaid Act were found in the Kerr–Mills statute. These included requirements for statewide coverage; financial participation by the states; administration by a single state agency; opportunity for a fair hearing for those whose applications were denied or not acted on with reasonable promptness; proper and efficient plan administration (including merit-based personnel policies); reporting to the secretary of Health, Education and Welfare; confidentiality safeguards; and establishment and maintenance of institutional standards. The list of services covered under Kerr–Mills also resembles closely that found in the later Title XIX.[152] Indeed, since the last category covered by Kerr–Mills was "any other medical care or remedial care covered under state law," as a practical matter the two are identical. While many of these requirements were found in earlier public assistance legislation, Kerr–Mills also imposed new requirements on participating states, including a condition that state plans include both institutional and noninstitutional services and prohibitions against state-imposed durational residency requirements or the imposition of liens on the property of recipients.[153] Perhaps most important, however, Kerr–Mills carried forward the key principle of federal matching funds to support state vendor payments, which had characterized the 1950 legislation. It refined this principle also, providing for different levels of federal matching funds varying between 50% and 80%, depending on the per capita income of the state. A similar formula continues to be used in the Medicaid program.

Kerr–Mills caught on slowly. By the time President Dwight D. Eisenhower left office in 1960, only six states had Kerr–Mills plans, several of which were established by simply transferring recipients from the old vendor payment plans that had a lower federal match.[154] Only 36 states had adopted Kerr–Mills plans by 1963, with legislatures rejecting the program in some states, governors vetoing legislation in others.[155] By July 1963, only 148,000 people received Kerr–Mills assistance, which was less than 1% of the nation's elderly, and 88% of all funds were going to five states.[156]

States that adopted the program were far from generous. Several states imposed deductibles or enacted laws allowing the state to make a claim against a recipient's estate at death.[157] A dozen states investigated the resources of children of the applicant as part of the eligibility process, while some states illegally charged enrollees "enrollment fees."[158] When Medicaid was created a half decade later, however, it was considered to be merely an expanded version of Kerr–Mills. Indeed, the section of the Senate report dealing with Medicaid was entitled "Improvement and Extension of Kerr–Mills Medical Assistance Program," and the language of the 1965 Medicaid Act resembles Kerr–Mills much more closely than it does the current Title XIX.[159]

## Efforts to Create Universal Social Health Insurance in the United States

As health-care coverage for the poor moved slowly forward, repeated attempts to create a universal social health insurance continued to stall. After World War II, the nature of public health insurance programs in Europe had began to change. Britain's Beveridge Commission Report had proposed moving beyond the British social insurance program (which had been established in 1911 and provided public health insurance for workers) to create a national health service that would cover the entire British population.[160] With the creation of the National Health Service (NHS) following the war, Britain's remaining private charitable hospitals became public hospitals and specialists became employees of the NHS; general practitioners remained in private practice under contract with the NHS.[161] Even before the establishment of the British NHS, New Zealand had created a national health service in 1938, followed in short order by similar services created in Costa Rica and Mexico. After the war, Japan, Norway, Sweden, Hungary, and Chile also established national health services.[162] During the same period, Germany and some central European countries expanded their social health insurance systems to cover most of their populations.

Although President Harry S. Truman campaigned for a national health insurance program more vigorously than had Franklin Roosevelt before him, the United States turned rightward following the war, electing a Republican congressional majority.[163] The only parts of Truman's program that survived congressional debate were the Hill–Burton hospital construction program (which between 1947 and 1971 disbursed $3.7 billion in federal funds for hospital construction, contributing to 30% of all hospital projects during the period), new federal funding for mental health care, and a heavy federal commitment to funding health-care research.[164] These programs were not entitlement programs, however, even though vague provisions in the Hill Burton program obligating grantees to serve their communities and to provide a "reasonable volume" of uncompensated care were relied on by the courts in later years to impose on hospitals an enforceable obligation to provide services to indigents.[165]

The rabid anticommunism of the late 1940s and early 1950s put on hold any further attempts to expand government funding of health-care services. For a generation after the war, organized medicine successfully raised the specter of socialism whenever proposals to expand coverage were mooted.[166] Throughout the 1950s, Congress was controlled by the Republican Party, which generally opposed a larger role for government.[167] President Eisenhower is quoted as saying "If all that Americans want is security, they can go to prison. They'll have enough to eat, a bed, and a roof over their heads."[168] More important, the Democrats in Congress during this time were dominated by conservatives from the South, who opposed programs that might undermine the racial and economic caste systems of that region.[169] Nevertheless, pressure for national health insurance was quietly building among organized labor and the elderly.[170] Advocates of national health insurance, moreover, adapted strategically so that by 1950 they limited their immediate goals to cover only Social Security beneficiaries with social health insurance, and by 1960, to the coverage of inpatient hospital care.[171]

With the election of President John F. Kennedy in 1960, efforts to provide health care for the elderly were redoubled. Proposed legislation enjoyed more support in Congress, but it continued to stall in the key House Ways and Means Committee, dominated by Congressman Wilbur Mills, who presided over a majority of Republicans and conservative Democrats. Only the landslide election of President Lyndon B. Johnson and of a liberal Democratic Congress (and the clear rejection of the conservative "choice, not an echo" represented by Barry Goldwater) in 1964 made some form of national health insurance finally inevitable.

Traditional advocates of national health insurance, disciplined by decades of disappointment, chose initially to hold to the strategy they had pursued for the previous decade, pushing only for hospital insurance for the elderly based on a contributory, social insurance model.[172] Republicans in Congress, realizing that some expansion of federal health insurance was inevitable, made a strategic retreat, proposing a subsidized voluntary health insurance program to cover the cost of doctors' services and drugs, with the federal government paying two-thirds of the cost and subscribers the other one-third in premiums.[173] Organized medicine—for the first time facing the realistic possibility of an expanded federal role in health insurance—pushed its own "Eldercare" program, a means-tested program that would amend the Kerr–Mills program to provide federal assistance to states that would subsidize the purchase of private insurance by indigents.[174]

These three proposals, of course, mirrored the three models discussed at the outset of this chapter. By this time, the Social Security old age insurance program was three decades old and a popular and well-established program.[175] Backers of national health insurance hoped that a contributory social insurance program for the elderly would form the basis for eventual expansion of health-care social insurance to the general population.

The American Medical Association's "Eldercare" plan[176] would have required federal matching funds to be provided to states that, in turn, would contract to purchase private insurance policies to cover hospital, doctor, and drug costs.[177] Beneficiaries would contribute toward premium payments, with contributions based on their income. From the conservative perspective of the AMA, the plan had both the virtue of being administered through private insurers, thus minimizing government oversight of medical practice, and of being means-tested, thus limiting eligibility and potential future expansion.

The Republican Byrnes bill[178] also called for a federally administered voluntary health insurance plan to cover hospital and medical costs, financed by graduated premiums based on ability to pay and matched by federal contributions.[179] Other Republicans submitted similar bills, including S. 395, proposed by Sen. Leverett Saltonstall (which would have allowed persons over 65 with incomes below $3,000 a year to choose between one of three private insurance plans in a program administered by the states and funded by the state and federal government and beneficiary contributions); and H.R. 1031, proposed by Congressman Charles S. Gruser (which would have provided federal funds to help states buy private insurance for the elderly, who would have a choice of four plans).[180] Other plans provided for federal tax subsidies for the purchase of private health insurance (H.R. 21, sponsored by Rep. Frank T. Bow) or tax deductions for medical bills (H.R. 2614).[181]

By 1965, tax subsidies had been available for group health insurance policies for over two decades and had resulted in widespread coverage of employees.[182] The medical profession, which had initially resisted private insurance as limiting its prerogatives, had come to terms with the existence of private indemnity insurance, which provided doctors with generous incomes but imposed minimal constraints on medical practice.[183] Several states had worked together with private insurers to offer low-cost health insurance plans to elderly persons, but even these plans cost more than most elderly persons could afford and received few takers.[184]

Public subsidization of private insurance seemed like a noncontroversial approach to broadening insurance coverage. As early as 1949, the Flanders–Ives bill (sponsored by Representative Richard Nixon, among others), had proposed partial federal reimbursement for state subsidies for private nonprofit health insurance.[185] In 1954, President Eisenhower had proposed a plan to offer federal reinsurance for private insurers with usually heavy health insurance losses.[186] Other bills sponsored by liberal Republicans John Lindsay and Jacob Javits would have created a social insurance–based program, like Medicare, but would have offered beneficiaries the alternative of a cash payment to purchase private insurance.[187] The American Association of Retired Persons (AARP), which began as an association of retired teachers partially funded by the Continental Casualty Insurance Company, backed Javits's bill for a time.[188]

Although the Kennedy administration was willing to consider Javits's proposal, the plan was opposed by Nelson Cruikshank, who represented the interests of the American Federation of Labor in the negotiations leading up to the creation of Medicare. Cruikshank argued that private insurance company administration would impose too high administrative costs, leaving as little as 39 cents on the dollar to actually pay for health care.[189] There was also a concern that allowing insureds to opt out of Medicare for private insurance would lead to cherry picking and undermine the financial base of Medicare.

What emerged from Congress in 1965 was the aforementioned "three-layer cake" of Medicare and Medicaid.[190] Under the direction of Wilbur Mills, the brilliant politician who headed up the House Ways and Means Committee, the Johnson administration's contributory hospital insurance program became Part A of Medicare, a trimmed-down and reworked Byrnes bill became Part B, and the AMA's Eldercare expansion of Kerr–Mills became Medicaid.[191] Both the House and Senate passed the legislation, which was signed into law by President Johnson on July 31, 1965, in Independence, Missouri, the home of President Truman, who had been denied the chance to sign such legislation two decades earlier.[192]

Part A, the Hospital Insurance (HI) program, covered inpatient hospital, skilled nursing, and home health services.[193] Part A was funded, like Social Security, by payroll taxes assessed against employers, employees, and the self-employed and by interest income on its trust fund.[194] Part B (Supplemental Medical Insurance, or SMI) benefits helped pay for physicians' services, outpatient hospital services, physical therapy, home health services, durable medical equipment, surgical dressings, splints and casts; ambulance services, prosthetics and orthotics; and some diagnostic tests.[195] Part A and Part B were to be administered under contract by private entities (usually Blue Cross and Blue Shield plans) referred to as "intermediaries" for Part A and "carriers" for Part B. Providing a role for private insurers in the administration of the program as a way of mollifying opposition to Medicare had been a part of Kennedy and Johnson administration proposals since the early 1960s.[196]

Medicaid, or Title XIX, carried considerably further the means-tested, state-administered model of providing public health insurance found in Kerr–Mills. The key difference between Kerr–Mills and Medicaid was that Medicaid expanded Kerr–Mills to cover all persons who received federally supported cash assistance—not just the aged but also the blind, the disabled, and dependent children. Medicaid also replaced the 1950 legislation, which had continued to provide much more limited federal medical assistance to families of dependent children and to the blind and disabled who were receiving state assistance under the federal/state cash assistance programs after Kerr–Mills had been adopted. States that participated in Medicaid were now required to cover all persons who received cash assistance under any of these programs, in addition to persons covered under Kerr Mills.[197]

Title XIX, like Kerr–Mills before it, permitted the states to offer medical assistance to persons who were not receiving cash assistance but who were in the categories otherwise eligible for cash assistance and whose income and resources were insufficient to cover the cost of needed medical services, a group known as the medically needy.[198] With respect to these persons, the states had to establish reasonable standards to take into account income and assets.[199]

Title XIX brought about not just an expansion in the groups covered by Kerr–Mills but also amelioration of its more burdensome eligibility requirements. States could no longer hold adult children responsible for their parent's medical costs, a characteristic of many state Kerr–Mills programs that had posed a substantial deterrent to elderly participation.[200] States also had to remove all residency requirements, ending centuries of the "settlement" tradition in welfare benefits.[201]

Although the services covered by Title XIX were nearly identical to those covered by Kerr–Mills, states were now required to cover a specified range of services, including hospital and physician care, which exceeded the services provided by most states under Kerr–Mills.[202] Further, § 1903(e) of Title XIX provided that the Department of Health, Education and Welfare (HEW) was not to make payments to states unless they were making "efforts in the direction of broadening the scope of care and services made available under the plan and in the direction of liberalizing the eligibility requirements for medical assistance, with a view toward furnishing by July 1, 1975 comprehensive care and services to substantially all individuals" who were financially eligible for services. This aspiration of comprehensiveness faded away in later years; the requirement was first delayed until 1977 and then repealed. Nevertheless, it represented an initial commitment to bring welfare medicine into the mainstream and to extend it to all American poor.

## Statutory Entitlements in the Medicare and Medicaid Legislation

As noted in Chapter 2, entitlement is a recurrent theme in the Medicare and Medicaid statutes. Entitlement language is used repeatedly in Parts A and B of Title XVIII in describing the rights of beneficiaries to coverage and is also found in Title XIX. Each of the three components of the new health insurance program also had its own administrative and judicial review provisions, reflecting the vision of entitlements in recipients and beneficiaries grounding each program. The Medicare Part A program simply adopted the administrative and judicial review provisions of the Social Security program by cross reference.[203] In 1972, Congress created the Provider Reimbursement Review Board (PRRB) to afford providers a means of review for reimbursement disputes. Consistent with the principle that rights under social insurance programs are earned, or exchange-based, rights, administrative and judicial review was fully available, subject only to efficiecy constraints where petty sums were involved.

Medicare Part B, the SMI program, afforded much more limited opportunities for review. Questions of eligibility for Part B services were reviewable by an ALJ and by the courts, just as were Part A eligibility decisions.[204] Denials of benefits, however, were reviewable only by the "carrier," the private entities through which Part B was to be administered.[205] No judicial review was provided for Part B benefit denials.[206] Apparently, Congress believed that claims under Part B would be both more numerous and for smaller amounts than claims under Part A, and that judicial review would be both less necessary to protect claimants and more burdensome on the government.[207]

The denial of federal administrative and judicial review of SMI claims was also consistent with the view that SMI was a subsidized voluntary insurance program rather than a social insurance program. One would not expect that federal administrative law judges and courts would be available to review the decisions of private insurers but was never really accurate to characterize SMI as a voluntary program. By the time that the SMI program became operational in 1966, virtually all (16 million of the 17 million) Americans eligible to participate had signed up.[208] Federal general revenue funds initially paid 50% of the program's cost (now 75%), and few of the elderly could afford to pass up this subsidy. Medicaid paid Part B premiums for the medically indigent, thus these persons were brought into the program as well. Persons who became eligible for the program had to sign up within three years after the close of the first enrollment period in which they could have enrolled, which discouraged adverse selection.[209] Moreover, because private insurance cannot compete with the deal Medicare SMI offers, private insurance as an alternative for the elderly became simply not available. Almost from the beginning, therefore, SMI was in fact an adjunct to the Medicare social insurance program, not a truly private insurance program. Nevertheless, legal remedies available under Part B did not for some time approximate the generosity of those available under Part A.

Medicaid, like Medicare and like the previous Kerr–Mills program, was established as a budgetary entitlement program. Section 1901 of the statute authorized, for each fiscal year, appropriations sufficient to pay the federal medical assistance percentage and thus to fund approved state plans. Section 1903(d), indeed, referred to the amounts to which the states are "entitled." In essence, Title XIX simply committed the federal government to match funds that states were willing to put up for funding medical assistance.

Moreover, the Medicaid statute expressly created federal rights for individual participants. Section 1092(a)(3), for example, required state plans to provide an "opportunity for a fair hearing before the State agency to any individual whose claim for medical assistance under the plan is denied or is not acted upon with reasonable promptness." Section 1902(a)(8) required participating states to "provide that all individuals wishing to make application for medical assistance under the plan shall have opportunity to do so, and that such assistance shall be furnished with reasonable promptness to all eligible individuals." The statute also imposed specific obligations on the states. Section 1902(a)(10) required states to make aid available to different categories of the categorically needy that was equal in "amount, duration, and scope." It also required states to make medical assistance available to all persons who were receiving cash assistance.

Title XIX further recognized (to a limited extent) the rights of providers. Section 1092(a)(13), for example, required that the states provide "for payment of the reasonable cost (as determined in accordance with standards approved by the Secretary and included in the plan) of inpatient hospital services provided under the plan." This essentially imported into Medicaid the reasonable-cost payment standard for insitutitional services applied by Medicare, which, in turn, had imported it from the prevailing Blue Cross standard.

While Congress explicitly created federal rights in the Medicaid program for participants and providers, the mechanism through which these rights were to be protected was less clear. The only reference in the statute itself to recipient remedies was the provision for an opportunity for a fair hearing for recipients who had been denied assistance or whose applications were not acted on in reasonable promptness, a provision that had been in the federally funded assistance program statutes since 1935.[210] The only other remedy Title XIX provided to protect recipient rights was a provision permitting the secretary of HEW to terminate further payments to a state (after reasonable notice and hearing) when a state plan became so altered that it no longer complied with Title XIX or when "in the administration of the plan there [was] a failure to comply substantially with" Title XIX.[211]

These remedies were by and large ineffective. Several states did not permit challenges to the legality of state laws or regulations under the Social Security Act in the fair hearing process.[212] Even where it was possible to press these issues through judicial review of state administrative decisions, the issues had to be raised on a case by case basis, as class actions were not available for review of state administrative decisions.[213] Given the fact that then, as now, welfare recipients rarely had access to counsel, this made it very difficult to bring about changes in illegal state Medicaid provisions. Litigating the interpretation of the Social Security statute in state court could also have led to inconsistent interpretations of the federal law, with the possibility of Title XIX providing different protections to recipients in different states. Finally, to the extent that the resolution of a challenge to a state Medicaid provision required relief against the federal government, state courts might prove impotent to protect recipients.

The federal conformity hearing provisions of the statute, permitting HEW to hold hearings to review the conformity of state plans with federal requirements, also afforded little protection for recipients. In the first 30 years of administration of the Social Security Act, HEW ordered only 16 conformity hearings.[214] The department had a stated policy of not bringing a conformity hearing "until after reasonable effort [had] been made by regional and central office representatives to resolve the questions involved by conference and discussion with State Officials."[215] More important, recipients had no means of initiating conformity proceedings. A formal request for action brought by Georgia and Arkansas welfare recipients, the only attempt by recipients to initiate a hearing, received no response.[216] Finally, it was far from clear that judicial review was available to recipients from a decision in a conformity hearing favorable to the state.[217] In sum, the statute provided very little protection for the entitlement created by Title XIX.

## Access to Judicial Review under Medicare and Medicaid

### Medicare

The limitations imposed by the Medicare statute on administrative and judicial review soon began to impose hardships on Medicare beneficiaries and providers who were denied either services or payment under Part B, without recourse to review beyond the carrier, or who were required to endure long and often costly delays while exhausting Part A remedies. For the first decade and a half of the program, the lower courts rather freely flouted the jurisdictional limitations of the Medicare statute, providing relief to beneficiaries and providers in sympathetic cases under 28 U.S.C. § 1331 (the general federal question jurisdiction statute); 28 U.S.C. § 1491 (the Court of Claims jurisdictional statute); 5 U.S.C. § 702 (the Administrative Procedures Act); or 28 U.S.C. § 1361 (the "All Writs" Act which provided for writs of mandamus). The lower courts also readily waived the exhaustion requirement in cases in which the claimant seemed to merit immediate relief.

Beginning in the decade following the adoption of Medicare, the Supreme Court attempted, in a series of Social Security Act cases—including Medicare cases—to rein in the lower courts. The first of these cases, *Weinberger v. Salfi* (a Title II Social Security benefits case) rejected general "federal question" jurisdiction in Social Security Act cases.[218] *United States v. Erika*, a Medicare case, rejected Court of Claims jurisdiction in Part B cases.[219] *Califano v. Sanders*,[220] another non-Medicare Social Security Act case, rejected independent federal court jurisdiction under the federal Administrative Procedures Act. In combination, these cases restricted judicial review of Social Security Act cases, including Medicare decisions, solely to judicial review of final administrative decisions, and then only where permitted by Congress.[221]

The Supreme Court's decisions during this period also required strict compliance with the procedures prescribed by the Medicare statute and regulations for administrative decisionmaking and review. In *Heckler v. Community Health Services of Crawford County*,[222] the Court rejected a provider's claim of estoppel based on the provider's asserted reliance on the oral representations of an intermediary employee, observing that the provider should have sought from the secretary a formal interpretation of the manual provisions at issue.[223] In *Heckler v. Ringer*,[224] the Court insisted on exhaustion of Part A remedies, even though under the circumstances at issue it was not possible for one of the beneficiary claimants to submit a claim that could be exhausted. In *Schweicker v. McClure*,[225] the Court found that the provisions of Medicare limiting Part B appeals to hearing officers chosen by the carriers did not violate the due process clause.

In only two instances did the Supreme Court stray from this course of limiting and channeling administrative and judicial review. In *Bethesda Hospital Association v. Bowen*[226] the Court permitted providers to omit the purely formal step of contesting the validity of Medicare regulations at the first, intermediary level of review—recognizing that the intermediary had absolutely no authority to consider a challenge to the regulations—as long as the provider properly raised the regulatory issue when it obtained agency review subsequently at the PRRB level.[227]

More surprisingly and significantly, in *Michigan Academy of Family Physicians v. Blue Cross and Blue Shield of Michigan*, the Supreme Court held that federal courts had jurisdiction to review the "method" under which Part B benefits were determined, even while acknowledging the statute's absolute preclusion of jurisdiction to review Part B benefit determinations themselves.[228]

*Michigan Academy* is unique in Supreme Court Social Security Act jurisprudence in rejecting congressional limitations on judicial review—in actually taking seriously a "strong presumption that Congress intends judicial review of administrative action."[229] *Michigan Academy* was almost immediately finessed by Congress, which adopted a provision explicitly permitting judicial review of Part B decisions.[230] In *Shalala v. Illinois Council on Long Term Care*, the Court effectively abandoned *Michigan Academy*, limiting its application to situations where administrative review was totally precluded by statute.[231] *Michigan Academy* did result, however, in bringing remedies available under Part B into rough parity with those available under Part A, more firmly establishing Part B as a social insurance program in the process.

In the end, the Supreme Court's campaign to limit and channel review of Medicare decisions has been very effective. By the 1990s, lower federal courts were in most instances accepting Medicare cases for review only when administrative remedies had been thoroughly exhausted and were rejecting most claims for direct intervention in Medicare disputes. In turn, these limitations contributed to a dramatic reduction in the interference of the courts in Medicare administration; they also had had the effect of concentrating judicial review on the highly specific and technical issues that emerge from application of policy in the administrative context, avoiding the broad, shotgun, challenges to regulatory policy possible in preenforcement review actions.[232] The Benefits Improvement and Protection Act of 2000 also reformed and streamlined the Medicare appeals process and coverage determination processes to make them more functional.[233] Even though the Medicare entitlement is facially absolute, therefore, it is in fact primarily an entitlement to an administrative process, with judicial review only available in extraordinary cases.

## Medicaid

Early attempts to challenge the actions of states administering welfare programs like Medicaid in federal court, and thus to establish Medicaid firmly as a federal entitlement, foundered, in part, on the venerable belief that welfare benefits were gratuities rather than rights.[234] In the years immediately following the creation of the Medicaid program, however, the Supreme Court decided a series of cases that firmly established the right of welfare recipients under federal/state programs, including Medicaid recipients, to remedies in the federal courts.

Between 1968 and 1975 the Supreme Court decided 18 cases involving the Aid to Families with Dependent Children (AFDC) program.[235] These cases were brought through a concerted effort of welfare reform advocates, spearheaded by the Columbia Center for Social Welfare Policy and Law (CSWPL) and by Edward Sparer, the first director of the legal services backup center that grew out of CSWPL.[236] Its agenda was to radically change the nature of federal cash assistance programs from welfare to social insurance programs through the development of substantive constitutional law. While this agenda succeeded only in part, the cases brought during this period firmly established federal jurisdiction over welfare claims.

The first of these cases to reach the Supreme Court was *King v. Smith*.[237] This case challenged an Alabama regulation that disqualified children from receiving AFDC if their mothers "cohabited" with a man who was not the children's parent as contrary to the Social Security Act and the U.S. Constitution. In unanimously affirming the three-judge district court judgment striking down the regulation, the Supreme Court held that the Alabama policy violated the

Social Security Act, but declined to reach the constitutional issue. In making its decision, the Court established several very important principles.

First, the Court recognized that federal law established under Congress' spending power is the supreme law of the land. In footnote 34 the Court stated:

> There is of course no question that the Federal Government, unless barred by some controlling constitutional prohibition, may impose the terms and conditions upon which its money allotments to the States shall be disbursed, and that any state law or regulation inconsistent with such federal terms and conditions is to that extent invalid.[238]

Three years later, in *Townsend v. Swank*,[239] the Court elevated this footnote into text, stating:

> *King v. Smith* establishes that, at least in the absence of congressional authorization for the exclusion clearly evidenced from the Social Security Act or its legislative history, a state eligibility standard that excludes persons eligible for assistance under Federal AFDC standards violates the Social Security Act and is therefore invalid under the Supremacy Clause.[240]

Second, the Court held that AFDC applicants were not required to exhaust the remedy of a state "fair hearing" before filing an action under 42 U.S.C. § 1983. Section 1983 is a Reconstruction-era civil rights law that provides a private remedy for actions taken by state officials that violate federal rights. Building on a series of civil rights cases that had excused plaintiffs from exhausting remedies in cases raising constitutional issues under § 1983, the Court rejected the exhaustion requirement, at least in § 1983 cases raising constitutional claims. Two years later, in *Rosado v. Wyman*,[241] the Court also excused plaintiffs in welfare rights cases from exhausting federal remedies—that is, from having to request HEW conformity hearings—noting that recipients had no means for triggering or participating such hearings.[242]

Although the Court decided *King v. Smith* on statutory grounds, it reserved judgment on whether § 1983 suits could be brought, challenging state AFDC provisions solely on the basis of nonconformity with the Social Security law absent a constitutional claim.[243]

The existence of a right of action for statutory violations under § 1983 was not finally established until over a decade later, when the Supreme Court in *Maine v. Thiboutout*,[244] squarely decided that the language of § 1983 allowing redress for violation of the "Constitution and laws" included violations of the Social Security Act.[245] In reaching this decision, however, the Court cited seven prior Social Security Act cases in which it had assumed that § 1983 provided the cause of action for suits challenging violations of the Social Security Act.[246]

The decision in *Maine v. Thiboutout* was important because a half decade earlier, *Edelman v. Jordan*[247] had rejected the argument that the Social Security Act itself provided an implied private right of action for public assistance recipients.[248] In reaching this result, however, *Edelman* had stated that *Rosado v. Wyman* had "held that suits in federal court under § 1983 are proper to secure compliance with the provisions of the Social Security Act on the part of participating states,"[249] though nowhere in *Rosado* is § 1983 mentioned. However, *Thiboutout* established, once and for all, the availability of a federal cause of action to enforce Social Security Act program rights under § 1983.

A final important development in the Supreme Court's early welfare jurisprudence was the rejection of the right-privilege distinction, which had limited the rights of welfare recipients since the earliest days of American welfare law. *Goldberg v. Kelly*,[250] which recognized the constitutional right of welfare recipients to notice and pretermination hearings, established welfare benefits as "statutory entitlements" and expressly rejected the argument that public assistance benefits were "a privilege" and not "a right."[251]

While all of these cases involved cash assistance, other cases in the early 1970s involved Medicaid. In particular, in a series of cases in the late 1970s and in 1980, the Supreme Court held that the federal and state governments had no obligation to fund abortions under the Medicaid program.[252] Although the plaintiffs in these cases generally lost, they lost on the substantive legal issues they were asserting. The right of recipients to Medicaid as an entitlement protected by federal law was never questioned.

Although the Supreme Court settled the question of a recipient's right to sue under the provisions of the Medicaid program in the late 1960s and early 1970s, the question of an explicit right of action under Medicaid for providers was settled much later in *Wilder v. Virginia Hospital Association*.[253] *Wilder* involved the Boren Amendment, which required states to pay nursing homes and hospitals based on rates that were "reasonable and adequate to meet the costs which much be incurred by efficiently and economically operated facilities"; it was one of a series of cases that challenged the conformity of state hospital or nursing home plans with this requirement.

*Wilder* is significant because it came after a decade of backpedaling from the furthest extension of § 1983 in *Maine v. Thiboutout*. *Thiboutout* had decided that § 1983 provided a remedy for violation of federal statutes unless "the statute [had] not created enforceable rights, privileges, or immunities within the meaning of § 1983" or "Congress has foreclosed such enforcement of the statue in the enactment itself."[254] In 1981, however, the Court in *Pennhurst v. Halderman*,[255] had suggested that the obligations of states to comply with federal restrictions in spending programs might be qualified. Justice Rehnquist stated for the Court:

> Legislation enacted under the spending power is much in the nature of a contract: in return for federal funds, the States agree to comply with federally im-

posed conditions. The legitimacy of Congress' power to legislate under the spending power thus rests on whether the State voluntarily and knowingly accepts the terms of the "contract." . . . There can, of course, be no knowing acceptance if a State is unaware of the conditions or is unable to ascertain what is expected of it. Accordingly, if Congress intends to impose a condition on the grant of federal money, it must do so unambiguously.[256]

Although Rehnquist proceeded to cite the "reasonable promptness" requirement of the Social Security Act (SSA) at issue earlier in *Smith* (and also found in the Medicaid statute) as an example of an explicit condition imposed by Congress, the holding of *Pennhurst* that the "appropriate treatment" and "least restrictive" environment requirements of the Developmentally Disabled Assistance and Bill of Rights Act did not meet these clarity requirements threatened to limit dramatically the effectiveness of spending clause litigation.

*Wilder* (written by Brennan, who had dissented in *Pennhurst*, with a dissent by Rehnquist, who had written the majority opinion in *Pennhurst*) returned to the language of *Thiboutout*, limiting *Pennhurst* to cases where the federal statute "reflects merely a 'congressional preference' for a certain kind of conduct rather than a binding obligation on the governmental unit."[257] *Wilder* concluded that the Boren Amendment created an enforceable "federal right" on the part of the Medicaid provider, noting that the statue used mandatory rather than precatory terms ("must . . . provide for payment").[258] The Court also recognized, however, that providers had been suing state Medicaid agencies under § 1983 for years and that Congress had been well aware of this before adopting the Boren Amendment.

In making this point, the Court explored at some length the history of congressional action in the mid-1970s following the Supreme Court's decision in *Edelman v. Jordan* that the Eleventh Amendment barred retroactive relief (damages) in SSA cases.[259] In 1975 Congress amended the Social Security Act to require states to waive their Eleventh Amendment immunity in suits for violations of the SSA. The amendment required HEW to withhold 10% of the Medicaid funds due to any state that refused to do so. This provision launched a storm of protest and was repealed by Congress in the next session. But, to quote *Wilder*:

> Congress explained that it did not intend the repeal to "be construed as in any way contravening or constraining the rights of the providers of Medicaid services, the State Medicaid agencies, or the Department to seek prospective, injunctive relief in a federal or state judicial forum. Neither should the repeal of [the waiver section] be interpreted as placing constraints on the rights of the parties to seek such prospective, injunctive relief."[260]

Thus, the Supreme Court expressed in *Wilder* its satisfaction that the requirements of the Medicaid statute met the unambiguous clarity requirement of the *Pennhurst* test.

*Wilder* also rejected the assertion of the defendants that Congress had intended to displace the § 1983 remedy through provisions for federal approval of state plans and federal compliance review processes or the state fair-hearing processes. Reaffirming its earlier holdings in *King* and *Rosado*, the Court noted that the federal conformity processes were rarely used and provided no mechanism for individuals to trigger a hearing, while the state administrative procedures did not allow providers to challenge the overall method by which rates were determined and were not intended by Congress to replace § 1983.[261] Earlier holdings that exhaustion of administrative remedies was not required under § 1983 were thus reaffirmed.

In two instances in the 1990s, Congress confirmed first, its intent to provide a private remedy under § 1983 to Medicaid recipients and providers and, second, its belief that it had already done so. In 1992 the Supreme Court decided in *Suter v. Artist M.*[262] that the Adoption Act could not be enforced under § 1983 by private parties because its only requirement was that a state must have the secretary approve a plan with listed features. All of the Social Security Act welfare programs, of course, require in the first instance that the states have in place an approved plan, so *Suter* had the potential of overruling all previous SSA cases (although in *Suter* the Court did go to pains to distinguish *Wilder*, which had relied on specific requirements of the Boren Amendment, in addition to the more general state plan requirement).

Congress acted swiftly and decisively, adopting § 1130A of the SSA (42 U.S.C. § 1320a–10) which provides:

> In an action brought to enforce a provision of this chapter [i.e. the Social Security Act], such provision is not to be deemed unenforceable because of its inclusion in a section of this chapter requiring a State plan or specifying the required contents of a State plan. This section is not intended to limit or expand the grounds for determining the availability of private actions to enforce State plan requirements other than by overturning any such grounds applied in *Suter v. Artist M.* . . . but not applied in prior Supreme Court decisions respecting such enforceability.

In explaining this amendment, the Conference Report stated:

> The conference agreement follows the intent of the House bill provision, which is to assure that individuals who have been injured by a State's failure to comply with the Federal mandates of the State plan titles of the Social Security Act are able to seek redress in the federal courts to the extent they were able to prior to the decision in *Suter v. Artist M.*[263]

Thus Congress explicitly adopted the holdings of *Thiboutout*, *Wilder*, and other cases that the requirements of Social Security Act programs can be enforced against the states through a private rights of action under § 1983.

Then in 1995 and 1996 Congress attempted to repeal the private right of action available under Medicaid, thereby explicitly acknowledging the existence of the right of action. Their efforts were turned back by presidential veto, thus preserving the private right to action. Here we are getting ahead of the story, however, which will be picked up in Chapter 7 in this volume.

Before moving on, it is important to note that the Supreme Court's § 1983 jurisprudence has continued to become more restrictive since *Wilder*, and *Suter* was one step in this process. The Supreme Court's latest decision on § 1983 jurisdiction, *Gonzaga University v. Doe*, represents a further ominous development in this trend. In this case (alleging a § 1983 cause of action under the Family Educational Rights and Privacy Act), Justice William Rehnquist, writing for the Court, rejected the possibility of a § 1983 remedy except in situations where Congress created a right under the underlying substantive law "in clear and unambiguous terms."[264] *Gonzaga* distinguished *Wilder*, and did not overrule it, but illustrates dramatically the Court's reluctance to permit plaintiffs to challenge state actions under federal statutes that establish spending programs. At least one district court has held that the Medicaid statute does not authorize a cause of action under § 1983, but that controversial and well-publicized decision was later reversed.[265] The future of a federal cause of action to protect Medicaid providers and recipients currently stands on uncertain and shifting sands.

## Employment-Related Health Insurance Benefits: Beneficiary Rights under ERISA

Although the exclusions and deductions provided by the federal tax law constitute the fundamental entitlement extending insurance to employed Americans, the actual right of employees to actual health benefits is governed primarily by the Employee Retirement Income Security Act (ERISA). A history of the rise of American health-care entitlements would not be complete, therefore, without a brief account of employee rights to benefits under ERISA.[266]

ERISA was adopted in 1974. Before then, employment-related group health plans, like insurance plans generally in the United States, were governed by state law. State law, of course, meant contract law, and insurance contract law was generally very favorable to the insured. ERISA was adopted primarily to deal with problems with the administration of pension plans; however, it also brought employee benefit plans under the scope of federal regulation.[267] Two sections of ERISA have had a particularly important influence on the rights of employee benefit plan members—§ 502,[268] which provides plan members a federal cause of action to recover benefits, enforce rights, and clarify future rights under a health plan or to enforce compliance by plan fiduciaries with fiduciary responsibilities; and § 514,[269] which preempts all state laws that "relate to" an ERISA plan, subject to several exceptions, the most important of which is an exception for state laws regulating insurance (§ 514 further provides that ERISA plans themselves are not to be construed as being "engaged in the business of insurance," the so-called deemer clause).

ERISA's preemption provisions are far from clear and were clearly not well thought out. A series of Supreme Court cases in the 1980s, however, read them very broadly to preempt virtually any rights that insured employees might have against employment-related health plans under state law. The most important of these cases, *Pilot Life Insurance Co. v. Dedeaux*,[270] read § 514 to expressly preempt state common law tort remedies for bad faith breach of contract, but also read § 502 both to preempt impliedly any state court remedies against plans for benefit denials and to completely preempt any state court jurisdiction over ERISA plans in cases involving benefits. Contemporaneous cases also interpreted the deemer clause broadly to exclude self-funded ERISA plans entirely from state regulation and state law claims[271] and refused to permit the recovery of extracontractual damages under § 502.[272] Finally, although the Supreme Court's 1989 opinion in *Firestone Tire & Rubber Co. v. Bruch*[273] rejected the position taken by a number of lower courts that an ERISA plan's decisions were subject to review only for arbitrary and capricious action, stating instead that the courts were to review plan decisions de novo, the Court did allow plans to contract out of the de novo review standard by giving "the administrator or fiduciary discretionary authority to determine eligibility for benefits or to construe the terms of the plan."[274]

In sum, by 1990, the entitlement enjoyed by employment-related group health plan members had shriveled considerably. Employees could no longer sue to enforce their rights against health plans under state law, but they also had very limited rights under federal law.

Since the mid-1990s, however, the rights of ERISA plan beneficiaries have begun to expand again. In 1995, the Supreme Court finally found the limits of ERISA preemption, holding that a state law regulating the rates that hospitals charged ERISA plans only had an "indirect economic influence" on ERISA plans.[275] In 2000, the Court, while refusing to treat ERISA plan HMOs as fiduciaries in their medical decision making, suggested that members could sue plans under state malpractice law for negligent mixed eligibility and treatment decisions that resulted in harm, escaping ERISA preemption.[276] Finally, in its most recent venture into ERISA jurisprudence, the Court upheld a state statute subjecting the medical necessity decisions of insured ERISA plans to external review.[277] At the same time, the Department of Labor is implementing new regulations that will significantly increase the protection afforded benefit plan members in initial plan decision making and internal review processes.[278] Finally, as of this writing, Congress is considering the possibility of enacting a "patients bill of rights" that would enhance the protection offered ERISA plan members, though the adoption of such a law seen increasingly unlikely.

Many ERISA plan beneficiaries continue to lack the legal protection afforded Medicare, or even Medicaid, recipients. Members of self-insured plans that delegate unbridled discretion to plan administrators can still barely be said to enjoy an "entitlement." But the extremes of the 1980s seem to be over for now, and the courts, the Department of Labor, and perhaps even Congress all seem willing to recognize a more substantial entitlement for ERISA plan members.

## Conclusion

To summarize where we have come this far: Each of the three health insurance components of the Social Security Amendments of 1965 represented a different historical strand of entitlement thinking. Medicare Part A draws most directly on the social insurance tradition, whose roots are found in the American Civil War pensions and in the European social insurance tradition. Medicaid grew directly out of the Kerr–Mills program and traced its roots back to vendor payments made under the Social Security Act public assistance programs and to local public relief programs that preceded it. Medicare Part B grew out of proposals that emerged in the 1950s and 1960s to insure the elderly through supplementation of private insurance. Part B is related, therefore, to the other major entitlement program addressed by this book—the entitlement of working Americans to tax subsidies if their employer chooses to offer employment-related health insurance.

Social insurance is grounded squarely in a tradition of entitlement. A contributor to a social insurance program earns the right to withdraw from the fund when the insured risk (such as reaching age 65) comes to pass. In contrast public assistance was historically a gratuity, granted at the discretion of the state. Had Congress remained with this tradition, therefore, Medicaid would not have been an entitlement. But the Supreme Court interpreted the Medicaid statute, like other Social Security Act public assistance statutes, to create an entitlement protected in the federal courts. The idea of subsidized private insurance had less of a tradition to draw on. But Congress eventually extended federal administrative and judicial review to Medicare Part B, while ERISA created federal statutory remedies for persons who were insured through employment-related health insurance policies that had been adopted in response to the federal tax subsidy entitlement (although ERISA also limited state remedies for those insureds).

By 1990, therefore, all three programs addressed by this book had evolved into federal entitlements protected in the federal courts. But public entitlements have never rested totally secure in the United States, and even as the foundations of these programs were solidifying, the forces of disentitlement began to be arrayed against them. It is to disentitlement that we now turn.

## Notes

1. Theodore Marmor, *The Politics of Medicare*, 2nd ed. (New York: Aldine De Gruyter, 2000), 49–53; Sheri I. David, *With Dignity: The Search for Medicare and Medicaid* (Westport, Conn.: Greenwood, 1985), 129.

2. See Eric R. Kingson and Edward D. Berkowitz, *Social Security and Medicare: A Policy Primer* (Westport, Conn.: Auburn House, 1993), 22 (defining the characteristics of social insurance).

3. Edward D. Berkowitz, *America's Welfare State: From Roosevelt to Reagan* (Baltimore: Johns Hopkins University Press, 1991), 21.

4. Jerry R. Cates, *Insuring Inequality: Administrative Leadership in Social Security, 1935–54* (Ann Arbor: University of Michigan Press, 1983), 15.

5. Ibid., 14, 29. Cates rejects the position that humiliation is inherent in means-tested programs and argues, rather, that the leaders of the Social Security Bureau in the 1930s and 1940s intentionally enhanced the humiliation attendant in public assistance as a means to strengthen their favored social insurance approach to the problem of poverty.

6. Ibid., 29.

7. U.S. Senate, Sen. Robert A. Taft of Ohio speaking to the Subcommittee of the Labor and Public Welfare Committee on National Health Program for 1949, Hearings on S. 1106, S. 1456, S. 1581, and S. 1679, 81st Cong., 1st sess., 1949, 12.

8. See David, *With Dignity*, 61.

9. Cates, *Insuring Inequality*, 30.

10. See *Westside Mothers v. Haveman*, 133 F. Supp. 2d 549 (E.D. Mich. 2001), reversed in *Westside Mothers v. Haveman*, 289 F. 3d 852 (6th Cir. 2002). See Erwin Chemerinsky, "Ensuring the Supremacy of Federal Law: Why the District Court Was Wrong in *Westside Mothers v. Haveman*," *Health Matrix* 12 (2002): 157–179.

11. During the medieval period, support of the poor had principally been the responsibility of the church, although the church was effectively inseparable from the state as it existed at that time. See Walter Trattner, *From Poor Law to Welfare State: A History of Social Welfare in America* (New York: Free Press, 1999).

12. Sir George Nicholls, *A History of the English Poor Laws*, Vol. 1 (New York: G.P. Putnam's Sons, 1898), 182–193. The key law was 43 Elizabeth, chap. 2 (1601).

13. Ibid., 182. Included in the list of offenders were "all persons calling themselves scholars going about begging."

14. Trattner, *From Poor Law to Welfare State*, 11.

15. Ursula R. Q. Henriques, *Before the Welfare State* (London: Longman, 1979), 13–15.

16. On the 1834 Poor Law, see Henriques, *Before the Welfare State*, 39–41. On American developments, see Michael B. Katz, *In the Shadow of the Poorhouse: A Social History of Welfare in America* (New York: Basic Books, 1996).

17. Trattner, *From Poor Law to Welfare State*, 22–25.

18. Ibid., 26–27. Apparently little public relief of any sort was available to Native Americans or African Americans.

19. Trattner, *From Poor Law to Welfare State*, 40; Katz, *In the Shadow of the Poorhouse*, 15.

20. Trattner, *From Poor Law to Welfare State*, 50-55.

21. Ibid., 55.

22. Ibid., 54–56.

23. Katz, *In the Shadow of the Poorhouse*, 8–10.

24. Trattner, *From Poor Law to Welfare State*, 59.

25. Nicholls, *A History of the English Poor Laws*, Vol. 2, 242, quoting Report.

26. Trattner, *From Poor Law to Welfare State*, 59–61; Katz, *In the Shadow of the Poorhouse*, 26–36.

27. Trattner, *From Poor Law to Welfare State*, 92–96.

28. Katz, *In the Shadow of the Poorhouse*, 68–83.

29. Trattner, *From Poor Law to Welfare State*, 101.

30. Hace Sorel Tishler, *Self-Reliance and Social Security, 1870–1917*, 66–67 (Port Washington, N.Y.: National University Publications, Kennikat Press, 1971), 9–10. By contrast, in England after 1792, applicants for relief had the right to appeal denials to local justices of the peace (who supervised relief operations); the justices could order the grant of relief (Nicholls, *History of the English Poor Laws*). This power came to be used fairly often, even though in form it was closer to administrative than to judicial review because of the justices' supervisory role.

31. See Trattner, *From Poor Law to Welfare State*, 98, and Ann Orloff, "The Political Origins of America's Belated Welfare State," in *The Politics of Social Policy in the United States*, edited by Margaret Weir, Ann Orloff, and Ann Theda Skocpol (Princeton, NJ: Princeton University Press, 1988), 49–50.

32. Berkowitz, *America's Welfare State,*, 45.

33. Katz, *In the Shadow of the Poorhouse*, 96.

34. Quoted in Ibid., 72.

35. Berkowitz, *America's Welfare State*, 16.

36. Ibid., 17.

37. Theda Skocpol, *Social Policy in the United States: Future Possibilities in Historical Perspective* (Princeton, N.J.: Princeton University Press, 1995), 42.

38. Ibid., 42–43.

39. Ibid., 45–46.

40. Ibid., 55–58.

41. Theda Skocpol, *Protecting Soldiers and Mothers: The Political Origins of Social Policy in the United States* (Cambridge, Mass.: Belknap Press, 1992), 132.

42. Ibid., 128.

43. Ibid., 118–119. However, decisions were often based on the testimony of applicants and their neighbors and friends heard in informal proceedings. Attempts in the late 1870s to regularize the process, creating a medical examiner's office and judicial-type proceedings, were largely rejected by Congress, which seems to have seen the pension program as a base for party patronage. Ibid., 118–128.

44. See Charles Tiefer, "Budgetized" Health Entitlements and the Fiscal Constitution in Congress's 1995–1996 Budget Battle," *Harvard Journal on Legislation* 33 (1996): 411.

45. Tishler, *Self-Reliance and Social Security*, 19.

46. Ibid., 137–138.

47. Ibid., 136.

48. Skocpol, *Protecting Soldiers and Mothers*, 142.

49. Ibid.

50. See Detlev Zöllner, "Germany," in *The Evolution of Social Insurance, 1881–1981*, edited by Peter A. Köhler and Hans F. Zacher (London: Frances Pinter, 1982), 13.

51. Zöllner, "Germany," 10–17; Gerhard A. Ritter, *Social Welfare in Germany and Britain: Origins and Development* (New York: Leamington Spa, 1986), 33–48.

52. Bismarck stated the following to Dr. Mortiz Busch in 1881: The contentment of the unpropertied classes . . . was well worth the great expense involved. . . . And if we use the result [of increased taxes] to safeguard the future of our workers, whose insecurity is the main cause of their hatred of the state, we are only guaranteeing our own future. That is a good investment for us as well. It enables us to thwart a revolution which could break out 50 years from now, or even ten—a revolution which, even if it was successful for only a few months, would directly and indirectly run up quite different costs from our pre-emptive strategy in terms of its disruption of business and trading." (Busch's diary entry in Bismarck, *Gesammelte Werke*, Vol. 8, Berlin 1926, 396, quoted in Ritter, *Social Welfare in Germany and Britain*, 34.)

53. Ritter, *Social Welfare in Germany and Britain*, 51; Richard Freeman, *The Politics of Health in Europe* (Manchester: Manchester University Press, 2000), 20–21; Peter Flora and Arnold J. Heidenheimer, eds., "The Historical Core and Changing Boundaries of the Welfare State," in *The Development of Welfare States in Europe and North America* (New Brunswick, Conn.: Transaction Books, 1981), 17, 18.

54. Zöllner, "Germany," 28–29. This sum equaled about three times the average worker's income in 1882 and resulted in 4.3 million workers being insured by 1885, which was about 40% of all persons employed and 10% of the total population.

55. Replacement pay was covered at 50% of wages from the third day of incapacity to the thirteenth week. Ibid., 29.

56. Ibid. The funds also provided maternity benefits for 4 weeks after delivery.

57. Ibid., 31.

58. Issac Max Rubinow, *Social Insurance* (New York: Henry Holt, 1913), 21; Barbara Nachtrieb Armstrong, *Insuring the Essentials* (New York: MacMillan, 1932).

59. Tishler, *Self-Reliance and Social Security*, 66–67.

60. Ibid., 56–58.

61. Skocpol, *Protecting Soldiers and Mothers*, 456–457; Trattner, *From Poor Law to Welfare State*, 228.

62. Skocpol, *Protecting Soldiers and Mothers*, 432–456.

63. Tishler, *Self-Reliance and Social Security*, 108–140; Katz, *In the Shadow of the Poorhouse*, 197–202.

64. Domenico Gagliardo, *American Social Insurance* (New York: Harper and Brothers, 1955), 48–52.

65. Tishler, *Self-Reliance and Social Security*, 159–160, 165.

66. Paul Starr, *The Social Transformation of American Medicine* (New York: Basic Books, 1982), 244; Tishler, *Self-Reliance and Social Security*, 164.

67. In particular, as Germany prepared for war, it was believed that the strength of its armed forces was attributable in part to the health of its soldiers, who had received regular medical care. Tishler, *Self-Reliance and Social Security*, 162.

68. Ibid., 166–172.

69. Ibid., 167–169; Ronald L. Numbers, *Almost Persuaded: American Physicians and Compulsory Health Insurance* (Baltimore: Johns Hopkins University Press, 1978), 1912–1920.

70. Robert Stevens and Rosemary Stevens, *Welfare Medicine in America: A Case Study of Medicaid* (New York: Free Press, 1974), 9.

71. Peter A. Corning, *The Evolution of Medicare: From Idea to Law* (Washington, D.C.: U.S. Department of Health, Education and Welfare, 1969), 16; Tishler, *Self-*

*Reliance and Social Security*, 180–185; Starr, *The Social Transformation of American Medicine*, 249–250.

72. Starr, *The Social Transformation of American Medicine*, 250–252; Tishler, *Self-Reliance and Social Security*, 188–191.

73. Numbers, *Almost Persuaded*; Starr, *The Social Transformation of American Medicine*, 252.

74. Starr, *The Social Transformation of American Medicine*, 252: Corning, *The Evolution of Medicare*, 17.

75. Starr, *The Social Transformation of American Medicine*, 253.

76. Trattner, *From Poor Law to Welfare State*, 66.

77. Ibid., 66–67.

78. Ibid., 67.

79. Skocpol, *Protecting Soldiers and Mothers*, 69–71, 256–226, 410–411.

80. *Helvering v. Davis*, 301 U.S. 619 (1937); Robert M. Cover, "Social Security and Constitutional Entitlement," in *Social Security: Beyond the Rhetoric of Crisis*, edited by Theodor R. Marmor and Jerry L. Mashaw (Princeton, N.J.: Princeton University Press, 1988), 70–72; Eric M. Patashnik, *Putting Trust in the United States Budget: Federal Trust Funds and the Politics of Commitment* (Cambridge: Cambridge University Press, 2000), 65–66; Cates, *Insuring Inequality*, 31–32. The constitutional issues are set out in Barbara Nachtrieb Armstrong, "The Federal Social Security Act and Its Constitutional Aspects," *California Law Review* 24 (1036): 247. Armstrong, one of the three members of the Committee for Economic Security's subcommittee on old age insurance, which drafted the 1935 Social Security Act, was the first full-time female professor at an accredited American law school. See Beth Hollenberg and Barbara Nachtrieb Armstrong, at The Women: Pioneer Profiles: Armstrong, Barbara Nachtrieb, http://www.stanford.edu/group/WLHP/profiles/ArmstrongBarbara.shtml (cited June 27, 2002).

81. Tishler, *Self-Reliance and Social Security*, 114–115.

82. Katz, *In the Shadow of the Poorhouse*, 217, 221.

83. Ibid., 222–223.

84. Ibid., 234; Trattner, *From Poor Law to Welfare State*, 284–288.

85. Katz, *In the Shadow of the Poorhouse*.

86. Ibid., 243–244.

87. Ibid., 243; Gagliardo, *American Social Insurance*, 53–54; J. Douglas Brown, *An American Philosophy of Social Security: Evolution and Issues* (Princeton, N.J.: Princeton University Press, 1972), 6–7.

88. Katz, *In the Shadow of the Poorhouse*, 243–244.

89. Ibid., 244–250; Cates, *Insuring Inequality*, 15–17, 27–49; Patashnik, *Putting Trust in the United States Budget*, 64–67; William H. Simon, "Rights and Redistribution in the Welfare System," *Stanford Law Review* 38 (1986): 1431, 1448–1452.

90. Edwin E. Witte, "Social Security: A Wild Dream or a Practical Plan?" in *Social Security Perspectives*, edited by Edwin E. Witte and Robert J. Lampman (Madison: University of Wisconsin Press, 1962), quoted in Cates, *Insuring Inequality*, 11.

91. An illustrative table of payment amounts is found in Armstrong, "The Federal Social Security Act and Its Constitutional Aspects," 253. See also Ann Shulz Orloff, "Political Orgins," in *The Politics of Social Policy in the United States*, edited by Margaret Weir, Ann Shulz Orloff, and Theda Skocpol (Princeton, N.J.: Princeton University Press, 1988), 78.

92. Orloff, "Political Origins," 74.

93. Ibid.

94. Berkowitz, *America's Welfare State*, 56.

95. Eveline M. Burns, *The American Social Security System* (Boston: Houghton Mifflin, 1949), 66; Patricia E. Dilley, "The Evolution of Entitlement: Retirement Income and the Problem of Integrating Private Pensions and Social Security," *Loyola Los Angeles Law Review* 30 (1997): 1063, 1137–1137; Berkowitz, *America's Welfare State*, 47–49; Simon, *Rights and Redistribution*, 1454–1457.

96. See Robert M. Ball, "The Original Understanding of Social Security: Implications for Later Developments," in *Social Security: Beyond the Rhetoric of Crisis*, edited by Theodore R. Marmor and Jerry L. Mashaw (Princeton, N.J.: Princeton University Press, 1988).

97. Although the 1935 statute failed to provide for appeals or for judicial review to oversee the decisions made by this bureaucracy, the Social Security Board began as early as 1936 to devise "fair hearing" policies, and the 1939 amendments established a statutory right to appeal. Ernest R. Burton, "The Appeals System in Old-Age and Survivors Insurance," *Social Security Bulletin* 9 (July 1946): 4, 5. Within a half decade, appeals and review were becoming increasingly common. In 1944–1945, there were 1,307 requests for hearings. Ibid., 4. Between July 1, 1940, and December 31, 1940, there were 42 civil actions to obtain juridical review of Social Security Act decisions. Ibid., 9.

98. In Cates, *Insuring Inequality*, 31–38. Until this point it was believed that the Court might well hold the legislation unconstitutional if the taxes and benefits were too closely tied. See Armstrong, "The Federal Social Security Act," 266–274.

99. Martha Derthick, *Policymaking for Social Security* (Washington, D.C.: Brookings Institute, 1979), 247–251; Simon, *Rights and Redistribution*, 1452–1454. Only with the Supreme Court's later decision in *Flemming v. Nestor*, 363 U.S. 603 (1960), did it become entirely clear that the government's obligation under Social Security was not, in fact, contractual.

100. Tiefer, "Budgetized" Health Entitlements and the Fiscal Constitution," 416.

101. See also Gagliardo, *American Social Insurance*, 56; Social Security Act, Pub. L. 271 § 2, 49 Stat. 620, 620 (1935).

102. Burton, "The Appeals System in Old-Age and Survivors Insurance," 5, n. 2.

103. Starr, *The Social Transformation of American Medicine*, 266–270; Marmor, *The Politics of Medicare*, 6; Orloff, "Political Origins," 75–76.

104. Eugene Feingold, *Medicare: Policy and Politics—A Case Study and Policy Analysis* (San Francisco: Chandler, 1966), 91, cited in Marmor, *The Politics of Medicare*, 5–6.

105. Pub. L. 271, §§ 501–515; 49 Stat. 620, 629–633 (1935).

106. Trattner, *From Poor Law to Welfare State*, 19.

107. Starr, *The Social Transformation of American Medicine*, 181–184.

108. Ibid., 147–162, 169–177.

109. Ibid., 169–173.

110. Stevens and Stevens, *Welfare Medicine in America*, 16.

111. Starr, *The Social Transformation of American Medicine*, 72–73, 169.

112. Stevens and Stevens, *Welfare Medicine in America*, 27.

113. Ibid., 240; Corning, *The Evolution of Medicare*, 3.

114. Frank J. Thompson, *Health Policy and the Bureaucracy: Politics and Implementation* (Cambridge, Mass.: MIT Press, 1981), 187.

115. Ibid.

116. Starr, *The Social Transformation of American Medicine*, 348; Thompson, *Health Policy and the Bureaucracy*, 187.

117. Trattner, *From Poor Law to Welfare State*, 84.

118. Skocpol, *Protecting Soldiers and Mothers*, 494–522.

119. Institute of Medicine, *Employment and Health Benefits: A Connection at Risk*, ed. Marilyn J. Field and Harold T. Shapiro, (Washington, DC:, National Academy Press, 1993), 51–56.

120. Ibid., 68. See also, Robert Cunningham III and Robert M. Cunningham, Jr., *The Blues: A History of the Blue Cross and Blue Shield System* (Dekalb, Ill.: Northern Illinois University Press, 1997).

121. Melissa A. Thomasson, *The Importance of Group Coverage: How Tax Policy Shaped U.S. Health Insurance* (Cambridge, Ma.: National Bureau of Economic Research, 2000): 28.

122. Louis S. Reed, *Blue Cross and Medical Service Plans* (Washington, D.C.: U.S. Public Health Service, 1947): 59–60.

123. Ibid., 59, 62; J. F. Follmann, Jr., *Medical Care and Health Insurance* (Homewood, Ill.: Richard D. Irwin, Inc., 1963): 141; Report of the Committee on Labor and Public Welfare, U.S. Senate, *Health Insurance Plans in the United States*, 82nd Cong. 1st Sess. (1951):7–9, 14, 54.

124. Reed, *Blue Cross and Medical Service Plans*, 59–60.

125. Report of Committee on Labor and Public Welfare, *Health Insurance Plans in the United States*, 67,

126. Institute of Medicine, *Employment and Health Benefits*, 70.

127. Alicia H. Munnell, "Employee Benefits and the Tax Base," *New England Economic Review* (January/February 1984): 39, 46.

128. Institute of Medicine, *Employment and Health Benefits*, 70–71.

129. Follmann, *Medical Care and Health Insurance*, 142.

130. Internal Revenue Code, Pub. L. No. 254 § 213(b)(6), 40 Stat. 1057, 1066 (1919).

131. Revenue Act of 1942, Pub. L. 753, § 127, 56 Stat. 798, 825 (1942).

132. See "Taxation of Employee Accident and Health Plans Before and After the 1954 Code," *Yale Law Journal* (1954) 64: 222, 223–227.

133. Ibid., 239–243.

134. See *Yale Law Journal*, "Taxation of Employee Accident," 241, citing Special Ruling, 3 CCH 1943 Fed Tax Rep. ¶ 6587 (1943). The Service, however, continued to consider employer payments for individual insurance policies as taxable income, and did not resolve the taxability of employer contributions to private plans until 1953, *Ibid*. See also Jay A. Soled, "Taxation of Employer-Provided Health Coverage: Inclusion, Timing and Policy Issues," *Virginia Tax Review* 15 (1996): 447, 450–451. The Service viewed these premiums as investments in increased efficiency rather than as compensation. *Ibid*.

135. Thomasson, *The Importance of Group Coverage*, 18.

136. Ibid., 2–3.

137. See L. Raish, "Cafeteria Plans," *Tax Management Portfolio* 397-3d, A-26–A-34.

138. Gruber, *Taxes and Health Insurance* (Cambridge, Mass.: National Bureau of Economic Research, 2001), 4.

139. 26 U.S.C., § 162(l)(2)(A) and (B).

140. Ibid., § 220, established by the Health Insurance Portability and Accountability Act of 1996.

141. Ibid., § 7702B, also added by the Health Insurance Portability and Accountability Act.

142. Rev. Rul. 2002-41 (July 15, 2002).

143. Gabel, "Job-Based Health Insurance," 65.

144. See Paul Fronstin, "Trends in Health Insurance Coverage: A Look at Early 2001 Data," *Health Affairs* 21 (January/February 2002): 188–193.

145. See Jon Gabel et al., "Job-Based Health Insurance in 2001: Inflation Hits Double Digits, Managed Care Retreats," *Health Affairs* 20 (2001): 180–186.

146. Social Security Amendments of 1956, Pub. L. No. 734, §§ 303(a), 323(a), 343(a) and 351; 64 Stat. 477, 549, 551, 554, 557–58 (1950). See David, *With Dignity*, 35.

147. Pub. L. 734, § 302. 64 Stat. 477, 548–549. See also U.S. Department of Health, Education and Welfare (HEW), "History and Evolution of Medicaid," in *Medicaid: Lessons for National Health Insurance*, edited by Allen D. Spiegel and Simon Podair (Washington, D.C.: U.S. Department of Health, Education and Welfare, 1975).

148. HEW, "History and Evolution of Medicaid," 6.

149. David, *With Dignity*, 35–36.

150. Social Security Amendments of 1960, Pub. L. 86-778 § 601, 74 Stat. 924, 987 (1960). Pub. L. No. 86-778 § 601; 74 Stat. 924, 987. See, discussing the politics attending the creation of Kerr–Mills, David, *With Dignity*, 32–47.

151. Pub. L. 86-778 § 601(b); 74 Stat., 924, 987.

152. The only differences are services by nonphysician medical practitioners within their scope of practice and mental health and tuberculosis services for those over age 65.

153. HEW, "History and Evolution of Medicaid," 6.

154. David, *With Dignity*, 44.

155. Berkowitz, *America's Welfare State*, 170.

156. David, *With Dignity*, 97–98. Some 42% went to New York alone (Berkowitz, *America's Welfare State*, 170).

157. David, *With Dignity*, 45; Stevens and Stevens, *Welfare Medicine in America*, 35.

158. David, *With Dignity*, 97; Stevens and Stevens, *Welfare Medicine in America*, 35.

159. See Stevens and Stevens, *Welfare Medicine in America*, 51.

160. Sir William Beveridge, *Social Insurance and Allied Services* (New York: Macmillan, 1942), 158–163.

161. Carolyn Hughes Tuohy, *Accidental Logics: The Dynamics of Changing the Health Care Arena in the United States, Britain, and Canada* (New York: Oxford University Press, 1999), 40.

162. World Health Organization, *World Health Report 2000* (Geneva: WHO, 2000), 11–13.

163. Tuohy, *Accidental Logics*, 38–41, 45–47; Corning, *The Evolution of Medicare*, 53–69.

164. Starr, *The Social Transformation of American Medicine*, 338–350.

165. See *American Hospital Ass'n v. Schweiker*, 721 F. 2d 170 (7th Cir. 1983); Michael A. Dowell, "Hill–Burton: The Unfulfilled Promise," *Journal of Health Politics, Policy, and Law* 12 (1987): 153; Kenneth R. Wing, "The Community Service Obligation of Hill–Burton Health Facilities," *Boston College Law Review* 23 (1982): 577.

166. In 1950, for example, the American Medical Association (AMA) mounted a $1 million election advertising campaign that attacked socialist medicine (Feingold, *Medicare: Policy and Politics*, 98–100). The AMA kept up a steady drumbeat on this issue for the succeeding decade and a half. In 1961, for example, the AMA sponsored a multimedia campaign against the King–Anderson bill with posters entitled "Socialist Medicine and You" and articles in national magazines stating that "once medicine is socialized, socialism will spread to every other aspect of American life." Ibid., 56–58.

167. Marmor, *The Politics of Medicare*, 23–25.

168. Quoted in David, *With Dignity*, 13, from House Committee on Ways and Means, *Hearings on Unemployment Insurance Amendments*, 85th Cong., 2d sess, 1958, 8.

169. See Jill Quadagno, "From Old-Age Assistance to Supplemental Security Income: The Political Economy of Relief in the South 1935–1972," in *The Politics of Social Policy in the United States*, edited by Margaret Wier, Ann Shola Orloff, and Theda Skocpol (Princeton, N.J.: Princeton University Press, 1988), 235; David, *With Dignity*, 14.

170. Marmor, *The Politics of Medicare*, 18.

171. Robert M. Ball, "Reflections on How Medicare Came About," in *Medicare: Preparing for the Challenges of the 21st Century*, edited by Robert D. Reischauer, Stuart Butler, and Judith Lave (Washington, D.C.: National Academy of Social Insurance, 1997), 40–41; Marmor, *The Politics of Medicare*, 46; David, *With Dignity*, 54; Corning, *The Evolution of Medicare*, 71–72.

172. Tuohy, *Accidental Logics*, 58–59; Lawrence R. Jacobs, *The Health of Nations* (Ithaca, N.Y.: Cornell University Press, 1993), 210–211.

173. Marmor, *The Politics of Medicare*, 48; Feingold, *Medicare: Policy and Politics*, 141–142.

174. Marmor, *The Politics of Medicare*, 46; David, *With Dignity*, 124; Feingold, *Medicare: Policy and Politics*, 141.

175. Berkowitz, *America's Welfare State*, 64–65.

176. HR 3727, 3728.

177. Anonymous. "Social Security Medicare Program Enacted," *Congressional Quarterly Almanac* (1965): 248–249.

178. H.R. 4351.

179. Anonymous, "Social Security Medicare Program Enacted," 249; Feingold, *Medicare: Policy and Politics*, 141–142.

180. Anonymous "Social Security Medicare Program Enacted," 249.

181. Ibid., 249.; Feingold, *Medicare: Policy and Politics*, 118. The Bow proposal effectively proposed a tax credit of $125 for persons 65 and over who purchased health insurance.

182. By 1958 nearly two-thirds of the population had some coverage for hospital costs, including 78% of households whose main workers had fulltime employment. Only 43% of families headed by a retired person and 29% of families headed by a disabled person had private insurance, however (Starr, *The Social Transformation of American Medicine*, 334). On the history of tax subsidies for private insurance, see "Taxation of Employee Accident and Health Plans," 222.

183. Starr, *The Social Transformation of American Medicine*, 331–334.

184. Margaret Greenfield, *Medicare and Medicaid: The 1965 and 1967 Social Security Amendments* (Berkeley: University of California, 1968), 61–62; Berkowitz, *America's Welfare State*, 170. David, *With Dignity*, 93. In the 1950s a few insurers had also offered low-cost programs on their own for the elderly in an effort to demonstrate the lack of need for social insurance, but these programs had limited reach. David, *With Dignity*, 13–14.

185. Eugene Feingold, *Medicare: Policy and Politics*, 97.

186. Greenfield, *Medicare and Medicaid*, 92; Corning, *The Evolution of Medicare*, 83; David, *With Dignity*, 68.

187. David, *With Dignity*, 69.

188. Ibid., 70.

189. Edward D. Berkowitz, *Mr. Social Security: the Life of Wilber J. Cohen* (Lawrence, Kansas: University Press of Kansas, 1995), 172–173.

190. Marmor, *The Politics of Medicare*, 49–53; David, *With Dignity*, 129.

191. Marmor, *The Politics of Medicare*, 47–53; Henry Miles Somers and Anne Ram-

say Somers, *Medicare and the Hospitals: Issues and Prospects* (Washington, D.C.: Brookings Institute, 1967), 12–16.

192. Marmor, *The Politics of Medicare*, 56.

193. 42 U.S.C.A. § 1395d.

194. 42 U.S.C.A. § 1395i; 26 U.S.C.A. §§ 1401(b), 3101(b), and 3111(b).

195. 42 U.S.C.A. § 1395k; 42 C.F.R. § 410.3.

196. David, *With Dignity*, 76.

197. Social Security Amendments of 1965, Pub. L. 89-97, § 1902(a)(10); 79 Stat 286, 345 (1965).

198. Pub. L. 89-97, Pub. L. 89-97, § 1905(a); 79 Stat 351 (1965).

199. Pub. L. 89-97, Pub. L. 89-97, § 1902(a)(17); 79 Stat 346 (1965).

200. David, *With Dignity*, 148.

201. Ibid.

202. Ibid.

203. Pub. L. 89-97, § 1869; 79 Stat. 330, codified at 42 U.S.C. § 1395ff.

204. 42 U.S.C. § 1395ff.

205. 42 U.S.C. § 1395u(3)(C). The term *carrier* is defined in 42 U.S.C. § 1395(f) as a private entity that administers group health insurance arrangements.

206. See *United States v. Erika, Inc.*, 456 U.S. 201 (1982).

207. See Social Security Amendments of 1965 89th Cong., 1st sess 1965, S. Rept. No. 404, 54-55 (1965).

208. David, *With Dignity*, 146–147.

209. 42 U.S.C. § 1395p.

210. See, e.g. Pub. L. 271, § 2, 49 Stat. 620.

211. Pub. L. 89-97, § 1904.

212. Note, "Federal Judicial Review of State Welfare Practices," *Columbia Law Review* (1967): 92 n. 56.

213. Ibid., 93–94.

214. Ibid., 91.

215. United States Department of Health Education and Welfare, *Handbook of Public Assistance Administration*, Part 1, § 4300 (Washington, D.C.: DHEW, 1966), cited in ibid. 91.

216. Note, "Federal Judicial Review," 91.

217. See ibid., 109–115.

218. *Weinberger v. Salfi*, 422 U.S. 749, 756–763 (1975).

219. *United States v. Erika*, 456 U.S. 201 (1982).

220. *Califano v. Sanders*, 430 U.S. 99 (1977).

221. The statute only permits review of Part A and Part B decisions that involve $1,000 or more (42 U.S.C. §§ 1395ii(b) and 1395ff), and then only after administrative remedies are exhausted.

222. *Heckler v. Community Health Services of Crawford County*, 467 U.S. 51 (1984).

223. Intermediaries are the private insurance and claims processing companies that administer Part A of the Medicare program.

224. *Heckler v. Ringer*, 466 U.S. 602 (1984).

225. *Schweicker v. McClure*, 456 U.S. 188 (1982).

226. *Bethesda Hospital Association v. Bowen*, 485 U.S. 399 (1988).

227. More precisely, the Court recognized jurisdiction of the PRRB to consider costs "self-disallowed" by the provider in its initial cost report submitted to the Medicare intermediary because of regulations prohibiting payment for these costs.

228. *Michigan Academy of Family Physicians v. Blue Cross and Blue Shield of Michigan,* 476 U.S. 667, 674–678 (1986).

229. Ibid., 670.

230. Omnibus Budget Reconciliation Act of 1986, § 9341 (amending 42 U.S.C. § 1395ff).

231. *Shalala v. Illinois Council on Long Term Care,* 529 U.S. 1 (2000).

232. See Jerry L. Mashaw, *Greed, Chaos, and Governance: Using Public Choice to Improve Public Law* (New Haven, Conn.: Yale University Press, 1987), 178 (noting the broad challenges, and subsequent broader judicial interference in administrative governance, facilitated by preenforcement review).

233. See Eleanor Kinney, ed., *Guide to Medicare Coverage Decision Making and Appeals* (Chicago: American Bar Association, 2002).

234. See *Smith v. Bd of Comm'rs,* 259 F. Supp. 423 (D.D.C. 1966).

235. Shep R. Melnick, *Between the Lines* (Washington, D.C.: Brookings Institute, 1994), 83.

236. Ibid., 75.

237. *King v. Smith,* 392 U.S. 309 (1968).

238. Ibid., 332.

239. *Townsend v. Swank,* 404 U.S. 282 (1971).

240. Ibid., 286.

241. *Rosado v. Wyman,* 397 U.S. 397 (1970).

242. Ibid., 406.

243. Ibid.

244. *Maine v. Thiboutout,* 448 U.S. 1 (1980).

245. Ibid., 4.

246. Ibid., 4–6. The Supreme Court also relied in passing on four other prior Social Security Act cases brought under § 1983.

247. *Edelman v. Jordan,* 415 U.S. 651 (1974).

248. Ibid., 674–677.

249. Ibid., 675.

250. *Goldberg v. Kelly,* 397 U.S. 254 (1970).

251. Ibid., 262. In doing so, the Court included at footnote 8 an acknowledgment of Charles Reich's new property argument.

252. *Maher v. Roe,* 432 U.S. 464, 469 (1976); *Harris v. McRae,* 448 U.S. 297, 316–318 (1980); *Singleton v. Wulff,* 428 U.S. 106 (1976); *Williams v. Zbaraz,* 448 U.S. 358 (1980); *Beal v. Doe,* 432 U.S. 438 (1977).

253. *Wilder v. Virginia Hospital Association,* 496 U.S. 498 (1990).

254. Ibid., 508, citing *Wright v. Roanoke Redevelopment and Hous. Authority,* 479 U.S. 418 (1987).

255. *Pennhurst v. Halderman,* 451 U.S. 1 (1981).

256. Ibid., 17.

257. *Wilder v. Virginia Hospital Association,* 509.

258. Ibid., 512.

259. Ibid., 516–517.

260. Ibid., 517–518, quoting Social Security Act—Medical Assistance S. Rep. No. 94-1240 at 4, *U.S. Code,* Cong. and Admin. News 1976, 5651 (1976).

261. *Wilder v. Virginia Hospital Association,* 522–523.

262. *Suter v. Artist M.,* 503 U.S. 347 (1992).

263. H.R. Conf. Rep. 102-1034 (1992).

264. *Gonzagea University v. Doe*, 122 S.Ct. 2268, 2279 (2002).

265. *Westside Mothers v. Haveman*, 133 F. Supp. 2d 549 (E.D. Mich. 2001), reversed in 289 F. 3d 852 (6th Cir. 2002).

266. A complete description and analysis of the effect of ERISA on employment-related group health insurance benefits is far beyond the scope and ambition of this book. A longer introduction to the subject, and to the literature, is found in Barry Furrow et al., *Health Law: Cases, Materials and Problems*, 4th ed. (St. Paul, Minn.: West, 2001), 601–659.

267. See Rand E. Rosenblatt, Sylvia A. Law, and Sara Rosenbaum, *Law and the American Health Care System* (Westbury, N.Y.: Foundation Press, 1997), 173–177; Daniel M. Fox and Daniel C. Schaffer, "Health Policy and ERISA: Interest Groups and Semipreemption," *Journal of Health Politics, Policy and Law*, 14 (1989): 239.

268. 29 U.S.C. § 1132.

269. 29 U.S.C. § 1144.

270. *Pilot Life Insurance Co. v. Dedeaux*, 481 U.S. 41 (1987).

271. *FMC Corporation v. Holliday*, 498 U.S. 52 (1990).

272. *Massachusetts Mutual Life Insurance Co. v. Russell*, 473 U.S. 134 (1985).

273. *Firestone Tire & Rubber Co. v. Brach*, 489 U.S. 101 (1989).

274. Ibid at 956–957.

275. *New York State Conference of Blue Cross and Blue Shield Plans v. Travelers Ins., Co.*, 514 U.S. 645 (1995).

276. *Pegram v. Herdrich*, 530 U.S. 211 (2000).

277. *Rush Prudential HMO Inc. v. Moran*, 122 S.Ct. 2151 (2002).

278. 29 C.F.R. Part 2560.

# 5

# Experiments with Privatization: Medicare and Medicaid Managed Care

THE emergence of managed care is certainly one of the most important developments in our public health-care entitlement programs over the past two decades. One of the central goals of the Medicare and Medicaid programs at their creation was to bring elderly and impoverished Americans into the mainstream of American medical care. In 1965, of course, this meant fee-for-service medicine. At the outset, therefore, Medicare and Medicaid were strictly fee-for-service programs. In the early twenty-first century, Medicare remains largely a fee-for-service program. But fee-for-service medicine is no longer mainstream medicine in the United States. Most insured individuals in the private sector are covered through managed care.[1] Recent attempts to encourage the expansion of managed care within the Medicare and Medicaid programs, therefore, are in a sense consistent with the historic philosophy of the program.

While the growth of managed care in Medicare and Medicaid arguably represents simply the "normalization" of these programs, it also has been a step toward their privatization. Those who argue for privatization of public programs—a form of disentitlement discussed at length in Chapter 6—contend that public programs could be operated more efficiently, perhaps even more equitably, through private insurers and managed-care organizations. Many privatization advocates go further, arguing as well for individualization—recommending vouchers for individual consumers, allowing them to choose among private financing entities in organized markets for purchasing individual insurance policies.

The Medicare and Medicaid managed-care programs offer us a real-time opportunity to examine the effects of privatization and individualization on public programs. To the extent that Medicare and Medicaid managed care can be judged to have been unbridled successes—to have brought down program costs, increased beneficiary satisfaction and quality of care, and improved equity of care accessibility—the advocacy of privatization and individualization of health care should be encouraged. To the extent that Medicare and Medicaid managed care have not succeeded, the rest of us should find reason to approach their proposals with greater caution.

In this chapter I examine first Medicare and then Medicaid managed care. I survey the history of these programs and analyze their successes and failures. I conclude that, although these programs have certain achievements, particularly in the Medicaid program, on the whole they have not saved money and have a mixed record on improving accessibility and quality. The Medicare and Medicaid managed-care experience, therefore, gives us more reason to be cautious than to be enthusiastic about privatization and individualization of public health-care entitlements.

## The History of Medicare Managed Care

Medicare began to experiment with managed care almost from the beginning of the program.[2] The 1972 Social Security amendments authorized Medicare to contract with health maintenance organizations (HMOs) on a "risk" (capitated) basis, although it only permitted contracting with established plans, subjected the plans to retrospective cost adjustments, and limited the amount of profit (but not losses) that plans could make.[3] Not surprisingly, there was little interest among plans in contracting on this basis, and by 1979 only one plan had signed up.[4]

The Tax Equity and Fiscal Responsibility Act (TEFRA) of 1982—supported by the Reagan administration and driven by the need to do something about the rapid escalation of Medicare costs—permitted for the first time true risk contracting with HMOs without retrospective adjustment.[5] Managed-care plans were also permitted to participate in Medicare on a cost basis, or to deliver part B services only (the Health Care Prepayment Plan [HCPP] option).[6] The Medicare risk program began on a demonstration basis but was fully operational by 1985.[7]

Growth in the managed-care program was slow through the first half decade of the program's existence; indeed, a number of plans withdrew from the program in the late 1980s.[8] Beginning in the early 1990s, however, the program took off, growing at double-digit rates through the mid-1990s.[9]

It is not difficult to understand why Medicare managed care grew so quickly in the 1990s. Under TEFRA, Medicare risk-based plans were paid 95% of the adjusted average per capita cost (AAPCC) of medical expenditures for Medicare fee-for-service beneficiaries in the county in which the beneficiary was located.[10] The 95% figure was based on the belief that Medicare managed-care organizations (MCOs) could deliver care more efficiently than the fee-for-service program, and thus should save the program money.[11] In fact, however, Medicare paid managed-care organizations significantly more to care for its beneficiaries than it would have paid for the same beneficiaries in the fee-for-service sector.

This happened because the beneficiaries who signed up for managed care—and, perhaps more important, those who stayed with managed care—were on average healthier and less costly to care for than those who stayed in the fee-for-service sector.[12] Payments to managed-care organizations were crudely adjusted for risk, considering age, gender, entitlement (disability or age) status, institutional status, and Medicaid eligibility, but most of the variation in health status among individuals remained unaccounted for by this risk adjustment.[13] Medicare managed-care organizations apparently attracted healthier beneficiaries to begin with, probably because really sick beneficiaries were reluctant to change providers or to lose access to specialists who were readily available in the fee-for-service programs and because younger beneficiaries were more familiar with managed care and more comfortable with it.[14] The HMOs also seem to have marketed their services and tailored their benefits to younger and healthier recipients, despite prohibitions against cherry picking.[15] This was relatively easy to do, since Medicare HMOs were marketed to individuals rather than to groups. Finally, beneficiaries often disenrolled from HMOs and returned to fee-for-service once their health deteriorated.[16] The General Accounting Office (GAO) estimated that in 1998, Medicare paid plans an average of 13.2% more for covering its beneficiaries than it would have spent had the same beneficiaries remained in the fee-for-service sector.[17]

Medicare HMOs were not simply able to pocket the difference between what they got from Medicare and what they spent for care for their beneficiaries. HMOs were (and still are) responsible for annual reporting of their adjusted community rates (ACR)—the amount that they estimate it will cost to provide medical services to their beneficiaries and cover their administrative costs.[18] The difference between a plan's ACR and its Medicare payment (after reductions to account for Medicare fee-for-service copayments and deductibles, which the plans were authorized to collect in the form of premiums), had to be returned to the program or to its beneficiaries through extra benefits, lower premiums, or contributions to a benefit-stabilization fund.[19] Most HMOs applied their overpayments for extra benefits or lower premiums. Some, indeed, provided extra benefits to their subscribers beyond what was required by the law simply to attract subscribers.[20]

Extra benefits provided by MCOs most commonly included outpatient prescription drugs, ear and eye examinations, routine physicals, and immunizations; less commonly, they included health education, dental coverage, foot care, eyeglasses, and hearing aids.[21] As of 1996, the average risk plan enrollee obtained $96 in extra benefits every month, with the value of the extra benefits growing over time and being greater in areas where plans were paid more.[22] Many HMOs also provided services without premiums (other than the normal Part B premium) or with minimal premiums, and spared beneficiaries from the cost sharing obligations they would have owed in fee-for-service Medicare.[23] These benefits and reduced cost-sharing were obviously of substantial value to Medicare beneficiaries and were otherwise available only through the purchase of costly supplemental policies. The attractiveness of these extra benefits and premium savings accounted for the substantial growth in Medicare managed care during the 1990s.

In practice, however, Medicare managed care simply provided some Medicare beneficiaries (usually those who were younger and healthier) with extra benefits that were not available to other beneficiaries. Moreover, because HMO payment rates were based on local fee-for-service payments, beneficiaries in areas with low fee-for-service costs got fewer extra benefits from Medicare HMOs or faced higher cost sharing.[24] Medicare risk plans were simply not available in many rural areas, so beneficiaries who lived in rural areas were denied even the possibility of the extra benefits.[25]

Beneficiaries who received extra benefits were not the only persons who profited from Medicare managed care. The plans themselves also did quite well. Although effectively they were limited to charging Medicare the amount that they charged for their commercial plans, the administrative costs on which their reported ACRs were based were not subject to any statutory or regulatory allowability limits, nor were they effectively regulated.[26] This continues to be true.[27] The Office of Inspector General (OIG) has frequently examined Medicare managed-care organization ACRs in recent years and has repeatedly found that (1) the estimated administrative costs on which reimbursement formulas are based exceed actual costs eventually incurred; (2) administrative costs that would not have been allowable under fee-for-service cost accounting have been charged to the program (including, for example, travel and entertainment costs and lobbying costs); (3) costs are charged to the Medicare program that should have been charged to commercial business, and (4) administrative costs included in the ACRs often cannot be documented under proper accounting principles.[28] Some MCOs also seem to have profited from adjustments to their rates that were intended to compensate for the added costs of institutional care, which were claimed for beneficiaries who were not in true nursing homes and which were excessive in terms of the actual expenses of institutionalized residents.[29]

## Medicare+Choice

The 1997 Balanced Budget Act (BBA) brought about dramatic changes in the Medicare managed-care program, which it renamed the Medicare+Choice (M+C) program. The legislation was driven by four major motivations, which account for the balancing—and sometimes contradictory—characteristics of the final legislation.

The primary influence driving the bill was the ideology of markets: privatization and individualization. Conservatives had long been unhappy with Medicare as a social insurance program, and two years earlier, Newt Gingrich's Contract with America Congress had tried to eliminate Medicaid as an entitlement, had cut Medicare dramatically, and had pressured Medicare beneficiaries into managed-care programs.[30] Although this effort had been blocked by President Bill Clinton's veto pen (in fact, the same pen with which Lyndon Johnson had signed the Medicare and Medicaid legislation in 1965), the drive to create markets within the Medicare program continued.[31] Pro-market conservatives played a major role in shaping the BBA.

First, market advocates were able to expand the menu of alternatives available to Medicare beneficiaries far beyond the risk- and cost-based HMOs that had been available since TEFRA. New options included preferred provider organizations (PPOs), point of service (POS) plans, provider-sponsored organizations (PSOs), and private fee-for-service plans.[32] Medical savings accounts (MSAs) with catastrophic coverage, the darling of conservative Republicans, were also permitted. The BBA recognized MSAs, but only on an experimental basis, permitting only up to 390,000 participants.[33] MSA plan beneficiaries were to be covered under the BBA by a catastrophic insurance plan with a deductible of $6,000, adjusted for inflation.[34] MSA plan beneficiaries would also receive from Medicare the difference between the premium of the high-deductible plan and the amount that Medicare would pay for other M+C plans, which would be deposited in a tax-free MSA from which medical expenses can be paid and from which money could eventually be withdrawn for other purposes.[35]

Second, some of the limitations historically imposed on Medicare managed care were lifted to make participation by new plans easier. TEFRA managed-care plans had only been permitted to participate in Medicare if half of their members were from the commercial sector, a requirement that avoided Medicare-only HMOs and guaranteed that only HMOs that were competitive in commercial markets would participate in Medicare.[36] Another protection that had been afforded Medicare managed-care recipients before the BBA was passed was the right to disenroll from HMOs or to switch plans at any time.[37] This allowed beneficiaries to abandon plans that proved unsatisfactory (creating a powerful incentive for plans to attend to their members), but it also made it difficult for HMOs to plan and created enrollment instability. It also made it easier for plans to encourage particularly costly members to disenroll. The BBA did not abandon this requirement initially, but it limited open enrollment and disenrollment after the first six months of 2002 to the first three months of each subsequent year, and it allowed only one change during the open enrollment period of each year (except for institutionalized individuals.)[38]

The statute also authorized provision of Medicare services through PSOs under a federal waiver from state licensure requirements under certain circumstances. PSOs are organized and operated by health-care providers or groups of affiliated health-care providers to offer a substantial proportion of health-care items and services themselves; the provider must be at substantial financial risk with respect to such items and services and have a majority financial interest in the entity.[39] Congress had become convinced that the states were imposing unreasonable licensure requirements on PSOs, and the BBA permits PSOs to participate in Medicare without state licensure (for up to three years) in situations where the state delays processing a licensure application unduly, applies discriminatory standards or conditions to the PSO, or applies solvency standards different from those imposed by Medicare, although waivered organizations are still subject to nondiscriminatory state consumer protection and quality standards.[40]

The BBA also established a small-scale competitive pricing demonstration project to explore the possibility of price and quality competition among M+C organizations[41] and another competitive bidding project for Part B services.[42] Competitive bidding represented another attempt to bring market discipline to the Medicare program.

Finally, market advocates wrote into the BBA a number of mechanisms for increasing information available to beneficiaries about the rich array of alternatives that the BBA's sponsors expected would become available as the BBA was implemented. In particular, plans are required under the BBA to provide information annually on a variety of topics, such as the plan's service area, benefits, providers, out-of-area coverage, emergency coverage, supplemental benefits, prior authorization rules, plan grievance and appeal procedures, and quality-assurance programs.[43] M+C organizations are responsible for providing their members with detailed descriptions of specified plan provisions.[44] The plans are also required to disclose information to beneficiaries upon request about the plan's utilization and expenditure control procedures, aggregate information about grievances and appeals, and summary descriptions of provider compensation arrangements.[45] Finally, the Department of Health and Human Services must provide beneficiaries with information on plan options and must maintain a toll-free number and Internet site for this purpose.[46]

A second major motivation of the BBA was the desire to save money. By 1997 it had become very difficult to deny that Medicare HMOs were overpaid, and that this overpayment was largely due to favorable risk selection.[47] There-fore, the BBA mandated that the Health Care Financing Administration (HCFA) (then in charge of administering the M+C program), develop a bet-ter risk-adjustment system to take into account the actual health status of insured beneficiaries.[48] This would result in smaller payments for Medicare managed-care organizations that in fact attracted healthier beneficiaries. As im-plemented by HCFA, however, it also meant that many of the Medicare MCOs would have to start keeping track of information (primarily encounter data) that they had not necessarily been keeping track of earlier, thus increasing their administrative costs.[49] Moreover, before the BBA was enacted, MCO payments had not taken into account the fact that the Medicare fee-for-service program not only pays for medical care for its recipients, but also subsidizes medical educa-tion. Because Medicare HMOs did not pass these subsidies on to educational in-stitutions, they were overpaid in comparison to the fee-for-service program. The BBA reduced M+C reimbursement to exclude medical education subsidies.[50]

A third goal of the M+C program, closely related to the first two, was to achieve greater equity in the program and to improve accessibility to MCOs in areas that had been historically underserved by the program. The BBA at-tempted to raise payment levels dramatically in counties where rates had been low—mainly rural counties—by putting a floor under reimbursement pay-ments, while at the same time holding down payments in high-paid, mainly ur-ban, counties by phasing in a blended rate that would take account of both na-tional and regional rates and by limiting increases to a fixed amount of 2% per year.[51] The whole system was to be budget-neutral with respect to the previ-ous payment formula, however; thus increases for poorly paid MCOs had to be balanced out with constraints on better paid MCOs.[52] Attempts to improve risk adjustment, of course, were also directed toward achieving greater equity.

A final factor influencing the legislation was a desire to protect Medicare managed-care recipients from managed-care abuses, which were becoming in-creasingly apparent in the private sector. Although the BBA must be seen by and large as a triumph for pro-market forces, those skeptical of the ability of managed care to serve Medicare beneficiaries were able to secure a number of provisions in the bill to protect beneficiaries. Many of these provisions, in fact, were carry-overs from the legislation that had previously governed man-aged care, although some new provisions were added.

For example, the BBA imposes a number of requirements to ensure that M+C organizations are viable business arrangements. Also, under the BBA, M+C organizations must have at least 5,000 members in urban areas and 1,500 in rural areas; PSOs can have smaller numbers.[53]

The BBA also included certain provisions to limit biased selection and im-proper marketing. It requires M+C organizations to accept any beneficiary who applies as long as the organization has the capacity to accept additional members.[54] M+C organizations must submit marketing material to HCFA for review 45 days before use, and they are not allowed to offer cash or rebates as inducements to get beneficiaries to enroll, to discriminate in marketing, to solicit beneficiaries door to door, or to engage in misleading or confusing marketing activities.[55]

M+C plans must offer at least the basic benefits that are covered by Parts A and B of Medicare, whether directly, through arrangement, or by payment.[56] As before, they must also cover supplemental benefits (or provide reduced premiums or cost sharing, or both) to the extent that their M+C payment exceeds their costs.[57] Coordinated-care plans (HMOs, PPOs, and PSOs) must pay out-of-plan providers for emergency services; for urgently needed services, and for renal dialysis when beneficiaries are temporarily out of the service area; and for poststabilization care services that are either preapproved or not disapproved within an hour of an approval request for their plan members.[58]

M+C coordinated-care plans must provide access to providers 24 hours a day, seven days a week; they must furnish services that are "culturally competent," ensure that hours of operation of providers are convenient and nondiscriminatory, provide adequate and coordinated specialist treatment for persons with complex or serious medical conditions, and allow women enrollees direct access to women's health specialists.[59] They must have an ongoing quality assurance and performance improvement program,[60] and they must have in place mechanisms to detect both under- and overutilization. Most types of plans must make provision for independent quality review. Organizations accredited by approved national accreditation agencies can be deemed to meet quality requirements.[61]

M+C plans are required under the BBA to charge the same premiums and cost sharing to all plan members in the service area.[62] M+C HMOs, PPOs, and PSOs may not charge enrollees more for premiums, deductibles, copayments, or coinsurance for basic benefits than the actuarial value of beneficiary cost sharing for traditional Medicare, and they cannot charge more for supplemental benefits than they charge their commercial populations.[63]

HCFA must make a new determination each year as to whether an M+C organization may continue in the program. Terminated or nonrenewed programs are entitled to due process protections.[64] Plans that violate plan requirements are also subject to civil fines.[65]

In sum, the BBA represented a careful balance of provisions that were intended to encourage the growth of Medicare managed care with provisions intended to protect Medicare beneficiaries from managed-care abuses that were becoming increasingly apparent in the late 1990s in commercial managed care.

## Medicare+Choice: A Balance Sheet

Although the BBA was primarily intended to nurture Medicare managed care, in fact, it has seriously damaged—perhaps destroyed—it.

Although the HCFA and those responsible for assisting it in providing information to beneficiaries carried out a massive (and expensive) educational effort to inform beneficiaries of all of the new managed-care alternatives that would be available under the BBA, few plans showed up to offer those alternatives.[66] Even though the MSA alternative should have been attractive to healthier beneficiaries, as it enabled them to divert Medicare funds into their own medical savings accounts, no insurers stepped forward to offer these plans. As should have been obvious, Medicare beneficiaries are too risk averse to self-insure themselves, and the few that had interest in the program were too scattered to create a market for an insurer.[67] The entire Medicare supplement industry, of course, is a testimony to this risk adversity.

The PSO and PPO alternatives also proved unattractive. PPOs basically exist in the commercial sector to service the employees of self-insured employers, and risk-bearing PPOs are not the norm. PPOs were not interested in becoming risk-bearing under the even more risky Medicare program.[68] PPOs also found it difficult to comply with the M+C care-management and quality requirements, which were designed for more tightly structured HMOs.[69] Moreover, few PSOs have shown an interest in the program, because hospitals, the natural sponsors of PSOs, can only make a profit as risk-bearers by holding down hospitalizations, and thus they face an inherent and unresolvable conflict of interest when accepting risk through capitation.[70] Even beyond the M+C program, the number of hospital-based PSOs seems to be declining.[71]

Much more surprising, however, was the reaction of traditional HMOs to the BBA. Soon after the BBA was adopted, HMO plans started withdrawing from the Medicare market. In 1999, 95 plans withdrew or reduced their service areas, affecting 407,000 enrollees, while in 2000, 99 plans withdrew, affecting 327,000 enrollees.[72] Plan withdrawals and reductions in 2001 affected 934,000 enrollees, while 500,000 enrollees were affected by 2002 plan contract terminations and service area reductions and probably another 200,000 will be affected in 2003.[73] Between January of 1999 and January of 2002, the number of plans participating in M+C dropped 57%, and withdrawals affected 2.2 million Medicare beneficiaries.[74] In many instances, moreover, plans that remained with the program reduced their service areas, eliminated optional benefits, or raised their premiums. The percentage of plans that provided a zero premium option dropped from 80% in 1999 to 46% in 2001, while the percentage of plans offering prescription drug coverage dropped from 84% to 70%.[75] The mean premium for plans rose from $6 a month to $23, while the percentage of plans that offered drug coverage with a cap of $500 or less rose from 11% to 28%.

Many beneficiaries, faced with reduced MCO benefits or increased premiums, returned to the traditional fee-for-service program, where at least they had free choice of physician. The number of Medicare beneficiaries in Medicare risk or M+C plans peaked in 1999 at 6.3 million, had dropped by February 2002 to about 5 million, and will probably decline to 4.1 million by 2005 if the current law is not changed.[76] Many of those who stayed, moreover, either lost the additional benefits that they had enjoyed under the previous Medicare MCO program or had to buy supplemental policies at a much higher price to continue to enjoy those benefits.

The reasons for the post-BBA HMO withdrawals are complex. The HMO industry and their surrogates and advocates complained loudly that the BBA rates had cut their payments too deeply and that they were being asked to provide services to Medicare beneficiaries for rates below commercial market or Medicare fee-for-service rates.[77] They also complained that the new regulatory requirements imposed by the BBA and by HCFA were excessive and unnecessary.[78] They protested that the new risk-adjustment refinements were unfair, and that implementing them required collection of new data elements not otherwise available or necessary, at great expense.[79] In particular, the competitive bidding demonstration projects were staunchly opposed and ultimately thwarted.[80] This controversy presented the almost comic picture of some of the strongest congressional advocates of markets suddenly turning against real competition when it threatened the economic interests of their constituents.[81]

The protests of the managed-care industry and of M+C beneficiaries were heard by responsive ears in Congress, which in 1999 passed the Medicare, Medicaid, and the State Children's Health Insurance Program Balanced Budget Refinement Act (BBRA) of 1999, slowing the implementation of scheduled M+C payment reforms and offering a new entry bonus payment in areas where M+C plans were not available.[82] In 2000, Congress passed the Benefit Improvement and Protection Act (BIPA), which increased M+C payments as of March 1, 2001.[83] To date, however, these efforts have had little effect, as managed-care plans continue to withdraw from the program, and most of those that remain with Medicare have directed the new money to provider payments rather than to improving benefits.[84] Of the 118 M+C plans that had planned withdrawals or service area reductions in 2001, only four decided to return because of BIPA.[85]

In the end, the reasons for plan withdrawals and service area reductions are more than a simple matter of underpayment and overregulation. Some plans that faced reduced growth in payments left the program, but many plan withdrawals were from areas where payments had been sharply increased under the BBA.[86] Further, because of an error made in computing initial M+C rates, and because of the extraordinary success of BBA cost-containment efforts in the fee-for-service sector (and the influence of other factors like fraud and abuse enforcement), rates paid to M+C plans continued to exceed the amounts paid for fee-for-service beneficiaries until 2001.[87] Although the quality and consumer protection requirements of the BBA certainly imposed additional burdens on plans, they are not excessive when compared to the "patient bill of rights" requirements imposed by many states, or even to recently promulgated ERISA rules.

Business-cycle patterns certainly seem to offer a partial explanation for plan withdrawals: many plans that withdrew or reduced service areas in 1999–2001 were plans that had entered new markets or had expanded significantly in the late 1990s during the period of rapid growth in the program, and thus simply became more realistic about plan participation.[88] Most of them were smaller plans, with smaller enrollments and less generous benefits than the plans that remained.[89] Moreover, managed care generally, which had appeared to be very successful in holding down health-care costs throughout the mid-1990s, faced sharply increased costs at the end of the period as provider consolidation and backlash against managed care strengthened the bargaining hand of providers.[90] Even the Federal Employees Health Benefits Program (FEHBP), long touted by market advocates as a model for Medicare, faced dramatically increased costs and plan withdrawals in the late 1990s and early 2000s.[91] Managed care generally seemed threatened by consumers who chafed under its restrictions, and the most restrictive forms of managed care seemed to be losing popularity.[92] Managers of many plans undoubtedly calculated that the Medicare population was not worth taking on unless the program offered rates significantly above what Medicare paid in the fee-for-service program.

## The Outlook for Medicare Managed Care

In retrospect, it is surprising that anyone should have been surprised by the failure of M+C. M+C represents the triumph of ideology over reality. As is explored more fully in Chapter 6, Medicare has tremendous market power as a buyer and can negotiate prices as low as or lower than can managed-care organizations, and Medicare experiences far lower administrative costs than MCOs. M+C plans should be able to control utilization better than the traditional Medicare program, but aggressive attempts to ration care by M+C organizations would simply drive beneficiaries back into fee-for-service Medicare. Therefore, it is difficult to see how M+C could save the program money, and it is not surprising that it failed to do so. If continued use of managed care in the Medicare program is to be justified, it must be on another basis than cost savings. Four possibilities commend themselves.

First, it is argued that providing beneficiaries with choice of plan is in itself a virtue, regardless of cost.[93] Although die-hard free-market advocates will take this position as a last-ditch defense, it is not one likely to commend itself to the taxpayers who will have to foot the bill. Moreover, if choice is important to beneficiaries, it is most likely choice of doctor or provider rather than choice of health plan that is of interest.[94] Managed care, of course, restricts rather than enlarges these choices.

The second and third justifications are closely related. One is that Medicare managed care provides beneficiaries with higher-quality care. The other is that it provides beneficiaries with better-coordinated care. The evidence on the first point is ambiguous, though not promising. A host of studies have now been conducted comparing quality of care, access to care, and beneficiary satisfaction in managed care and in traditional fee-for-service medicine. At best they can be characterized as establishing that managed care is not superior to fee-for-service medicine in terms of quality, access, and satisfaction.[95] Moreover, a recent study specifically comparing Medicare with private insurance (now predominantly managed care), found that Medicare beneficiaries were more likely to rate their insurance as "excellent," less likely to have complaints about their insurance, more confident in their future access to care, less likely to encounter access to care based on cost, and more satisfied with the quality of their medical care than privately insured individuals.[96]

In recent hearings on the M+C program, the main argument made by its advocates was that it provides beneficiaries with better-coordinated care, more preventive services, and better care management.[97] This may be true, and it certainly should be true if managed care means anything at all. The ultimate question, however, is whether the M+C program is so superior to fee-for-service Medicare in this dimension as to justify its substantial additional cost. A vital consideration in making this judgment is that Medicare could simply pay for care coordination as an additional covered service if it is important enough, or create special care coordination programs for populations in particular need of it, as is currently being done under the Program for All-inclusive Care for the Elderly (PACE) program.[98] It is difficult to make the case for retaining an entire, costly M+C program to this end.

Fourth and finally, it can be argued that it is worth retaining a small market-based program to provide a benchmark for price setting under Medicare-administered price systems.[99] Again, the judgment here must be whether the light is worth the candle. This is particularly true as a large commercial managed-care market exists, and it should provide considerable price information for Medicare price setting.

It is time to recognize that the Medicare managed-care experience offers little support for the superiority of privatization and individualization as strategies for reforming public health insurance programs. The program was conceived to save money for the Medicare program and to expand choices and improve care for Medicare beneficiaries. It has become dramatically clear that managed care does not save the Medicare program money; indeed, it costs more than fee-for-service medicine. It is also not at all clear that it offers better medical care, although it may do so for some recipients in some cases.

## Medicaid Managed Care

Medicare managed care can be judged to have failed, but it is harder to reach a final conclusion about Medicaid managed care. In part, this is because there is not just one Medicaid managed-care program, but many. All but two of the states now have managed-care programs, and a number of states have separate programs for different categories of recipients.[100] Some of these programs can be judged to be relatively successful, such as the Arizona program, which has survived for 20 years and has been reviewed positively by those who have examined it.[101] Other programs, such as the Ohio 1115 waiver program never got off the ground.[102] Most programs have varied over time, with periods of relative success or failure, as seems to be true of the California and Tennessee programs.[103]

It is also difficult to evaluate the success of Medicaid managed care because the Medicaid fee-for-service program that it replaced was deeply flawed. Before the coming of managed care, most state Medicaid programs were characterized by poor physician payment rates, usually resulting in poor physician participation rates.[104] Medicaid fee-for-service reimbursement rates averaged half that of commercial insurance, and one-quarter of physicians treated three-quarters of Medicaid patients, while another one-quarter did not participate at all.[105] In turn, this resulted in excessive reliance on hospital emergency rooms for primary care and in lack of adequate preventive care.[106] It is also widely believed that Medicaid fee-for-service care suffered from lack of coordination and indiscriminate and episodic seeking of care ("doctor shopping").[107] If managed care resulted in only a modest expansion of access to primary care or improvement of care coordination, therefore, it could be judged an improvement.

A further issue that complicates an evaluation of the contribution of Medicaid managed care is that the period immediately before the dramatic expansion of managed care in the 1990s was quite atypical. First, it was marked by major eligibility expansions, from 5.6% of the national population under the age of 65 in 1984 to nearly 11% in the late 1990s.[108] Congress extended Medicaid coverage to a number of new groups in the late 1980s and early 1990s, including, most important all children born after September 30, 1983, who lived in families with incomes below the poverty level.[109] The Supreme Court's decision in Sullivan v. Zebley rejecting the Reagan administration's restrictive definition of disability also expanded Medicaid coverage of the disabled, a very expensive population.[110] In turn, these eligibility expansions contributed to dramatic increases in the cost of Medicaid programs, which grew at a compound average rate of 19% per year between 1988 and 1993.[111]

At the same time, program costs were being driven upward by state manipulation of federal financial participation. The states had realized in the late 1980s that by imposing phony "taxes" on (or accepting contributions from) providers, obtaining federal funds to match those funds, and then paying the providers back through targeted "disproportionate share hospital" payments, they could attract large sums of federal money without putting state money at risk.[112] State manipulation of federal financial participation resulted in dramatic growth in Medicaid program costs, even though this program cost growth often did not impose a real cost on the states. Medicaid managed care blossomed just as federal eligibility expansions were slowing and federal financial participation manipulation was being checked. Therefore, it is difficult to evaluate how much of the subsequent reduction in Medicaid cost growth was attributable to managed care and how much to other factors.

The primary driving force for most states in adopting managed care was cost control.[113] Fee-for-service payment is generally regarded as the most inflationary form of payment for health-care services. It was hoped that managed-care firms would be more successful at containing health-care costs than state Medicaid agencies had been. However, whether or not managed care actually resulted in reducing health-care inflation, it would at least, it was hoped, make health-care costs more predictable by shifting the risk of cost growth from state governments to managed-care organizations.

A second aspiration was that managed care would result in better coordination of care, and perhaps even in bringing Medicaid recipients truly into the mainstream of American health care for the first time.[114] As has already been noted, Medicaid had never really been successful in attracting mainstream primary care physicians. By the mid-1990s, managed care had already become the mainstream of American medicine, and it was hoped that managed care would make available to Medicaid recipients the same providers and professionals that served commercial managed-care plan members. Managed-care advocates also hoped that improved access to primary care would result in better care coordination and less dependence on hospitals and emergency rooms.[115]

## A History of Medicaid Managed Care

Early experiments in Medicaid managed care were not encouraging. Beginning in the late 1960s, attempts by Governor Reagan to move California Medi-Cal recipients into HMOs resulted in scandal: deceptive marketing, poor-quality care, inadequate access to providers, inadequate capitalization, fraud, and profiteering characterized the program.[116] Reforms adopted by Congress in 1976 by and large put an end to the California experiments. These reforms limited Medicaid recipients to HMOs that were commercially competitive by prohibiting Medicaid contracting with HMOs whose membership consisted of more than 50% Medicaid recipients. The reforms also limited Medicaid full-risk contracts to federally qualified HMOs.[117] These reforms put later Medicaid HMO plans on a more stable footing.

The first successful major experiment with Medicaid managed care was the Arizona Health Care Cost Containment System, established in 1971.[118] Arizona had long remained the only state to resist the temptation of federal money and forego the establishment of a Medicaid program, relying instead on its counties to provide indigent care.[119] When it finally adopted a Medicaid program, the program was based on managed care. Rather than establishing a program within the confines of the Medicaid HMO program, as it then existed, however, Arizona requested a waiver from the Department of Health and Human Services under § 1115 of the Social Security Act, which permits experimental demonstration programs.[120] The Arizona program got off to a rocky start (it had to abandon private administration of the program a year after the program began), but it has generally come to be recognized as a model program, reasonably low in cost with adequate quality of care and member satisfaction.[121]

During the 1990s, Medicaid managed care became much better accepted. First, a number of states initiated managed-care programs within the constraints of the Medicaid statute. Many of these programs were HMO programs, although primary care case-management programs—fee-for-service programs in which the recipient's care is managed by a primary care gatekeeper physician—were also common, especially in the early years.[122] As the Medicaid statute permitted mandatory assignment of recipients to managed-care organizations only when the state was granted a waiver, these programs were often far from universal.[123] Second, some programs were established pursuant to so-called 1915(b) waivers, under which the Department of Health and Human Services allowed states to operate managed-care programs free from certain legal constraints, most notably the freedom-of-choice requirement of the Medicaid statute.[124] Section 1915(b) waiver programs were otherwise required to comply with federal Medicaid program requirements. Finally, a few states followed Arizona's example and obtained 1115 waivers, freeing them comprehensively from program constraints and permitting them to chart their own course, subject to HHS oversight.[125]

Two states, Tennessee and Oregon, took particularly radical approaches to reforming Medicaid. Both attempted to use managed care to cut program costs, like all other states, but also proposed in turn to expand program coverage.[126] The federal government signed off on these expansions with the understanding that the program would be revenue-neutral for the federal government: that is, it would not cost the federal government more than a traditional Medicaid program would have.[127] Tenncare was implemented largely through executive action before effective opposition could be fully marshaled.[128] Tennessee lacked a developed and sophisticated managed-care industry at the time Tenncare was initiated, and the first year of the program was chaotic.[129] By including a large group of otherwise uninsured residents, as well as traditional Medicaid recipients, however, Tennessee created a pool of recipients large enough to appeal to commercial managed-care organizations. Tenncare's largest MCO, Blue Cross/Blue Shield, initially required physicians who served state employees to also serve Tenncare patients, a policy that came to be known as "cram down" and resulted in an initial loss of about one-fifth of network physicians, although many later rejoined the plan.[130]

The Tennessee program got off to a rocky start, and has hit some rough spots since, but it expanded coverage and for a time garnered relatively good marks for quality of care and satisfaction.[131] In the recent past, however, a federal court has adjudged the program to have violated its obligations to provide screening, diagnosis, and treatment services to children and appointed a master to supervise a separate program for Medicaid children.[132] Tenncare has also encountered serious financial problems, and Tennessee has recently renegotiated its Medicaid waiver with the federal government to split the program into separate programs for Medicaid eligibles and for other uninsureds.[133]

In the early 1990s, Oregon proposed to expand its Medicaid program to cover all persons under the poverty line, increasing by 120,000 the 243,000 persons then covered by Medicaid. It proposed to do this by ranking 688 health services in terms of cost effectiveness and denying coverage for low-ranked procedures. It requested a waiver from a number of the requirements of the Medicaid program to implement this proposal.

The first George Bush administration denied the Oregon waiver request in 1992 because of concerns that the proposed Oregon program would violate the Americans with Disabilities Act by denying coverage for some services to persons with certain disabilities. For example, the rationing program originally proposed by Oregon would have denied liver transplants for alcoholic cirrhosis or life support for extremely low-birth-weight babies under 23 weeks' gestation. The Clinton administration approved a revised waiver request in 1993. The waiver was approved on the condition that Oregon would meet certain requirements to lessen the effect of considerations of disability on prioritizing treatments.

Oregon's program seems to have been largely successful. It has expanded a fairly generous coverage package to 130,000 persons that were not previously covered. It has done so, however, primarily by increasing funding from general revenues and a tobacco tax and by holding the line on expenses through managed care. The "rationing" list has proved to be primarily of value as a political tool to refocus political debate on what will be covered rather than on who will receive benefits.[134]

The 1997 Balanced Budget Act made it much easier for states to establish Medicaid managed-care programs. The 1997 amendments permitted states to require Medicaid recipients (other than Medicare beneficiaries, Native Americans, or certain special-need children) to enroll with a Medicaid managed-care organization or primary care case manager.[135] States are generally required under the BBA to permit recipients a choice of two or more Medicaid managed-care plans, but this requirement is loosened for rural areas.[136] Medicaid recipients who do not exercise their choice, moreover, may be assigned by the state through a default enrollment process, and states may establish enrollment priorities for plans that are oversubscribed.[137] Recipients may terminate (or change) enrollment in a Medicaid managed-care program for cause at any time, but may only do so without cause during the 90-day period after enrollment and once a year thereafter.[138]

The 1997 amendments imposed certain restrictions to encourage competition among plans and to discourage risk selection. Medicaid managed-care plans are not permitted to discriminate on the basis of health status or requirements for health service in enrollment, reenrollment, or disenrollment of recipients.[139] Medicaid managed-care plans are required to make information available to enrollees and potential enrollees with respect to the identity, location, qualifications, and availability of participating providers; enrollee rights and responsibilities; grievance and appeal procedures; and covered items and services.[140] States are required to provide recipients annually, and upon request, with comparative information regarding benefits, cost sharing, service area, and quality and performance.[141]

The 1997 BBA also provides certain protections for plan beneficiaries. Beneficiaries must be afforded access to services to evaluate and stabilize emergency medical conditions without prior authorization requirements or provider participation limitations.[142] The statute prohibits Medicaid managed-care organizations from interfering with communications between health-care providers and beneficiaries, and it requires plans to have grievance procedures in place.[143] Medicaid managed-care plans are required to offer an appropriate range of services and a sufficient number, mix, and geographic distribution of providers.[144]

States that operate Medicaid managed-care plans are required to develop and implement a quality-improvement strategy that complies with standards developed by the CMS and that addresses timely access to care, continuity of care, and quality and appropriateness of care and services.[145] Medicaid managed-care organizations must also have contracts providing for an annual (as appropriate) external independent review of quality outcomes and of access to items and services, and the results of this review must be available to providers, enrollees, and potential enrollees.[146]

A variety of fraud and abuse prohibitions also apply to Medicaid managed-care organizations. Medicaid managed-care organizations must have their marketing material approved by the state; they may not include false or materially misleading information in the materials, must distribute the material through their entire service area, and may not conduct door-to-door, telephonic, or other "cold call" marketing.[147]

States must have available "intermediate sanctions" for dealing with Medicaid managed-care organizations that fail to comply with program requirements.[148] Intermediate sanctions include civil penalties of up to $25,000 ($100,000 for discrimination in enrollment and false statements); the appointment of temporary management for continued egregious behavior that poses a substantial risk to the health of enrollees; permitting disenrollment without cause by members of problem plans; suspension of enrollment; suspension of payment, and, with notice and hearing, contract termination.[149]

The BBA also made it much easier for states to establish and maintain experimental managed-care plans under § 1115 waivers, which the BBA deemed to be approved unless turned down by HHS within six months.[150] Even before the BBA, the Clinton administration had already been much more welcoming to state waiver proposals than earlier administrations, and by 2001, 18 states had established managed-care plans under waiver authority.[151]

## Medicaid Managed Care: An Evaluation

Few states provide all Medicaid services for all Medicaid recipients through managed care. Most states now cover children and their families under managed care, but only about one-quarter of Medicaid recipients with disabilities are covered by managed care.[152] Disabled and elderly populations are very different from the population that is normally covered by commercial managed care—employees and their families. The elderly and disabled are more expensive to cover, and they present managed-care organizations with greater risks. They also tend to be more politically protected by advocacy and provider groups than are families and children on welfare, and they have been more successful in resisting managed care.[153] Only six states enroll over three-quarters of their state's disabled Medicaid beneficiaries in managed care, and 15 states do not enroll any disabled beneficiaries in managed care at all.[154]

Medicaid managed-care plans often do not cover all services. Medicaid programs offer a much broader range of services than do most employee benefit plans—in part because they cover services like dental and vision care, which is paid for out of pocket by most employees but is unaffordable to many Medicaid recipients—and in part because they cover chronic health-care services like nursing home care or home health care that are rarely needed by beneficiaries of employment-related plans and often not covered by them.[155] Some states "carve out" these services and contract with separate managed-care plans (like behavioral health plans) to cover them; other states simply cover them directly through fee-for-service payments.[156]

In fact, covering populations with special needs, particularly the mentally disabled, has proved to be one of the greatest challenges to Medicaid managed care.[157] These populations are very expensive to serve adequately, and easy to underserve, and some states have come up short. The federal government revoked New Mexico's Medicaid behavioral managed-care program for a time because of serious deficiencies in the program,[158] while Pennsylvania's Medicaid program was sued for delays in providing behavioral health care to children.[159]

Another major challenge presented to managed care is the preservation of safety-net providers. Because we lack a national health program in the United States, a complex web of institutions has been created to serve the medically indigent. These institutions include public hospitals, academic medical centers, and federally qualified health-care centers.[160] These institutions are funded through a variety of sources, but many have depended heavily on Medicaid payments. In recent years, Medicaid programs have funneled large sums of money to safety-net hospitals that care for indigents through disproportionate share payments. Disproportionate share payments cover the cost of the care these institutions provide to Medicaid recipients, and they subsidize the cost of the care they provide to uninsured indigents.[161] Since 1989, Medicaid programs have also been required under federal law to pay federally qualified health centers on a cost basis.[162]

Commercial Medicaid managed-care plans, however, may refuse to contract with safety-net providers, leaving safety-net providers in the lurch.[163] Moreover, academic medical centers that do participate in Medicaid managed care often end up the victims of adverse selection, serving the sickest and most costly patients without the resources to care for them.[164] The change to Medicaid managed care, therefore, has posed a major threat to the viability of safety-net institutions, which have depended on Medicaid subsidies to serve the 40 million Americans who are uninsured.

In some communities, managed-care organizations that have been built around safety-net providers are proving to be the most reliable managed-care partners for Medicaid programs.[165] Despite early interest by commercial managed-care plans in Medicaid managed care, many have subsequently dropped the program.[166] Medicaid is simply too different from their normal lines of business. Medicaid usually offers a more needy population, plagued by more chronic and expensive problems. Medicaid pays parsimoniously, but demands a great deal in terms of program requirements. Medicaid requires coverage of services that many commercial plans do not otherwise cover, and it covers many recipients who live in places where commercial plans do not have providers. Moreover, providers that contract with commercial plans are often reluctant to have Medicaid recipients in their waiting rooms. Increasingly, commercial plans have been abandoning Medicaid and leaving the market to safety-net plans that are experienced in dealing with Medicaid recipients.

In the end, however, managed care has worked out better for Medicaid than for Medicare. In most states managed care has not saved Medicaid programs a great deal of money, but neither has it added to program cost.[167] Several studies show that it has decreased dependence of Medicaid recipients on emergency rooms, but most studies show that recipient access to care has otherwise been unaffected. In some states, however, money has been saved and access and quality have improved. The bottom line seems to be that in most states Medicaid was such a poor program before it embraced managed care that improvement was an easy target, which in some states has been achieved.

On the other hand, the Medicaid managed-care experience does not offer much comfort to those who argue for privatization and individualization of government programs. In fact, the Medicaid experience with private, commercial MCOs has not been particularly positive, and many have left the Medicaid program. Many of the most successful Medicaid managed-care organizations are sponsored by public hospitals or clinics and thus resemble somewhat integrated public providers in other countries, such as Sweden or even Great Britain. Individual choice of Medicaid plan, along the lines of the competitive models pushed by market advocates, has not played a major role in state Medicaid managed-care programs. Indeed, many recipients have been assigned to plans by state enrollment brokers when they have failed to make their own choice. In sum, Medicaid managed care, though not a total failure, does not seem to provide us with a blueprint for the future development of a privatized, choice-driven, health-care program for the poor.

# Notes

1. In 2001, 93% of insured employees were enrolled in Health Maintenance Organizations, Preferred Provider Organizations, or Point of Service plans, and only 7% were in conventional plans, even though most of these have managed-care features such as utilization review. See Jon Gabel et al., "Job-Based Health Insurance in 2001: Inflation Hits Double Digits, Managed Care Retreats," *Health Affairs* 20 (September/October 2001): 180, 184.

2. Lawrence D. Brown, *Politics and Health Care Organizations: HMOs as Federal Policy* (Washington D.C.: Brookings Institute, 1983).

3. Social Security Amendments of 1972, Pub. L. 92-603, § 226, 86 Stat 1329, 1391 (1972) adding § 1876 to the Social Security Act.

4. Jonathan B. Oberlander, "Managed Care and Medicare Reform," *Journal of Health Politics, Policy, and Law* 22 (1997): 595, 598.

5. Ibid., 598. See also John Iglehart, "Medicare Turns to HMOs," *New England Journal of Medicine* 312, no. 2 (1985): 132.

6. Charlotte W. Collins, "Medicare Managed Risk Contracting before 1999," in *Risk Contracting and Medicare+Choice*, edited by Winfield Towles and Charlotte Collins (New York: McGraw-Hill, 2000), 3–6.

7. Oberlander, "Managed Care and Medicare Reform," 598.

8. General Accounting Office (GAO), *Medicare Managed Care Plans: Many Factors Contribute to Recent Withdrawals; Plan Interest Continues*, Pub. No. GAO/HEHS-99-91 (Washington, D.C.: GAO, 1999), 6.

9. Marsha Gold, "Medicare+Choice: An Interim Report Card," *Health Affairs* 20 (July/August 2001): 122.

10. See Alison Cherney, "Payment Methodology," in *Risk Contracting and Medicare+Choice*, edited by Winfield Towles and Charlotte Collins (New York: McGraw-Hill, 2000), 84.

11. Oberlander, "Managed Care and Medicare Reform," 606.

12. Ibid., 606–607.

13. The Prospective Payment Assessment Commission (ProPAC) estimated that these adjusters only accounted for about one percent in variation. ProPAC, *Medicare and the American Health Care System, Report to Congress* (Washington, D.C.: ProPAC, June 1997).

14. Oberlander, "Managed Care and Medicare Reform," 607.

15. Ibid., 607–608.

16. One study found that beneficiaries who disenrolled from HMOs cost the program 160% as much as did the average beneficiary in the six months following disenrollment. Cherney, "Payment Methodology," 85.

17. General Accounting Office (GAO), *Medicare+Choice, Payments Exceed Cost of Benefits in Fee-for-Service, Adding Billions to Spending*, Pub. No. GAO-HEHS-00-161 (Washington, D.C.: GAO, 2000) 11.

18. This amount is based on the costs of providing services to commercial enrollees, adjusted for higher use by Medicare enrollees. Prospective Payment Advisory Commission (ProPAC), *Medicare and the American Health Care System, Report to Congress* (Washington, D.C.: ProPAC, 1997), 44.

19. Ibid.

20. GAO, *Medicare+Choice: Payments Exceed Cost of Benefits*, 14.

21. Office of Inspector General (OIG), Department of Health and Human Services, *Medicare+Choice HMO Extra Benefits: Beneficiary Perspectives*, Pub. No. OEI-02-99-00030 (Washington, D.C.: DHHS, 2000), 7. See also Kathryn Langwell, Christopher Topoleski, and Daniel Sherman, *Analysis of Benefits Offered by Medicare HMOs, 1999: Complexities and Implications*" (Washington, D.C.: Kaiser Family Foundation, 1999).

22. ProPac, *Medicare and the American Health Care System*, 44.

23. OIG, *Medicare+Choice*, 10. A study by the OIG reported that lower cost sharing was a more important reason for joining Medicare HMOs for most beneficiaries than were extra benefits. Ibid., 10.

24. ProPAC, *Medicare and the American Health Care System*, 44–45.

25. Ibid., 39–41.

26. See Office of Inspector General (OIG), Department of Health and Human Services, *Review of the Administrative Cost Component of the Adjusted Community Rate*

*Proposal at Nine Medicare Managed Care Organizations for the 1997 Contract Year,* Pub. No. A-03-98-00046 (Washington, D.C.: DHHS, 2000), 6.

27. See Office of Inspector General (OIG), Department of Health and Human Services, *Review of the Administrative Costs Component of the Adjusted Community Rate Proposal for Contract Year 2000,* Pub. No. A-03-01-00002 (Washington, D.C.: DHHS, 2001), 1.

28. In addition to the reports listed in notes 26 and 27, see Office of Inspector General (OIG), Department of Health and Human Services, *Review of Administrative Costs Included in the Adjusted Community Rate Proposals for a Missouri Medicare+Choice Organization,* Pub. No. A-07-00-00114 (Washington, D.C.: DHHS, 2001); OIG, *Review of the Administrative Cost Component of the Adjusted Community Rate Proposal for a New York Medicare+Choice Organization,* Pub. No. A-02-00-01034 (Washington, D.C.: DHHS, 2001); OIG, *Review of the Administrative Cost Component of the Adjusted Community Rate Proposal for a Northwest Medicare+Choice Organization for Contract Year 2000,* Pub. No. A-10-00-00013 (Washington, D.C.: DHHS, 2001), and others.

29. See General Accounting Office (GAO), *Medicare HMO Institutional Payments: Improved HCFA Oversight, More Recent Cost Data Could Reduce Overpayments,* Pub. No. HEHS 98-153 (Washington, D.C.: GAO, 1998); Office of Inspector General (OIG), *Audit of Medicare Payments to PacifiCare of California for Beneficiaries Classified as Institutional during the Period October 1, 1996 through December 31, 1999,* Pub. No. A-09-00-00104 (Washington, D.C.: DHHS, 2001).

30. Theodore Marmor, *The Politics of Medicare,* 2nd ed. (New York: Aldine De Gruyter, 2000), 137–141; Cathie Jo Martin, "Markets, Medicare, and Making Do: Business Strategies after National Health Care Reform," *Journal of Health, Politics, Policy, and Law* 22 (1997): 556, 574–576.

31. Martin, "Markets, Medicare, and Making Do," 587.

32. 42 U.S.C. § 1395w-21(a)(2).

33. 42 U.S.C. § 1395w-28(b)(4).

34. 42 U.S.C. § 1395w-28(b)(3).

35. 42 U.S.C. § 1395w-23(e).

36. Barry Furrow et al., *Health Law* 1st ed. (St. Paul, Minn.: West Publishing, 1995), 174.

37. Ibid., 176.

38. 42 U.S.C. § 1395w-21(e)(2). It also permitted disenrollment outside of the normal open enrollment period under special circumstances, such as the termination of the plan or violation by the plan of contract requirements in § 1395w-21(e)(4).

39. 42 U.S.C. § 1395w-25(d); § 422.350(b).

40. 42 U.S.C. § 1395w-25(a)(2).

41. Balanced Budget Act of § 4011. 1997 Pub L. 105-33 111 Stat 251.334 (1997). Section 4015 of the BBA also provided for payment to the Department of Defense (DOD) for treatment of Medicare-eligible military retirees and dependents in a DOD managed-care plan using military treatment facilities at 95% of M+C rates under the Medicare subvention demonstration project for three years. Other sections of the BBA established a variety of other demonstration projects.

42. 42 U.S.C. § 1395w-3.

43. 42 U.S.C. § 1395w-22(c).

44. 42 U.S.C. § 1395w-22(c); 42 C.F.R. § 422.111.

45. 42 U.S.C. § 1395w-22(c)(2).

46. 42 U.S.C. § 1395w-21(4).

47. This point had been made by the GAO and by the Prospective Payment Advisory Commission. GAO, "Medicare HMOs: HCFA Can Promptly Eliminate Hundreds of Millions in Excess Payments," GAO/HEHS-97-16 (Washington, D.C.: GAO, 1997); Prospective Payment Advisory Commission, *Medicare and the American Health Care System: Report to Congress* (Washington, D.C.: ProPAC, 1997), 36–39.

48. 42 U.S.C. § 1395w-23(a)(3).

49. Bruce Merlin Fried and Janice Ziegler, *The Medicare+Choice Program: Is It Code Blue?* (Washington, D.C.: ShawPittman, 2000), 13.

50. 42 U.S.C. § 1395w-23(c)(3)(B).

51. Medicare Payment Advisory Commission (MedPAC), "Reconciling Medicare+Choice Payments and Fee-for-Service Spending," *Report to Congress: Medicare Payment Policy* (Washington, D.C.: MedPAC, 2000), 19.

52. Ibid.

53. 42 U.S.C. § 1395w-27(b).

54. 42 U.S.C. § 1395w-21(g)(1) and (2).

55. 42 U.S.C. § 1395w-21(h).

56. 42 U.S.C. § 1395w-22(a)(1).

57. 42 U.S.C. § 1395w-24(f)(1)(A).

58. 42 C.F.R. § 422.100(b).

59. 42 U.S.C. § 1395w-22(d); 42 C.F.R. § 422.112.

60. 42 U.S.C. § 1395w-22(e); 42 C.F.R. §§ 422.152–.154.

61. 42 U.S.C. § 1395w-22(e)(4); 42 C.F.R. §§ 422.156–158.

62. 42 U.S.C. § 1395w-24(c).

63. 42 U.S.C. § 1395w-24(e).

64. 42 U.S.C. § 1395w-27(h); 42 C.F.R. §§ 422.641–422.698.

65. 42 U.S.C. 1395w-27(g)(2); 42 C.F.R. §§ 422.750, 422.752, 422.758.

66. The new plans included a PSO in New Mexico, a private fee-for-service plan, and two PPOs. Robert A. Berenson, "Medicare+Choice: Doubling or Disappearing?" *Health Affairs Web Exclusive* available at http://www.healthaffairs.org/WebExclusives/Berenson_Web_Excl-112801.htm

67. Medicare Payment Advisory Commission (MedPAC), *Medical Savings Accounts and the Medicare Program: Report to Congress* (Washington, D.C.: MedPAC, 2000).

68. Nora Super Jones, *Medicare+Choice: Where Do We Go from Here?* Issue Brief No. 758 (Washington, D.C.: George Washington University National Health Policy Forum, 2000), 9.

69. Ibid.

70. Gold, "Medicare+Choice: An Interim Report Card," 126.

71. Jones, "Medicare+Choice: Where Do We Go from Here?" 10.

72. Gold, "Medicare+Choice: An Interim Report Card," 122.

73. Ibid., 123; Berenson, "Medicare+Choice: Doubling or Disappearing?" W66. American Association of Health Plans, "Memorandum Medicare+Choice Participation in 2003," available at http://www.aahp.org/Content/Navigation/About_AAHP/News_Room/Press_Releases/Medicare+Choice_Participation_in_2003_(9_9_2002).htm (cited October 24, 2002).

74. Brian Biles, et al., *Medicare+Choice After Five Years: Lessons for Medicare's Future* (Washington, D.C.: The Commonwealth Fund, 2002): 2.

75. Gold, "Medicare+Choice: An Interim Report Card," 125.

76. Kenneth Thorpe and Adam Atherly, "Medicare+Choice: Current Role and Near-

Term Prospects," *Health Affairs Web Exclusive,* available at http://www.healthaffairs. org/WebExclusives/Thorpe_Web_Excl_071702.htm (cited August 8, 2002); Lori Achman and Marsha Gold, *Medicare+Choice 1999–2001: An Analysis of Managed Care Plan Withdrawals and Trends in Benefits and Premiums* (New York: Commonwealth Fund, 2002), 14.

77. Fried and Ziegler, *The Medicare+Choice Program*; Alejandra Arguello Carmerlengo, "Medicare in Red," in *CATO Today's Commentary,* available at http://www.cato. org/dailys/07-14-99.html (cited 14 July 2000); *Health Insurance Association of America* "Low Payments and Excessive Regulation Are Undermining the Medicare HMO Program," available at http://www.hiaa.org/search/content.cfm?ContentID=397 (cited 29 June 2000); James Forgue, Richard Smith, Alissa Fox, Jane Stokes Trautwein, and Victoria Craig Bunce, "Overhauling Medicare: What It Will Take to Attract Private Providers," *Heritage Lectures* (Washington, D.C.: The Heritage Foundation, May 18, 2001): 704.

78. Fried and Ziegler, *The Medicare+Choice Program.*

79. Ibid., 9.

80. Barbara S. Cooper and Bruce C. Vladeck, "Bringing Competitive Pricing to Medicare," *Health Affairs* 19 (September/October 2000): 49.

81. Ibid.

82. Balanced Budget Refinement Act, Pub. L. 106-113, App. F, §§ 511 and 512; 113 Stat. 1501, 1501A-380 and 1501A-382 (1999).

83. Benefit Improvement and Protection Act, Pub. L. 106-554, App. F, § 601 (2000); 114 Stat. 2763, 2763A-554.

84. General Accounting Office (GAO), *Medicare+Choice: Recent Payment Increases had Little Effect on Benefits or Plan,* Pub. No. GAO-02-202 (Washington, D.C.: GAO, 2001); Achman and Gold, *Medicare+Choice 1999–2001.*

85. Achman and Gold, *Medicare+Choice 1999–2001,* 8.

86. General Accounting Office (GAO), *Medicare+Choice: Plan Withdrawals Indicate Difficulty of Providing Choice While Achieving Savings,* Pub. No. GAO/HEHS-00-183 (Washington, D.C.: GAO, 2000).

87. See Office of Inspector General (OIG), Department of Health and Human Services, *Adequacy of Medicare's Managed Care Payments after the Balanced Budget Act,* Pub. no A-14-00-00212 (Washington, D.C.: DHHS, 2000); GAO, *Medicare+Choice: Payments Exceed Cost of Benefits.*

88. GAO, *Medicare+Choice: Plan Withdrawals Indicate Difficulty,* 18–22.

89. Achman and Gold, *Medicare+Choice 1999–2001,* 6.

90. Gold, "Medicare+Choice: An Interim Report Card."

91. GAO, *Medicare+Choice: Plan Withdrawals Indicate Difficulty,* 19.

92. Debra C. Draper, Robert E. Hurley, Cara S. Lesser, and Bradley C. Strunk, "The Changing Face of Managed Care," *Health Affairs* 21(January/February 2002): 11.

93. See, e.g., John Bertko, "Medicare Managed Care: Preserving an Option for the Future," in *Health Affairs Online,* available at http://www.healthaffairs.org/WebExclusives/Bertko_Perspectives_Web_EXCL_112801_html (cited November 28, 2001); Ronald M. Klar, "Medicare+Choice: A Time for Hibernation," in *Health Affairs Online,* available at http://www.healthafairs.org/WebExclusive/Klar_Perspectives_Web_Excl_112801.htm (cited November 28, 2001).

94. Theordore Mamor and Jonathan Oberlander, "Rethinking Medicare Reform," *Health Affairs* 17 (January/February 1998): 52.

95. Robert Miller and Harold Luft, "HMO Plan Performance Update: An Analysis of the Literature, 1997–2001," *Health Affairs* 21 (July/August 2002): 63–86.

96. Karen Davis, et al., "Medicare Versus Private Insurance: Rhetoric and Reality," *Health Affairs*, Web Exclusive, http://www.healthaffairs.org/WebExclusives/Davis_Web_Excl_100902.htm (cited October 24, 2002).

97. Statements of Cheryl M. Scott, Michael J. O'Grady, and Victor E. Turvey, Hearings before the Subcommittee on Health, Committee on Ways and Means, House of Representatives, May 1, 2001. 107th Cong., 1st Sess. Serial No. 107-20.

98. See Robert A. Berenson, "Medicare+Choice: Doubling or Disappearing?"; Klar, "Medicare+Choice: A Time for Hibernation."

99. Berenson, "Medicare+Choice: Doubling or Disappearing?"

100. See "2001 Medicaid Managed Care Enrollment Report," available at www.hcfa.gov/medicaid/omc2001.htm (cited June 24, 2002); Colleen M. Grogan, *The Medicaid Managed Care Policy Consensus for Welfare Recipients: A Reflection of Traditional Welfare Concerns, Journal of Health Politics, Policy, and Law* 22 (1997): 815.

101. See Michelle A. Saint-Germain, "Arizona Health Care Cost Containment System," in *Medicaid Reform and the American States: Case Studies on the Politics of Managed Care*, edited by Mark Daniels (Westport, Conn.: Auburn House, 1998), 28; General Accounting Office (GAO), *Arizona Medicaid: Competition among Managed Care Plans Lowers Program Costs*, Pub. No. GAO/HEHS-96-2 (Washington D.C.: GAO, 1995).

102. James Boex, Laura C. Yancer, and Terry F. Buss, "OhioCare: The Waiver That Wasn't," in *Medicaid Reform and the American States: Case Studies on the Politics of Managed Care*, edited by Mark Daniels (Westport, Conn.: Auburn House, 1998), 202.

103. On California, see Michael S. Sparer, *Medicaid and the Limits of State Health Reform* (Philadelphia: Temple University Press, 1996). On Tenncare, see, James F. Blumstein and Frank A. Sloan, "Health Care Reform through Medicaid Managed Care: Tennessee (Tenncare) as a Case Study and Paradigm," *Vanderbilt Law Review* 53 (2000): 125; Anna Aizer, Marsha Gold, and Cathy Schoen, *Managed Care and Low-Income Populations: Four Years' Experience with Tenncare* (Washington, D.C.: Kaiser Family Foundation/Commonwealth Fund, 1999).

104. Grogan, "The Medicaid Managed Care Policy Consensus," 831; Stephen M. Davidson and Stephen A. Somers, "Understanding the Context for Medicaid Managed Care," in *Remaking Medicaid: Managed Care and the Public Good*, edited by Stephen M. Davidson & Stephen A. Somers (San Francisco: Jossey-Bass, 1998), 3, 10–11.

105. Sidney D. Watson, "Commercialization of Medicaid," *St. Louis University Law Journal* 45 (2001): 53, 55–56.

106. Grogan, "The Medicaid Managed Care Policy Consensus," 832.

107. Mark R. Daniels, "Introduction: The Inconsistency and Paradox of American Health Care," in *Medicaid Reform and the American States: Case Studies on the Politics of Managed Care*, edited by Mark Daniels (Westport, Conn.: Auburn House, 1998), 5.

108. James W. Fossett and Frank J. Thompson, "Back-off Not Backlash in Medicaid Managed Care," *Journal of Health Politics, Policy, and Law* 24 (1999): 1159.

109. 42 U.S.C. § 1396a(a)(10)(A)(i)(VII), (1)(1)(D), and (1)(2)(C).

110. *Sullivan v. Zebley*, 493 U.S. 521 (1990).

111. Fosett and Thompson, "Back-off Not Backlash," 1160.

112. Blumstein and Sloan, "Health Care Reform through Medicaid Managed Care," 151–166; John Holahan and David Liska, "The Slowdown in Medicaid Spending Growth: Will It Continue?" *Health Affairs* 16 (March 1997): 157–158.

113. Grogan, "The Medicaid Managed Care Policy Consensus," 829–830; General Accounting Office (GAO), *Medicaid: States Turn to Managed Care to Improve Access and Control Costs*, Pub. No. GA/HRD93-46 (Washington, D.C.: GAO, 1993).

114. Grogan, "The Medicaid Managed Care Policy Consensus," 830–833.

115. Ibid., 832; Daniels, "Introduction: The Inconsistency and Paradox of American Health Care," 4.

116. Sparer, *Medicaid and the Limits of State Health Reform*, 157.

117. Ibid.

118. Saint-German, "Arizona Health Care Cost Containment System," 22–33.

119. Ibid., 28–29.

120. Ibid., 31.

121. See ibid.; See also Nelda McCall, "The Arizona Health Care Cost Containment System," in *Remaking Medicaid: Managed Care for the Public Good* edited by Stephen M. Davidson and Stephen A. Somers (San Francisco: Jossey-Bass), 127.

122. John Holahan, Suresh Rangarajan, and Matthew Schirmer, *Medicaid Managed Care Payment Methods and Capitation Rates: Results of a National Survey* (Washington, D.C.: Urban Institute, 1999), 3-4; Fossett and Thompson, "Back-off Not Backlash," 1161; Grogan, "The Medicaid Managed Care Policy Consensus," 819; John Holahan, Alison Evans, and Stephen Zuckerman, "Impact of the New Federalism on Medicaid," in *Remaking Medicaid: Managed Care and the Public Good*, edited by Stephen M. Davidson and Stephen Somers (San Francisco: Jossey-Bass), 51–52. A third option, pre-paid health plans or prepaid health services plans, based on safety-net providers, was also pursued by some states.

123. Holahan et al., "Impact of New Federalism," 53. In New York, for example, where Medicaid managed-care enrollment was largely voluntary until quite recently, it only covered about one-third of the population. Kent Gardner and David Bond, "New York: Medicaid Managed Care Coverage in the Empire State," in *Medicaid Reform and the American States: Case Studies on the Politics of Managed Care*," edited by Mark Daniels (Westport, Conn.: Auburn House, 1998), 194–195; Sparer, *Medicaid and the Limits of State Health Reform*, 175–177.

124. Section 1915(b) of the Social Security Act permitted waivers to be granted for two-year periods, and with the possibility for continual renewals from the prohibitions of § 1902(a)(23) on restriction of beneficiary provider choice (the "freedom of choice" waiver) and from the requirements of 1902(a)(1) that health-care delivery systems be uniform statewide (to allow local managed-care experiments) and of 1902(a)(10) that services be comparable for all recipients (to allow managed-care plans affecting only some recipients). Joyce Jordan, Alisa Adamo, and Tanya Ehrmann, "Innovations in § 1115 Demonstrations," *Health Care Financing Review* 22 (2000): 49. Section 1915(b) waivers were readily granted by HHS. Leighton Ku et al., "Medicaid Managed Care Programs in Hawaii, Oklahoma, Rhode Island, and Tennessee," in *Medicaid Reform and the American States: Case Studies on the Politics of Managed Care*, edited by Mark Daniels (Westport, Conn.: Auburn House, 1998), 147–148.

125. Section 1115 of the Social Security Act permits the secretary of HHS to waive compliance with any sections of the Medicaid Act to permit experimental, pilot, or demonstration projects. 42 U.S.C. § 1315(a)(1). See Blumstein and Sloan, "Health Care Reform through Medicaid Managed Care" 169–170.

126. See Blumstein and Sloan, "Health Care Reform through Medicaid Managed Care"; Aizer et al., *Managed Care and Low-Income Populations*; Jessica Mittler, Marsha Gold, and Barbara Lyons, *Managed Care and Low Income Populations: Four Years' Experience with the Oregon Health Plan*, (Washington, D.C.: Kaiser Family Foundation, Commonwealth Fund, 1999); Howard M. Leichter, "The Poor and Managed Care in the Oregon Experience," *Journal of Health Politics, Policy and Law* 24 (1999): 1173.

127. Blumstein and Sloan, "Health Care Reform through Medicaid Managed Care," 170–172.

128. Mark R. Daniels, "Medicaid Reform from the Executive Branch: Tennessee's Tenn Care Program," in *Medicaid Reform and the American States: Case Studies on the Politics of Managed Care*, edited by Mark Daniels (Westport, Conn.: Auburn House, 1998), 253–256.

129. Aizer et al., "Managed Care and Low-Income Populations," 10. Marsha Gold, "Markets and Public Programs: Insights from Oregon and Tennessee," *Journal of Health Politics, Policy and Law* 22 (1997): 633.

130. Ku et al., "Medicaid Managed Care Programs," 164.

131. Blumstein and Sloan, "Health Care Reform through Medicaid Managed Care."

132. *John B. v. Menke*, 176 F. Supp. 2d 786 (M.D. Tenn. 2001).

133. See Paula Wade, "Feds Sign off on Overhaul of Tenncare," *Commercial Appeal* (June 1, 2002), A1.

134. See Howard M. Leichter, "Oregon's Bold Experiment: Whatever Happened to Rationing?"; *Journal of Health Politics, Policy, and Law*, 24 (1999): 147. Lawrence Jacobs et al., "The Oregon Health Plan and the Political Paradox of Rationing," *Journal of Health Politics, Policy, and Law* 24 (1999): 161.

135. 42 U.S.C. § 1396u-2. Proposed regulations to implement the Medicaid managed-care sections of the BBA were published in *Federal Register* 63, 52,021ff (September 28, 1998): Interim final rules were published in the dying moments of the Clinton administration in *Federal Register* (January 19, 2001): 66, 6228, but they were withdrawn by the following Bush administration. Final rules were published by the Bush Administration on June 14, 2002, to take effect on August 13, 2002, with the states having one year further to come into compliance; see *Federal Register* 67, 40,989. See, summarizing the Rules, Families USA, "Medicaid Managed Care Final Regulations Issued," available at www.familiesusa.org/mmc6Sept2002.pdf (cited October 22, 2002). Medicaid advocates criticized the Bush administration rules as having weakened recipient protections found in the Clinton rules, even though the Bush administration claimed that the rules expanded prior protections. See Families USA, "Bush Administration Issues Final Medicaid Managed Care Rule: Protections Much Weaker Than Clinton Version," available at www.famliesusa.org/BushAdministrationIssues.htm (cited June 14, 2002); and Department of Health and Human Services, "HHS Issues New Medicaid Managed Care Regulation to Guarantee Strong Patient Protections," available at www.hhs.gov/news/pres/2002pres_(vi/20020613a.html (cited July 3, 2002). It should be noted that many states operate their Medicaid managed-care programs under federal waivers, which permit considerable flexibility in variances from federal requirements.

136. 42 U.S.C. § 1396u-2(a)(3). For a report on the development of rural Medicaid managed care, see Rebecca T. Slifkin et al., "Medicaid Managed Care Programs in Rural Areas: A Fifty State Overview," *Health Affairs* 18 (November/December 1998): 217.

137. 42 U.S.C. §§ 1396u-2(a)(4)(C) and (D).

138. 42 U.S.C. § 1396u-2(a)(4)(A). The Medicaid managed-care plan must inform the beneficiary of this right. 42 U.S.C. § 1396b(m)(2)(A)(vi).

139. 42 U.S.C. § 1396b(m)(2)(A)(v).

140. 42 U.S.C. § 1396u-2(a)(5).

141. 42 U.S.C. § 1396u-2(a)(5)(C).

142. 42 U.S.C. §§ 1396b(m)(2)(A)(vii) and 1396u-2(b)(2).

143. 42 U.S.C. §§ 1396u-2(b)(3) and (4).

144. 42 U.S.C. §§ 1396u-2(b)(5) and (6).

145. 42 U.S.C. § 1396u-2(c)(1).

146. 42 U.S.C. § 1396u-2(c)(2). State quality oversight is optional for Medicare+ Choice organizations, and external review activities are not to duplicate accreditation reviews for accredited managed-care organizations. 42 U.S.C. §§ 1396u-2(c)(2)(B) and (C).

147. 42 U.S.C. § 1396u-2(d)(2).

148. 42 U.S.C. § 1396u-2(3)(1).

149. 42 U.S.C. §§ 1396u-2(e)(2), (3), and (4); 1396b(m)(5). See *MEDCARE HMO v. Bradley*, 788 F. Supp. 1460 (N.D. Ill. 1992) (providing a Medicaid HMO with a pretermination hearing).

150. 42 U.S.C. § 1315(e).

151. Jeanne Lambrew, *Section 1115 Waivers in Medicaid and the State Children's Health Insurance Program: An Overview* (Washington, D.C.: Kaiser Commission on Medicaid and the Uninsured, 2002).

152. Kaiser Commission on Medicaid and the Uninsured, *Medicaid's Disabled Population and Managed Care* (Washington, D.C.: Kaiser Commission on Medicaid and the Uninsured, 2001).

153. Fossett and Thompson, "Back-off Not Backlash," 1163–1164.

154. Kaiser Commission, 1. *Medicaid's Disabled Population.*

155. Sidney D. Watson, "Commercialization of Medicaid," *Saint Louis University Law Journal*, 45 (2001): 53, 68; Sara Rosenbaum and David Rousseau, "Medicaid at Thirty-Five," *St. Louis University Law Journal* 45 (2001): 7, 45–46.

156. Rosenbaum and Rosseau, "Medicaid at Thirty-Five," 45–56.

157. See Marsha Gold and Jessica Mittler, "Medicaid's Complex Goals: Challenges for Managed Care and Behavioral Health," *Health Care Financing Review* 22 (2000): 85; Marsha Regenstein and Stephanie E. Anthony, *Medicaid Managed Care for Persons with Disabilities* (Washington, D.C.: Urban Institute, 1998).

158. Anonymous "New Mexico: HCFA Again Permits Medicaid Program to Use Managed Care for Mental Health," *BNA's Health Care Daily Report* (March 2, 2001).

159. Anonymous "Pennsylvania: Settlement Addresses Long Waits for Behavioral Health Care by Poor Kids," *BNA's Health Care Daily Report* (March 9, 2001).

160. Watson, "Commercialization of Medicaid," 54; Institute of Medicine, *America's Health Care Safety Net* (Washington, D.C.: National Academy Press, 2000).

161. Watson, "Commercialization of Medicaid," 59. Medicare also funds safety-net institutions through disproportionate share and graduate medical education payments.

162. 42 U.S.C. § 1396. See Shelia D. Hoag, Stephen A. Norton, and Shruti Rajan, "Federally Qualified Health Centers: Surviving Medicaid Managed Care, but Not Thriving," *Health Care Financing Review* 22 (2000): 107.

163. Watson, "Commercialization of Medicaid," 68.

164. James E. Bailey et al., "Academic Managed Care Organizations and Adverse Selection under Medicaid Managed Care in Tennessee," *Journal of the American Medical Association* 282 (1999): 1067.

165. Watson, "Commercialization of Medicaid," 68–70.

166. Fossett and Thompson, *Back-off Not Backlash*, 1164–1169.

167. Robert Hurley and Stephen Zuckerman, *Medicaid Managed Care: State Flexibility in Action* (Washington, D.C.: Urban Institute, 2002).

# 6

# Medicare "Reform": Disentitlement through Privatization

M EDICARE is our most robust and secure public health insurance entitlement program. It is a popular program, accepted and supported by politicians across the political spectrum, and it is generously funded. If Medicare were to falter, the future of American health-care entitlements would be grim indeed. The greatest threat to contemporary American health-care entitlements, therefore, is the movement advocating the privatization of Medicare. This movement threatens to privatize both the delivery of Medicare services (through voucher or premium support proposals) and the financing of Medicare (through proposals to create individual investment accounts).[1] Either form of privatization would endanger Medicare as a universal social insurance program for the elderly and disabled.

Arguments for privatization are based on a particular story about the future of Medicare. Under this account, the Medicare program (like our other great social insurance program, Social Security), is moving inexorably toward disaster.[2] This story begins with the uncontroversial assertion that the American population is aging. There are really three potential issues here. First, the baby-boom generation, that extraordinary bulge in the American population born in the years after World War II, will be reaching age 65 beginning in 2011, swelling the ranks of those receiving Medicare for the following half century.[3] Medicare enrollment is expected to surge from a current 15% of the population to 20%

in 2025 and to 25% in 2073.[4] The cost of the Medicare program will inescapably increase as more and more boomers become eligible for Medicare coverage.

Second, however, because fertility rates dropped in the decades following the baby boom (from 3.6 children per couple in the late 1950s to about 1.8 in 1976 and to 2.0 today), fewer and fewer workers will be available to finance Medicare for the baby boomers as they move into retirement.[5] According to current projections, there will only be 2.4 workers per Medicare beneficiary in 2030, compared to 3.7 workers per beneficiary when the baby boomers begin to retire in 2010.[6] If we continue to finance Medicare on a pay-as-you go basis, current workers will need to bear an ever greater burden as the baby boomers retire.

Third, not only is the population as a whole aging as the baby boomers age, but also individuals are living longer. Between 1960 and 1999, the life expectancy of persons who reach age 65 increased by 3.4 years.[7] In 1999 there were 4.2 million Americans aged 85 and older, compared to only 929 thousand in 1960.[8] The aging of the population means that Medicare costs will inevitably increase as beneficiaries will be covered for a longer period of time.[9] It has also been argued that costs may increase because beneficiaries require more services as they age. In fact, however, although expenditures in the last two years of life increase with age of death, this increase is primarily due to the cost of nursing-home care for the very old, which is only covered by Medicare to a very limited extent. Medicare expenditures during the last two years of life decline from $37,000 for persons who die at age 75 to $21,000 for those who die at age 95.[10] But the simple fact that Medicare beneficiaries remain on the rolls longer will drive up costs, even if their care does not become more expensive with age.

As beneficiaries age and their numbers increase, the cost of health care per beneficiary is also steadily and independently increasing. Since the inception of the Medicare program, the cost of medical care purchased by the program has regularly increased at rates exceeding the rate of inflation generally. Medicare expenditures have increased since the inception of the program at a rate of 4.9% per year.[11] As growth of the gross domestic product (GDP) growth since World War II has averaged only 1.8% per year, Medicare costs have grown 3.6% per year faster than GDP growth.[12] This growth seems to be both a result of increasing prices for health-care goods and services, and of increasing volume and intensity of the use of these goods and services, although quantity increases dominate over price increases.[13] It is also in part a result of the increasing use of health-care services, not just to cure disease but also to restore functioning and improve quality of life.[14] In fact, over the history of the Medicare program, growth in health-care costs have played a much larger role in the increasing cost of the Medicare program than has the aging of the population.[15]

While growth in the rate of Medicare spending over the past 35 years has been impressive, if these rates of growth are projected over the next half century, the results are alarming. Over the next 75 years, for example, the proportion of the gross domestic product spent on Medicare is projected by the trustees of the Part A trust fund to grow from 2.24% to 8.6%.[16] Other analysts claim that by 2030, Medicare will consume one-quarter of the federal budget, up from 11% in 1995.[17]

Alarmist accounts of the financial instability of the Medicare program are often stated in terms of the imminent bankruptcy of the Part A trust fund.[18] As noted in earlier chapters in this volume, Medicare Part A is funded through a "trust fund" account into which payroll taxes are paid and out of which expenditures are made. Although Medicare is basically funded on a pay-as-you-go basis, modest reserves have been built up in the trust fund, in part because of the expected expansion of program obligations after the baby-boom generation begins to receive Medicare.

The Part A trust fund is overseen by the board of trustees of the Federal Hospital Insurance Trust Fund, which reports annually on the present and future financial status of the trust fund.[19] As the balance between Medicare costs and revenues has fluctuated over time, the trust fund has grown and shrunk. At times when Medicare revenue growth has not kept ahead of cost growth, the balance in the trust fund has dropped to relatively low levels, provoking concern for the "bankruptcy" of the program.[20] In 1970, for example, the Part A trust fund was projected to remain solvent for only two years; in 1997, solvency was projected through only 2001.[21] In their 2001 and 2002 reports, the trust fund trustees projected that the Part A trust fund would remain solvent for 28 years, the longest period of projected solvency in the past three decades.[22] The bottom line, however, is that Medicare, as a federal program, can no more go bankrupt than can the Defense Department or, for that matter, the Congress. The trust fund is primarily an accounting artifact. Nevertheless, the impending bankruptcy of the program has often served as a popular rallying cry for those who would like to shrink the program or to privatize it.

The trust fund also serves as the lightning rod for another criticism of the Medicare program. In fact, the trust fund is not an account in a financial institution or even a private investment fund; rather, it is an obligation of the U.S. government. When revenues raised through payroll taxes for the Medicare program exceed expenses, the revenue is loaned to the federal government in exchange for nonnegotiable government bonds.[23] The revenues are then spent by the federal government, generally for current obligations. The debt, however, is backed by the full faith and credit of the United States, bears interest at competitive rates, and is subject to the legal national debt ceiling set by Congress.[24] When, at some point in the future, this money will be required for program obligations, the U.S. government will have to pay back its debt, either through borrowing from private sources or through raising additional taxes. Although much is made of this characteristic of the trust fund by some of Medicare's critics, the fact that Medicare obligations are held by the federal government should not be too disquieting—U.S. savings bonds are not generally regarded as high-risk investments.

One final problem with Medicare financing is less frequently noted by Medicare's would-be reformers, but it should be considered to get a full picture of Medicare's financial setting. Medicare Part A is financed through payroll taxes. Part A revenues, therefore, are only drawn from a portion, about one-half, of the nation's income: wages, salaries, and self-employment income.[25] Thus, while the Trustees of the Part A trust fund projected in 2001 that Part A expenditures would grow from 2.7% to 10.7% of workers' earnings between 2000 and 2075, Part A expenditures would only grow from 1.3% to 4.7% of GDP over the same period of time.[26] Moreover, wages, salaries, and self-employment income subject to Medicare taxes are shrinking as a share of GDP, in large part because they are declining as a share of total compensation as nontaxable fringe benefits continue to grow in importance.[27] There are readily understandable historical and policy reasons why social insurance programs are funded through payroll taxes.[28] But payroll tax financing does mean that Medicare is funded by a limited and shrinking proportion of the national income (and is also funded quite regressively).

## Problems with the Current Medicare Program

Critics of the Medicare program also point out serious flaws in the program itself, beyond its financing, which were present at its founding but seem increasingly troublesome over time. The Medicare program is clearly a product of its time, and even in 1965 when it was created it was the result of political compromises and pleased no one fully. No one would design a health insurance program today that would look like the Medicare program.

One of its most glaring faults is its lack of outpatient prescription drug coverage. In 1965, when Medicare was launched, standard employment-based health insurance policies—in particular, the Blue Cross and Blue Shield policies after which Medicare was modeled—did not cover prescription drugs.[29] While this was no doubt attributable to historical reasons, in the 1960s drugs were also far less expensive and were efficacious for far fewer medical conditions than is now the case.[30]

Today, about 73% of Medicare recipients have drug coverage for at least some part of the year through individual Medicare supplement policies, employer retirement coverage, Medicaid, or Medicare+Choice HMOs, but this coverage is often accompanied by high cost sharing and low out-of-pocket maximums.[31] Drug coverage for Medicare beneficiaries is also unstable over time.[32] Indeed, at any one time, only about 62% of Medicare beneficiaries may have coverage, and coverage rates are much lower among beneficiaries living in rural areas, the near poor, and those 85 and older.[33] The average Medicare beneficiary paid $1,051 out of pocket for drugs in 2002, but the most costly 5% of Medicare beneficiaries paid $4,000 or more out of pocket during 2002.[34] Some beneficiaries, moreover, have to do without medically necessary drugs because they simply cannot afford them.[35] It is also believed that better access to prescription drugs might permit some Medicare beneficiaries to avoid surgery or institutionalization in nursing facilities, thus saving money for the program (though no one is under the illusion that a Medicare drug benefit will not require substantial additional program resources).[36]

Prescription drug coverage is not the only glaring omission in the current Medicare program, however. Medicare also affords poor coverage for long-term care. The Medicare skilled nursing facility benefit is limited to 100 days per spell of illness for post-hospital extended care services and is aimed primarily at short-term rehabilitation care.[37] It does not cover "custodial" care.[38] Nationally, Medicare finances only 16% of long-term care services, including 12% of nursing-home care and 25% of home health care.[39] Medicare also covers inpatient hospital care for only up to 90 days for any "spell of illness," plus up to 60 "life time reserve days" available on a one-time basis.[40] Medicare affords no out-of-pocket maximum limits, as has become common in group insurance policies generally.

Another antiquated feature of the Medicare program is its high and irrationally targeted cost sharing. Cost sharing is an essential component of most market-based proposals for health insurance reform, but to be effective in reducing health-care costs, cost sharing must be targeted at services that are in some sense discretionary. Medicare, however, imposes high deductibles ($812 for 2002) and copayments ($203 for days between 61 and 90), for hospital care, which beneficiaries often have little choice about consuming.[41] Most irrationally, until 1997 coinsurance for hospital outpatient care was based on charges, while Medicare payments were formula-based, causing coinsurance payments to average 47% for outpatient costs instead of the nominal 20%.[42]

The high cost-sharing obligations imposed by Medicare have been largely responsible for the flourishing of the Medicare supplement industry. Individual Medigap policies, which wrap around Medicare benefits to cover cost-sharing obligations and gaps in coverage (like pharmaceuticals), covered about 24.3% of Medicare beneficiaries in 1999, while an additional 33% of beneficiaries received supplemental coverage through their employers.[43]

Medicare supplement policies are difficult to justify from any rational policy perspective. They impose high administrative costs, paying out, on average, only 84% of their premiums for benefits.[44] The industry was attended by fraud and consumer abuses through much of its early history. This resulted, in turn, in heavy regulation at both the federal and the state levels, thereby increasing costs and limiting flexibility.[45] Medicare supplement companies are allowed to risk-underwrite after the first six months of a beneficiary's eligibility for Medicare, and most do.[46] Nevertheless, in part because supplement policies have in fact been purchased disproportionately by those who use them most, they have become increasingly expensive. Between 1998 and 2000, Medigap premiums increased 20.2% on average.[47] In 2000, premiums for policies that offered drug coverage averaged between $2347 and $3065 per year.[48]

In the end, however, the greatest fault of Medicare supplemental insurance in the eyes of market advocates is that it cushions the effects of Medicare cost sharing, depriving cost-sharing of the power that it might otherwise have had to dampen health-care costs.[59] The Congressional Budget Office has estimated that Medigap coverage increases service use by about 24%, while the Physician Payment Review Commission found that Medicare payments for beneficiaries without supplemental coverage equaled only 72.5% of payments for those with coverage after adjusting for other explanatory variables.[50] These effects have led to the ironic situation of market proponents advocating that the thriving market for Medigap be suppressed in order to allow market forces to operate more effectively on Medicare.[51]

Medicare not only fails to cover vital services and charges irrationally high cost sharing for those that it does cover, but it also does a poor job of coordinating the care that it offers. Medicare covers only a limited list of services and has little flexibility for covering other services. As Medicare payment policy has changed over the decades, it has created incentives and disincentives that have encouraged some forms of treatment and discouraged others without necessarily serving the best interests of its recipients.[52] The mere fact that Medicare Parts A and B are administered by separate entities creates a barrier to the effective coordination of care.

Finally, Medicare has been faulted for its approach to new medical technologies. Until recently, most decisions as to coverage of new technologies were made locally by local carriers and intermediaries.[53] National technology determinations were reached through a slow and cumbersome process.[54] Medicare has now moved to a more centralized process, involving an independent, expert advisory board, specific time frames, and clearer standards, as described in Chapter 3 of this volume.[55] The process is still moving slowly, however, and is limited in its ability to consider the costs of a new technology.[56] Perhaps most problematically, however, Medicare only covers technologies that fall within the categories of coverage offered by the program; thus, for example, new drugs used on an outpatient basis will not be covered, no matter how effective, or cost-effective, they may be.

## How Should Medicare Be Modernized?

It is beyond debate that Medicare needs to be modernized (though I take issue later in this chapter with some of the arguments made for its reform). In particular, some form of drug benefit, improved catastrophic coverage, and better care coordination are indicated. The fact that many recipients already receive some of these services through individual or retirement Medigap policies or Medicare HMOs, while others—particularly the near poor, those who live in rural areas, and the very old—are left out, makes the current situation even more objectionable from the standpoint of equity. The problem is, of course, that adding benefits or reducing recipient obligations can only make Medicare more expensive at a time when many perceive the program to already be unaffordable.

The solution many Medicare reformers propose is privatization. As noted earlier, privatization can take place in the provision of benefits or in the financing of the program. Most proposals to date have focused on the provision of benefits, so it is here that we begin.

### A Defined Contribution Program?

Proposals for privatization of Medicare services provision are generally based on the idea of moving Medicare from a defined benefit to a defined contribution program.[57] In recent years many employers have moved from defined benefit pension plans—where retired employees are guaranteed a specified income for a specified period of retirement based on some sort of rule or formula—to defined contribution plans, where the employer contributes a specified amount to an account managed by the retiree, but the actual payout depends on how that account performs over time.[58] Lately, employers have begun to also consider defined contribution health plans as a means to controlling their risk for health insurance costs (and their liability for managed-care decision making).[59]

There are many possible approaches to establishing a defined contribution plan for Medicare, of course. The most radical would simply be to give beneficiaries a voucher and set them loose in an unregulated individual insurance market to find coverage. Because this approach would undoubtedly leave many beneficiaries uncovered and lead to significant inequities in coverage, it is not advocated by serious health policy experts.

The best-known defined contribution proposal for Medicare is the premium support plan favored by a majority of the BBA Bipartisan Medicare Commission and represented in bills supported by Senator John Breaux and Congressmen Bill Thomas and Bill Frist.[60] Like most defined contribution proposals, it is based on the idea of managed competition, as originated by Alain

Enthoven of Stanford and propagated by the Jackson Hole group in the 1980s.[61] Managed competition also formed the basis of the Clinton Health Security Act, which was debated in 1993–1994 (leading to the ironic situation of many politicians who opposed managed competition for the general population when Clinton proposed it but who now advocate it for Medicare beneficiaries).

Under a premium support plan, private managed-care plans that meet program requirements would compete for Medicare beneficiaries in an organized market.[62] Under most proposals, these plans would offer at least the benefits presently covered by Medicare, plus perhaps a drug benefit and catastrophic coverage above some maximum level of beneficiary responsibility. Presumably, the plans would charge different premiums, depending on their business strategies and the advantages (including additional benefits) that they offered to Medicare beneficiaries. The Medicare fee-for-service program would have to compete with private plans for beneficiaries.[63] Medicare would pay some share of the premiums, set so that beneficiaries who opted for lower cost plans would have most or all of their premiums covered, while those who opted for higher premium plans would have to pay more out of pocket. Medicare's special payments for noninsurance purposes like medical education or safety-net hospitals would be funded from sources other than Medicare.

The great virtue of defined contribution approaches is that they could in fact be used to limit federal expenditures. The federal government would never have to pay more per beneficiary than the amount established for the federal contribution. Although most proposals would tie this amount to the premiums established through competitive bidding, once the notion of a defined contribution was accepted, the contribution could be limited to the amount considered politically affordable by Congress.

The problem, of course, is that if a defined contribution does no more than limit the federal share of Medicare costs, it will simply shift costs from the government to Medicare beneficiaries. Even though Americans over the age of 65 no longer suffer from the poverty they endured a half century ago (in part because of Medicare's health-care coverage), they are still far from wealthy. While 10% of Medicare households earned more than $75,000 in 1998, more than 50% had an income of less than $25,000 and some 33% earned less than $15,000.[64] The poorest 40% earned more than 80% of their income from Social Security in 1996.[65]

Yet beneficiaries already spend a substantial proportion of their income on medical care. Elderly households currently spend about 19% of their income on health care, while poor beneficiaries who do not receive Medicaid spend 49% of their income on health care.[66] It is projected that by 2025, Medicare beneficiaries will spend 29% of their income on health care and cover almost 26% of Medicare-related expenses, even if no changes are made in the current program.[67] Simply shifting costs to Medicare recipients, therefore, is not going to solve the problem of the high and rising cost of health care for the elderly.[68]

It is at this point that privatizers take a leap of faith. They assume, seemingly as a matter of simple belief, that if Medicare beneficiaries have to purchase insurance in a private market (be it structured through regulation or unstructured and unregulated), health-care cost increases will come down.

This belief flies in the face of empirical reality. As already discussed at length in Chapter 5, the Medicare+Choice program, an ambitious experiment in Medicare privatization, has shown that private managed-care plans cannot provide Medicare benefits less expensively than does the Medicare fee-for-service program. Following the 1997 Balanced Budget Act—as HHS began to implement a risk-adjustment formula that deprived Medicare managed-care plans of some of the substantial benefits of favorable selection that they had long enjoyed, and payment reform began to bring risk-adjusted managed-care plan payment levels down to a level approximating the cost of the fee-for-service program—managed-care plans started leaving the program in droves. The Medicare medical savings account (MSA) plan provided by the 1997 Balanced Budget Act never even got off the ground because there was no market for it.[69]

The belief that privatization could bring down Medicare costs is also contradicted by the real-world history of the relationship between comparative expenditure growth in Medicare and private insurance and managed-care markets. Over the decades Medicare cost increases have approximated cost increases in the private market, even though Medicare has remained largely fee-for-service as the private market has moved toward managed care.[70] Medicare costs grew more slowly than did private insurance costs during the 1980s, after Medicare began to take cost control seriously; then they grew faster during the mid-1990s, while the private sector began to take a more aggressive control to cost control; finally, Medicare costs grew more slowly again during the late 1990s and early 2000s, as the initial cost-control effects of managed care in the private sector began to wear off (Table 6–1).[71] This was true even though Medicare insures an older and less healthy population. In the recent past, moreover, Medicare cost increases have been well below those of the Federal Employees Health Benefits Program (FEHBP), a managed competition program that is often touted as a model for Medicare.[72] In fact, there is little empirical basis for believing that privatizing Medicare would save money.

The proposition that privatizing Medicare will save money also defies logic. Classical economics contends that competition will lower expenditures, a proposition that seems to hold true in most markets for goods and services. In the end, however, health-care expenditures are a function of four factors: the price of health-care goods and services; the quantity (volume and intensity) of

**TABLE 6–1.** Average Annual Growth (%) from Previous Year Shown

| ITEM | 1980° | 1990 | 1995 | 1996 | 1997 | 1998 | 1999 | 2000 |
|------|-------|------|------|------|------|------|------|------|
| National health expenditures | 11.7 | 11.7 | 5.7 | 5.0 | 4.9 | 5.4 | 5.7 | 6.9 |
| Private | 10.2 | 11.7 | 4.7 | 4.5 | 5.5 | 6.8 | 6.0 | 6.9 |
| Public | 14.8 | 11.7 | 6.9 | 5.6 | 4.3 | 3.7 | 5.4 | 7.0 |
| U.S. population | 1.1 | 1.1 | 1.0 | 0.9 | 0.9 | 0.9 | 0.9 | 0.9 |
| Gross domestic product | 8.7 | 6.6 | 4.9 | 5.6 | 6.5 | 5.6 | 5.5 | 6.5 |

°Average annual growth between 1960 and 1980.

*Source:* Center for Medicare and Medicaid Services, "Table 1: National Health Expenditures" available from http://www.cms.gov/statistics/nhe/historical/t1.asp (cited October 21, 2002).

health-care goods and services purchased; substitutions of more efficient (in terms of ratio between cost and benefit) services for less efficient ones; and administrative costs expended in providing coverage for health-care goods and services. Health-care costs can be decreased (or more realistically, cost increases can be moderated) by holding down the price of goods and services or the volume or intensity of goods and services received, substituting more efficient goods and services for less efficient ones, or cutting administrative costs.

It is obvious that the administrative costs of private plans are going to be higher than those of the Medicare program. Plans have marketing and underwriting costs not experienced by Medicare. For-profit plans must also make a profit. Any attempts by plans that undertake to limit the volume of health-care services provided will also add to administrative costs. In fact, Medicare consistently experiences administrative costs of under 2%, while private insurance administrative costs average closer to 10% and HMOs around 12%.[73] Therefore, private plans start well behind the Medicare program in cost competition.

Moreover, it is very unlikely that health plans will routinely pay lower prices than Medicare. Medicare's administered price systems are exceedingly complex, and it is likely that Medicare pays more for some services than would an insurer in an unconstrained private market. This may well be true where inertia holds Medicare back from dropping its payments fast enough in markets where the cost of services is falling after a new technology is introduced. Political pressure from providers of some goods and services also holds prices at artificially high levels.[74] But Medicare holds such a large market share for so many goods and services that it is often able to demand one of the lowest prices in the market. Historically, private payers have paid far higher prices for hospital care than Medicare pays. In 1992, for example, Medicare paid approximately 90% of actual cost for hospital care, while private payers paid on average 131% of actual cost. In recent years, Medicare payments have slowly risen while payments from private payers, through a decade of managed care, have slowly fallen. In 1999, however, private payers still paid 112% of hospital costs while Medicare paid 101%.[75] Medicare physician payments have also been historically well below physician rates, and many physicians have seen their Medicare payments fall after the 1997 Balanced Budget Act was passed.[76] In 2002, for example, Medicare reduced physician payments by 5.4%.[77]

It is also not at all obvious that private plans hold an edge over Medicare in speeding the adoption of lower-cost technologies or in blocking the use of ineffective higher-cost technologies. In fact, Medicare's limited coverage has probably meant that in some situations beneficiaries have received more-expensive services covered by Medicare (surgery in the hospital, for example) rather than less-expensive services not covered by Medicare (drug treatment, for example). This is a function of Medicare coverage, however, not of public payment, and a private plan that covered only the services Medicare covered would face the same problem. Medicare has also traditionally been tardy in providing coverage for some new technologies (a situation that is changing, as noted in Chapter 3). But because new technologies have tended to increase, rather than decrease, costs, by and large, this has not generally led to increased program costs.[78]

If private plans have any advantage, therefore, it is in their ability to hold down the volume and intensity of services provided to their members—to ration care. The mechanisms through which private managed-care organizations ration care are well known; generally, these include the use of gatekeepers and limited referral networks; provider-specific incentives, such as capitation or withhold or bonus plans; and utilization review.[79] As used by some plans for some types of care, these controls have been quite effective.[80] Medicare, in contrast, has been less stringent in controlling service utilization, and the increase in volume of services provided has been a primary factor in driving Medicare program cost growth.[81]

However, Medicare has not been wholly passive in controlling service volume. Prospective payment—first for inpatient hospital care in the early 1980s and now for nursing facilities, home health, and rehabilitation hospitals—controls Medicare's exposure for the cost of particular units of services, or even of episodes of care. Peer review organizations (PROs) have long overseen utilization of particular services.[82] Perhaps most important, high-profile fraud and abuse investigations and prosecutions have controlled abusive claims practices.[83]

Moreover, private health plans have been backing off the rigor by which they applied rationing in the mid-1990s. Consumer backlash against the restrictiveness of managed care and provider resistance to restrictive managed-care practices led to a movement to less-restrictive forms of managed care in the late 1990s and early 2000s, which, in turn, led to renewed increases in utilization.[84] Unless and until Americans are willing to put up with far more aggressive controls over health-care service utilization (and in particular, new technology adoption) than they currently endure, private plans will not be able to cover their higher administrative costs and compete with Medicare fee-for-service because of Medicare's advantages in holding down prices.

There are also very real concerns about the ability of Medicare recipients to function in an environment where they have to pick among competing health-care plans. At the very least, Medicare (or a Medicare contractor) would have to provide beneficiaries with comparative information on private health-care plans on a regular basis with rapid updating.[85] Of course, this would add to the cost of the program without providing health-care services. The program would also have to regulate the marketing practices of private plans and oversee the quality of care that they provided to protect beneficiaries from abuses, as it does now with Medicare+Choice plans.[86] Unless Medicare ceased to be an entitlement, the program would have to provide an appeal process so that beneficiaries could appeal care denials.[87]

But even with comparative information and regulatory protections, it is likely that many beneficiaries would function poorly in a competitive environment. Many beneficiaries are likely to poorly understand the basic nature of managed-care choices.[88] Many beneficiaries, particularly those most in need of insurance coverage, are in frail health and suffer from mental deterioration, so that the difficult comparative choices that attend plan selection might well overwhelm them. Unless more sophisticated risk adjusters are devised than those that presently exist, in all likelihood plans would avoid the highest-cost beneficiaries as well and court the healthiest.[89] A wealth of experience with private insurance around the world shows that it is very difficult to control such selection bias.[90]

Furthermore, many beneficiaries living in rural areas might not have plans available. This is certainly the case with Medicare+Choice.[91] If the program were structured to put traditional fee-for-service Medicare at a competitive disadvantage (as was true with the 1995 Republican Budget Reconciliation Act, which first put the defined contribution approach on the political agenda), beneficiaries in those areas might end up much worse than they now are, with neither competitive health plans nor a functioning Medicare fee-for-service system available. Finally, if the program only reimburses the premiums of the lowest-cost plan, there will be coverage problems if, as is likely, the lowest-cost plan does not have capacity to cover all who would elect it.

## Competitive Contracting

An alternative approach for privatizing Medicare might be to have private plans compete for contracts with Medicare rather than for beneficiary membership. This would allow Medicare to bring its full market power to bear in driving contracts with private health plans, while allowing plans, in turn, to use their assumed skill in controlling utilization and driving hard bargains with providers to bring down costs.

There are concerns, however, about the potential detrimental effects of such a program. For example, in all likelihood it would do serious economic damages to providers who were excluded from the plan that captured Medicare's business, and it would encourage stinting and underservice. It is telling that real-world experiments that, in fact, could have tested the ability of real competition to lower Medicare costs—such as competition for managed-care contracts with the Medicare program—have been repeatedly thwarted, both by potential competitors and by their political allies in Congress.[92] Each time competitive bidding has been attempted, potential bidders have been able to block the experiment, apparently aware of the fact that they cannot cut costs below Medicare levels without risking disaster. This experience should give us pause about embracing competition too enthusiastically.

## Proposals to Privatize Medicare Financing

To this point we have considered merely proposals that would privatize the claims payment and care-management functions of Medicare. Other proposals would privatize both the provision of benefits under Medicare and its financing.[93] They would allocate to each person who pays Medicare payroll taxes all or a proportion of their taxes as those taxes were paid for investment in individual medical benefit accounts.[94] Some of the money paid by higher-income members of society could be allocated to those who earn less if the program were adjusted to achieve some level of redistribution. These accounts would then be used at retirement as medical savings accounts and would be supplemented by catastrophic insurance policies.

The most thoroughly developed proposal is that of Andrew J. Rettenmaier and Thomas R. Saving.[95] Under their proposal, persons under 65 would contribute during their working lives to Private Retirement Insurance for Medical Expenditure (PRIME) accounts.[96] Funds accumulated in these accounts would be used at retirement to purchase prefunded high-deductible private insurance policies, which would cover the enrollees for the rest of their lives.[97] Some sort of mechanism would be worked out for achieving some level of equity within age cohorts, such as shifting funds from the accounts of wealthier persons to those with lower incomes (or simply taxing poorer people at higher rates during their working lives so that they would have the same amount of money available at retirement).[98] Current Medicare beneficiaries would continue to have their costs met through payroll taxes that would be paid in addition to PRIME account contributions (raising contribution rates for a time), but these would diminish as new retirees used their PRIME accounts rather than going onto traditional Medicare.[99]

Proposals such as these rely on several assumptions that are heroic, to say the least. The most basic assumption is that investing funds for health insurance in old age in private accounts will result in dramatic economic growth and high rates of return. It is likely that increased private investment would result in economic growth, although the returns might be quite modest.[100] But if the late 1990s and early 2000s have taught us anything, it is that private investments are not a sure thing. If in the 1990s individuals with private Medicare investment accounts had chosen to invest them into dot-com, Enron, or World-Com stock, there would be huge gaps in the current safety net. Even contributors who invested in funds that tracked the Dow Jones (or NASDAQ) would be facing serious problems if they were planning to retire as this book is going to press at the end of 2002. Further, it is possible that the massive increase in private capital stock that would result from prefunding Medicare would itself reduce historic returns on investment, by one estimate by 2%.[101]

These proposals leave many questions to be answered, moreover. What happens when individuals invest unwisely, or when returns are not as remunerative as expected? If Medicaid would have to fill the gaps at this point, we would simply be shifting from a payroll-taxed system to one financed by general revenues (and by the states). Also, keeping track of millions of individual accounts would result in high administrative costs. These costs might well consume much of the additional income gained through private investment.[102] And equity across income levels might be much more difficult to achieve if individuals developed a proprietary interest in their own accounts. Finally, one can only wonder which insurance companies are going to offer life-time coverage for a one-time, lump sum, premium which could last for 30 to 40 years after retirement, as contemplated by the Rettenmaier and Saving proposal, given the fact that medical costs are certain to keep escalating unpredictably for the foreseeable future. Considering the volatility of the health insurance industry over the past decade, moreover, one wonders who would want to buy such a contract.

A compromise here might be to allow the trustees of the Medicare Trust Fund to invest in the private sector. State and local pension funds do this, with considerable success. There is no reason why the federal government could not do so also, if private investment makes sense. Then all Medicare beneficiaries, not just lucky or unlucky ones, would gain or lose from private investment.

## Is "Reform" Really Necessary?

A more basic issue, however, is whether radical changes in the Medicare program are really necessary. The predicted doom of the Medicare program is based on a number of presuppositions, several of which are quite speculative. It is highly likely that the population is going to continue to age and that fertility will continue to decline. It is also a fair assumption, though not beyond debate, that a restrictive American immigration policy will continue, effectively, to keep younger immigrants from replacing the American workforce as it retires. We still have, however, one of the youngest populations of any developed nation, and countries with significantly older populations have been able to provide health care to their elderly (and their younger workers, incidentally) while holding their health-care costs well below ours.[103] A recent, thorough literature review noted that, while most studies of comparative health-care costs include population age structure as a variable, it is usually found to be an insignificant factor in cost variation.[104]

It is also likely that health-care costs will continue to increase. This is mostly due to the fact that the benefits that health care offers us are likely to continue to increase. The United States is investing far more than any other nation in the world in basic health science research.[105] American drug companies, supported by favorable intellectual property laws and few limitations on their prices, invest vast sums in developing (and marketing) new drugs.[106] Americans are in general more likely to identify themselves as "very interested" in new medical discoveries than are Europeans (66% of Americans to 44% of Europeans) and are more likely to believe that it is possible for public or private insurance to pay for all new medical technologies (47% of Americans to 36% of Europeans).[107] As long as we continue to put such stress on the development of more expensive medical technology, someone will have to pay for it.[108] If the technology is able to keep elderly people alive longer, or to make their old age more comfortable and fulfilling, then Medicare will continue to face higher bills. But, if we are spending more on health care because it improves the quality of our lives, who is to tell us that we should spend less?

This does not mean, however, that cost escalation will never end, or even that it will continue at current rates. At any point we can decide that the additional benefits of medical care do not equal their cost.[109] At that point, we can adopt approaches that will limit costs. We have no lack of examples from other countries that have been more successful than us in achieving this.[110] What we lack is evidence that competitively organized health-care systems are successful at limiting costs.[111] Indeed, competition may focus on offering more expensive technologies, not on controlling costs.

We should also not begin with the assumption, as did apparently the Bipartisan Medicare Commission, that raising taxes is out of the question as part of the solution for addressing rising Medicare costs. Medicare Part A payroll taxes currently consist of only 2.9% of taxable earnings total, including both employer and employee shares, and have not been raised since 1986.[112] A modest rise of 1% of taxable earnings, if adopted promptly, could keep Medicare Part A in balance through 2075.[113]

It might be wiser, however, to consider funding more of the Medicare program out of general revenues. To the extent that the 1997 BBA shifts home health costs from Part A to Part B, we have already begun this movement. The primary reason for shifting to general revenues is that all sources of income would share in funding program cost, not just the wages of workers, just as all of us (who become disabled or live to old age) share in the benefits of the program.[114]

Perhaps it may also become necessary to consider whether beneficiaries could contribute more to the program. This topic bears very careful deliberation. As noted here, many beneficiaries already spend a large proportion of their income on Medicare, and most beneficiaries are already living pretty close to the margin. Even if nothing else changes in the Medicare program, it is likely that beneficiaries will continue to spend an ever-increasing share of their income on health care. Moreover, the cost-sharing obligations of many poorer Medicare beneficiaries are covered by Medicaid. As these obligations increase, Medicaid expenditures will have to increase accordingly. This cost shift may help the federal government, which pays only 57% of Medicaid costs, but will impose an unwelcome burden on the states.

One obvious way to shift some costs to beneficiaries is to means-test Medicare in some way—to make it more like Medicaid. This could be done by increasing cost sharing or Part B premiums for higher-income beneficiaries, although this would be administratively costly and complex. It might also lead to the divisive politics that doomed the 1989 Medicare Catastrophic Care legislation, which attempted to pay for expanded Medicare benefits by shifting the cost to wealthier beneficiaries. Most countries have concluded that means-testing public health programs is ill-advised, but many countries do provide extra benefits, such as reduced cost sharing, for the poor.[115] Perhaps the best approach would be simply to adopt hypothecated income taxes dedicated to covering Medicare costs which would spread the cost of the program (or part of program costs, if a payroll tax were retained) over all forms of income and all income earners, including Medicare beneficiaries themselves.

The argument is often made that shifting more costs to beneficiaries would be more equitable because it is unfair to burden the next generation with the cost of their care. The issue of intergenerational equity is complex and will not be fully resolved here.[116] But consider a few points. First, revenue flows run both ways between generations, and the generation that would pay Medicare taxes to fund care for elderly baby boomers is also the generation whose childhood and education was funded by those now retiring. Moreover, as the baby-boom generation retires, the next generation will face a glut of housing and jobs and of investments that are being unloaded and in all likelihood will enjoy higher salaries and lower housing prices. Further, if we simply project increased worker productivity forward at 1.1% per year (compared to historic increases of 1.5% per year over the past 50 years), per worker GDP will expand from \$67,473 in 2000 to \$105,982 in 2035, in 2002 dollars. Even if per worker Medicare taxes grow from \$1,315 in 2000 to \$4,219 in 2035, as projected, the average per worker GDP will still be over half again as large as it is today: \$101,763 compared to \$66,158, in 2002 dollars.[117] This is hardly a crisis to panic about.

Most important, however, we must simply be cautious in approaching Medicare reform, following the ancient medical nostrum, *primum non nocere*. We have much to learn from the lessons of the past few years. In 1997, the Congressional Budget Office (CBO) estimated that the Part A Medicare Trust Fund would be bankrupt by 2001. By 2002, however, bankruptcy of the trust fund had receded to 2030.[118] In 1997, the Health Care Financing Administration (HCFA) estimated that Medicare would consume 8.38% of the GDP by 2070.[119] Three years later HCFA estimated that it would consume 5.19% by 2070.[120] By 2000, the annual federal deficit that seemed as if it would grow forever had disappeared, and the country in turn, began to worry about what to do with a huge predicted surplus. One of the ideas that both President Clinton and Congress seemed to agree on at that moment in time was to use part of the surplus to firm up the Medicare and Social Security programs.[121] However, the intoxication of actually having money to start paying down debts was too much for the politicians to bear; huge tax cuts followed, as well as an unexpected war, and before long, the surplus was gone. But one lesson remains: expect the unexpected. To make dramatic changes in the program based simply on pure speculation about what the world will look like in three-quarters of a century would be the most foolish thing we could do.

# Notes

1. The most widely discussed premium support plan is that supported by a majority of (though not officially endorsed by) the National Bipartisan Commission on the Future of Medicare, which was created by the Balanced Budget Act of 1997. In subsequent years this proposal was introduced in Congress by Senator John Breaux and Congressmen Bill Thomas and Bill Frist. The most widely discussed proposal for privatizing Medicare finance is that of Andrew J. Rettenmeir and Thomas R. Saving, which appears in its fullest form in *The Economics of Medicare Reform* (Kalamazoo Mich.: W. E. Upjohn Institute for Employment Research, 2000).

2. See, e.g., Saving and Rettenmeir, *The Economics of Medicare Reform*, 4–12; Gail Wilensky and Joseph P. Newhouse, "Medicare: What's Right? What's Wrong? What's Next?" *Health Affairs* 18 (January/February 1999): 92, 95–97; Peter J. Ferrara, "The Next Steps for Medicare Reform," *Cato Policy Analysis No. 305* (April 29, 1998), 5–10; Robert B. Helms, Introduction to *Medicare in the Twenty-first Century: Seeking Fair and Efficient Reform*, edited by Robert B. Helms (Washington, D.C.: American Enterprise Institute Press, 1999), 3–7. The most alarming version of this vision is that presented by Jagadeesh Gokhale and others in their work on generational accounting. They

conclude that the Medicare program must be cut immediately by 68% to achieve "generational balance" with respect to tax liabilities. See Jagadeesh Gokhale and Laurence J. Kotlikoff, "Medicare from the Perspective of Generational Accounting," in *Medicare Reform: Issues and Answers*, edited by Andrew J. Rettenmaier (Chicago: University of Chicago Press, 1999), 153, 170.

3. See David McKusick, "Demographic Issues in Medicare Reform," *Health Affairs* 18 (January/February 1999): 194.

4. Ibid., 196.

5. Ibid., 201.

6. Boards of Trustees, Federal Hospital Insurance, and Federal Supplementary Medical Insurance Trust Funds, *2002 Annual Report of the Boards of Trustees of the Federal Hospital Insurance and Federal Supplementary Medical Insurance Trust Funds* (Washington, D.C.: Federal Hospital Insurance, and Federal Supplementary Medical Insurance Trust Funds, 2002), 18.

7. National Center for Health Statistics (NCHS), *Health, United States*, 2001 (Hyattesville, Md.: NCHS, 2001), table 163.

8. Ibid., 127.

9. According to one recent estimate, the cumulative cost of Medicare-covered services plus cost sharing for a person who dies at 65 is $26,161; for a person who dies at age 100, it is $130,910. Brenda C. Spillman and James Lubitz, "The Effect of Longevity on Spending for Acute and Long-Term Care," *New England Journal of Medicine* 342 (2000): 1409, 1411.

10. Ibid., 1412.

11. Technical Review Panel on the Medicare Trustees Reports, *Review of Assumptions and Methods of the Medicare Trustees' Financial Projections*, (Baltimore, Md.: Health Care Financing Administration, 2000), 30.

12. Ibid.

13. David Cutler, "What Does Medicare Spending Buy Us?" in *Medicare Reform: Issues and Answers*, edited by Andrew J. Rettenmaier and Thomas R. Saving (Chicago: University of Chicago Press, 1999), 131.

14. James Lubitz, Linda G. Greenberg, Yelena Gorina, Lynne Wartzman, and David Gibson, "Three Decades of Health Care Use by the Elderly, 1965–1998," *Health Affairs* 20 (March/April 2001): 19, 26, 28–29. David Cutler estimates the value of improved health for the elderly over the past quarter of a century at $215,000, compared to a $50,000 increase in Medicare spending over the same period. Cutler, "What Does Medicare Spending Buy Us?" 142. Such estimates are highly speculative, of course.

15. One recent report estimates that if the age of the Medicare population had remained constant from 1978 to 1995, overall per capita spending on Medicare recipients would only have been 2.6% less in 1995. In other words, of Medicare per capita cost growth of 10.3% per year during that period, only 0.2 percentage points were attributable to population aging. Marilyn Moon, *Beneath the Averages: An Analysis of Medicare and Private Expenditures* (Washington, D.C.: Urban Institute, 1999), 12.

16. Boards of Trustees, Federal Hospital Insurance, *2002 Annual Report*, 9.

17. Wilensky and Newhouse, "Medicare: What's Right? What's Wrong? What's Next?" 97. This assumes that the federal budget remains a constant 21% of GDP.

18. Helms, "Medicare in the Twenty-first Century," 2.

19. Although the trustees' reports are widely cited as objective accounts of the status of the trust fund, it is important to realize that the board is itself a political body. Three of the trustees are the heads of the departments of Treasury, Labor, and Health

and Human Services, while a fourth is the commissioner of Social Security. Two other members are appointed by the president; one of them is currently a leading advocate of Medicare privatization. The administrator of the Center for Medicare and Medicaid Services serves as the secretary. Board of Trustees, Federal Hospital Insurance Trust Fund, *2001 Annual Report of the Board of Trustees of the Federal Hospital Insurance Trust Fund* (Washington, D.C.: Federal Hospital Insurance Trust Fund, 2001), 1. The trustees, therefore, effectively represent the governing administration and its ideology.

20. See Henry J. Kaiser Family Foundation, *Medicare Chart Book*, 2nd ed. (Washington, D.C.: Kaiser Family Foundation, 2001), 76.

21. Ibid.

22. Ibid.

23. Eric M. Patashnik, *Putting Trust in the U.S. Budget: Federal Trust Funds at the Politics of Commitment* (Cambridge: Cambridge University Press, 2000), 6.

24. Ibid.

25. Council of Economic Advisors, *The Economic Report of the President* (Washington, D.C.: Council for Economic Advisors, 2001), tables B-26 and B-28.

26. Board of Trustees, Federal Hospital Insurance, *2001 Annual Report*, 3.

27. Ibid., 21.

28. See Chapters 4 and 10 in this volume.

29. Century Foundation Task Force on Medicare Reform, *Medicare Tomorrow* (New York: Century Foundation Press, 2001), 48–49.

30. Ibid.

31. See National Bipartisan Commission on the Future of Medicare, "Private Supplemental Coverage Summary," available at http://thomas.loc.gov/medicare/K-P-1499.html (cited June 4, 2001).

32. Bruce Stuart, Dennis Shea, and Becky Briesacher, "Dynamics in Drug Coverage of Medicare Beneficiaries: Finders, Losers and Switchers," *Health Affairs* 20 (March/April 2001): 86.

33. Kaiser Family Foundation, "Medicare and Prescription Drugs Chartpack," figure 7, available from http://www.kff.org/content/2002/6048/6048v.1.pdf (cited October 21, 2002).

34. Ibid.

35. Stuart et al., "Dynamics in Drug Coverage of Medicare Beneficiaries."

36. Ibid.

37. 42 U.S.C. § 1395d(a)(2) and 1395x(j).

38. 42 U.S.C. § 1395y(a)(9).

39. Robert B. Friedland, "The Coverage Puzzle: How the Pieces Fit Together," presented at National Academy of Social Insurance, Annual Meeting, Washington, D.C., January 24–25, 2002.

40. 42 U.S.C. § 1395d(a).

41. Boards of Trustees, Federal Hospital Insurance, *2002 Annual Report*, 127.

42. This problem has been partially sorted out by the 1997 Balanced Budget Act, but the solution will not be fully phased in for another half century. See Medicare Payment Advisory Commission (MedPAC), *Report to Congress: Selected Medicare Issues* (Washington, D.C.: MedPAC, 2000), 45.

43. Laschober et al., "Trends in Medicare Supplemental Insurance," 133.

44. National Bipartisan Commission on the Future of Medicare, *Final Proposal: Breaux–Thomas Premium Support Model for Medicare* (Washington, D.C.: Bipartisan Commission 1999), 6.

45. See Barry Furrow et al, *Health Law* (St. Paul, Minn.: West Publishing, 1995), 27–28.

46. National Bipartisan Commission, *Final Proposal*, 5–6.

47. Weiss Ratings Inc., "Medigap Consumers Face Erratic Price Increases," available at www.weissratings.com (cited April 17, 2001).

48. Weiss Ratings, Inc., "Prescription Drug Costs Boost Medigap Premiums Dramatically," available from www.weissratings.com (cited 3 March 2001).

49. See, e.g., Mark V. Pauly, "Can Beneficiaries Save Medicare?" in *Medicare in the Twenty-first Century: Seeking Fair and Efficient Reform*, edited by Robert B. Helms (Washington, D.C.: American Enterprise Institute Press, 1999), 67, 81; Henry J. Aaron, "Medicare Choice: Good, Bad, or It All Depends," in *Medicare Reform: Issues and Answers*, edited by Andrew J. Rettenmaier (Chicago: University of Chicago Press, 1999), 57.

50. Congressional Budget Office, *Long-Term Budgetary Pressures and Policy Options*, Report to the Senate and House Committees on Budget (Washington, D.C.: CBO, May 1998); Physician Payment Review Commission, *Private Supplemental Insurance for Medicare Beneficiaries*, PPRC Update 13 (Washington, D.C.: Physician Payment Review Commission, 1997).

51. See, e.g., H. E. Frech III, "The Forgotten Opportunity of Reforming Fee-for-Service Medicare," in *Medicare in the Twenty-first Century, Seeking Fair and Efficient Reform*, edited by Robert B. Helms (Washington, D.C.: American Enterprise Institute Press, 1999), 115.

52. See Friedland, *The Coverage Puzzle*; Bruce Vladeck, "You Can't Get There from Here: Obstacles to Improving Care of the Chronically Ill," *Health Affairs* 20 (November/December 2001): 175.

53. Kathleen A. Buto, "How Can Medicare Keep Pace with Cutting Edge Technology?" *Health Affairs* 13 (summer 1994): 137. See also the discussion in Chapter 2, in this volume.

54. Buto, "How Can Medicare Keep Pace?"

55. See also Sean R. Tuni and Jeffrey L. Kant, "Improvements in Medicare Coverage of New Technology," *Health Affairs* 20 (September/October 2001): 83.

56. Alan M. Garber, "Evidence-Based Coverage Policy," *Health Affairs* 20 (September/October 2001): 62.

57. This was the basis of the proposal of the majority of the Bipartisan Commission, as noted here. National Bipartisan Commission, *Final Proposal*. See also Henry J. Aaron and Robert D. Reischauer, "The Medicare Reform Debate: What Is the Next Step?" *Health Affairs* 14 (winter 1995): 8–30; Wilensky and Newhouse, "Medicare: What's Right? What's Wrong? What's Next?" 92–106; Roger Feldman and Bryan Dowd, "Structuring Choice under Medicare," in *Medicare: Preparing for the Challenges of the 21st Century*, edited by Robert D. Reischauer, Stuart Butler, and Judith Lave (Washington, D.C.: National Academy of Social Insurance, 1998), 75–104; Stuart M. Butler and Robert E. Soffit, "The FEHBP as a Model for the New Medicare Program," *Health Affairs* 14 (winter 1995): 74.

58. See Paul Fronstin, *Defined Contribution Health Benefits*, Issue Brief no. 231 (Washington, D.C.: Employee Benefit Research Institute, 2001), 9–11.

59. See ibid.; Sally Trude et al., "Employer-Sponsored Health Insurance: Pressing Problems, Incremental Changes," *Health Affairs* 21 (January/February 2002): 66–75; Jon B. Christianson, Stephen T. Parente, and Ruth Taylor, "Defined-Contribution Health Insurance Products: Development and Prospects," *Health Affairs* 21 (January/February 2002): 49–64. Although there has been a great deal of discussion of defined con-

tribution health plans, major employers have not yet adopted them. The term is also still used loosely to cover a variety of arrangements, from situations in which benefits are simply cashed out and employees are left to the individual market through arrangements in which employees purchase insurance in an insurance market organized by an entity other than the employer (possibly using the Internet) to arrangements where the employer offers the employee a range of insurance plans and a limited premium. See Chapter 8 of this volume.

60. See National Bipartisan Commission, *Final Proposal*.

61. See Alain Enthoven, *Health Plan: The Only Practical Approach to the Soaring Costs of Medical Care* (Reading, Mass.: Addison-Wesley, 1980).

62. For a description of premium support plans, see sources listed in note 59, and Marilyn Moon, ed., *Competition within Constraints: Challenges Facing the Medicare Program* (Washington, D.C.: Urban Institute, 2000); National Academy of Social Insurance, *Structuring Medicare Choices* (Washington, D.C.: National Academy of Social Insurance, 1998).

63. President Clinton's proposal in response to the Bipartisan Commission would have ensured that every beneficiary would have access to traditional Medicare with no extra cost and would have limited premium support to alternatives. See Marilyn Moon, *An Assessment of the President's Proposal to Modernize and Strengthen Medicare* (Washington, D.C.: Urban Institute, 2000).

64. National Academy of Social Insurance (NASI), *Financing Medicare's Future* (Washington, D.C.: NASI, 2000), 13–14.

65. Ibid.

66. NASI, *Financing Medicare's Future*, 17; Jill Bernstein, *Should Higher Income Beneficiaries Pay More for Medicare?* (Washington, D.C.: National Academy of Social Insurance, 1999).

67. Marilyn Moon, *Growth in Medicare Spending: What Will Beneficiaries Pay?* (Washington, D.C.: Urban Institute, 1999).

68. As is noted later in this chapter, however, a considerable proportion of beneficiary expenditures is currently devoted to Medicare supplement policies. If this money could be redirected toward more comprehensive coverage through the Medicare program, beneficiary expenditures would not necessarily have to increase in total to achieve fuller coverage.

69. Medicare Payment Advisory Commission (MedPAC), *Medical Savings Accounts and the Medicare Program,* Report to Congress (Washington, D.C.: MedPAC, 2000).

70. Marilyn Moon, *Beneath the Averages: An Analysis of Medicare and Private Expenditures* (Washington, D.C: Kaiser Family Foundation, 1999).

71. Ibid. If one compares only costs common to both Medicare and private insurers (omitting thereby, nursing facility and home health costs, which made Medicare costs grow more quickly at the beginning of the 1990s, and prescription drug costs, which did the same for private insurance later in the decade), growth rates look even more similar.

72. FEHBP premiums increased 7.2% in 1998, 9.5% in 1999, 9.3% in 2000, and 10.5% in 2001; while Medicare costs increased in the same years: 1%, 1%, 2.9%, and 9.6%. Congressional Research Service (CRS), *Report to Congress: Health Insurance for Federal Employees and Retirees* (Washington, D.C.: CRS, 2002), 20; and Boards of Trustees, Federal Hospital Insurance, *2002 Annual Report*, 125. Over the past 20 years, however, the FEHBP program has had lower premium increases than Medicare; of course, FEHBP insures a population that is on average younger and healthier than the Medicare population.

73. See House Committee on Ways and Means, *Medicare and Health Care Chartbook*, 105th Cong. 1st Sess, (February 27, 1997), 138.

74. See Bruce C. Vladeck, "The Political Economy of Medicare," *Health Affairs* 18 (January/February 1999): 22–36.

75. Medicare Payment Advisory Commission (MedPAC), *Report to Congress: Medicare Payment Policy* (Washington, D.C.: MedPAC, 2001), 69.

76. See Moon, *Beneath the Averages*, 8; Julie A. Shocnman, Kevin J. Hayes, and C. Michael Cheng, "Medicare Payment Changes: Impact on Physicians and Beneficiaries," *Health Affairs* 20 (March/April 2001): 263–273.

77. Medicare Payment Advisory Commission (MedPAC), *Report to Congress: Medicare Payment Policy* (Washington, D.C.: MedPAC, 2002), 74.

78. See Penny E. Mohr et al., *The Impact of Medical Technology on Future Health Care Costs* (Bethesda, Md.: Project Hope, 2001), 21.

79. See Jacob S. Hacker and Theodore R. Marmor, "How Not to Think about 'Managed Care'," *University of Michigan Journal of Law Reform* 32 (1999): 661. They suggest that managed care should be conceptualized in terms of these approaches rather than using the traditional categories of HMO, PPO, POS, and so on.

80. The widespread belief that managed care was responsible for limited cost growth in the private health-care sector during the 1990s, however, is not uncontested. See Kip Sullivan, "On the 'Efficiency' of Managed Care Plans," *Health Affairs* 19 (July/August 2000): 139–148.

81. Between 1985 and 1992, for example, growth in volume and intensity of physician's services per beneficiary averaged almost 7% per year; since then, volume and intensity have grown more slowly. See Medicare Payment Advisory Commission (MedPAC), *Report to Congress; Medicare Payment Policy* (Washington, D.C.: MedPAC, 1999), 126.

82. Under the the seventh scope of work for Medicare Peer Review Organizations, the PROs are responsible for reviewing a random sampling of hospital admissions for medical necessity and for appropriateness of setting. Draft of Seventh Peer Review Organization Scope of Work, Version 6.0, (Washington, D.C. DHHS, Dec. 3, 2001).

83. See Timothy S. Jost and Sharon L. Davies, "The Empire Strikes Back: A Critique of the Backlash against Fraud and Abuse Enforcement," *Alabama Law Review* 51 (1999): 239–318.

84. See Debra A. Draper et al., "The Changing Face of Managed Care," *Health Affairs* 21 (January/February 2002): 11–23; Katharine Levit et al., "Inflation Spurs Health Spending in 2000," *Health Affairs* 21 (January/February 2002): 172–181; Stephen Heffler et al., "Health Spending Growth up in 1999: Faster Growth Expected in the Future," *Health Affairs* 20 (March/April 2001): 193–195.

85. NASI, *Structuring Medicare Choices*, 81–89; Institute of Medicine, *Improving the Medicare Market: Adding Choice and Protections* (Washington, D.C.: National Academy Press, 1996), 56–65.

86. NASI, *Structuring Medicare Choices*, 89–97.

87. Institute of Medicine, *Improving the Medicare Market*, 71–72.

88. Judith H. Hibbard et al., "Can Medicare Beneficiaries Make Informed Choices?" *Health Affairs* 17 (November/December 1998): 181–193.

89. NASI, *Structuring Medicare Choices*, 43. On the current state of risk adjustment, see Stuart Guterman, "Risk Adjustment in a Competitive Medicare System with Premium Support," *Competition within Constraints, Challenges Facing Medicare Reform*, edited by Marilyn Moon (Washington, D.C.: The Urban Institute, 2000), 119.

90. Timothy S. Jost, "Private or Public Approaches to Insuring the Uninsured: Lessons from International Experience with Private Insurance," *New York University Law Review* 76 (2001): 419.

91. Medicare Payment Advisory Committee (MedPAC), *Report to Congress: Medicare in Rural America* (Washington, D.C.: MedPAC, 2001), 115, 116.

92. Bryan Dowd, Robert Coulam, and Roger Feldman, "A Tale of Four Cities: Medicare Reform and Competitive Pricing," *Health Affairs* 19 (September/October 2000): 9–29; Len M. Nichols and Robert D. Reischauer, "Who Really Wants Price Competition in Managed Care?" *Health Affairs* 19, (July/August 2000): 30–43; Barbara S. Cooper and Bruce C. Vladeck, "Bringing Competitive Pricing to Medicare," *Health Affairs* 19 (September/October 2000): 49–54.

93. See Deborah J. Chollet, *Individualizing Medicare* (Washington, D.C.: National Academy of Social Insurance, 1999).

94. The main advocates of this approach are Andrew J. Rettenmaier and Thomas R. Saving. See Rettenmaier and Saving, *The Economics of Medicare Reform*. Other proposals are also available, however. See Martin Feldstein, "Prefunding Medicare," *National Bureau of Economic Research Working Paper Series*, Working Paper 6917, available at http://www.nber.org/papers/w6917 (cited January 1999).

95. Rettenmaier and Saving, *The Economics of Medicare Reform*. See also Philip Gramm, Andrew Rettenmaier, and Thomas Savings, "Medicare Policy for Future Generations: A Search for Permanent Solutions," *New England Journal of Medicine* 338 (1998): 1307–1311.

96. Saving and Rettenmaier, *The Economics of Medicare Reform*, 14.

97. Ibid., 104–118.

98. Ibid., 125.

99. Rettenmaier and Savings at least acknowledge that taxes would need to be raised to meet current program needs during a transition. Other proponents of financing privatization simply ignore this very significant issue. See Feldstein, "Prefunding Medicare."

100. Joseph White, *False Alarm: Why the Greatest Threat to Social Security and Medicare Is the Campaign to Save Them* (Baltimore: John Hopkins University Press, 2001), 73–98.

101. Chollet, *Individualizing Medicare*, 7.

102. Ibid.

103. Theodore Marmor and Jonathan Oberlander, "Rethinking Medicare Reform," *Health Affairs* 17 (January/February 1998): 55.

104. Ulf-G. Gerdtham and Bengt Jönsson, "International Comparisons of Health Expenditure: Theory, Data and Econometric Analysis," in *Handbook of Health Economics*, edited by Anthony J. Culyer and Joseph P. Newhouse (Amsterdam: Elsevier, 2000), 46.

105. In 1997, public expenditures on health research and development totaled $17.1 billion. By comparison, the U.K. spent $1.4 billion and Germany $422 million. Only Japan, at $7 billion came close. OECD 2001 Data (Paris: Organization for Economic Cooperation and Development, 2001).

106. In 1997, the U.S. pharmaceutical industry invested $17 billion in research and development, compared to $3.7 billion in the U.K. and $2.3 billion in Germany. OECD 2001 Data.

107. Kim Minah, Robert J. Blendon, and John M. Benson, "How Interested Are Americans in New Medical Technologies? A Multicountry Comparison," *Health Affairs* 20, no. 5 (September/October 2001): 194–201.

108. Michael Moran in *Governing the Health Care State* (Manchester: Manchester University Press, 1999) is particularly effective at demonstrating how American governmental policy encouraging the development of health-care technology runs counter to its policy of controlling health-care costs.

109. See White, *False Alarm*, 111–113.

110. See, e.g., Joseph White, "Targets and Systems of Health Care Cost Control," *Journal of Health Politics, Policy, and Law* 24 (1999): 653–696.

111. A recent study identifies technological advances as the primary factor driving cost growth today, and notes that managed care has not been significantly more successful than fee-for-service plans in limiting diffusion of technology. Len M. Nichols, *Can Defined Contribution Health Insurance Reduce Cost Growth?* (Washington, D.C.: Employee Benefit Research Institute, 2002): 7–8, 11–12.

112. Boards of Trustees, Federal Hospital Insurance, *2002 Annual Report*, 39.

113. Ibid., 24.

114. See, analyzing the options for funding Medicare, NASI, *Financing Medicare's Future*.

115. Some countries such as the Netherlands and Germany excuse or exclude the wealthy from participation in social insurance programs. Others, such as England and France cover cost-sharing obligations that are otherwise imposed by their public programs for poor beneficiaries.

116. The issue is thoroughly discussed in White, *False Alarm*, 117–140.

117. Marilyn Moon and Matthew Storeyguard, *Solvency or Affordability? Ways to Measure Medicare's Financial Health* (Washington, D.C.: Kaiser Family Foundation, 2002).

118. Boards of Trustees, Federal Hospital Insurance, *2002 Annual Report*, 3.

119. White, *False Alarm*, 101.

120. Ibid.

121. Ibid., 94–95.

# 7

# Health Insurance for the Poor: Disentitlement through Devolution

## History of Federal and State Relations within the Medicaid Program

### The Beginnings

From its beginning, the Medicaid program has been operated jointly by the federal and state governments. Its roots as a federal/state cooperative program run deep, emerging most immediately from the Kerr–Mills program that began in 1960, running back through the vestigial medical vendor payment program that first supplemented the federal/state cash-assistance programs in 1950, and originating in the Old Age Assistance and Aid to Dependent Children programs of the original Social Security Act. All of these programs (as well as the Sheppard–Towner Act, which came even earlier), were attempts to provide federal funds to undergird what was traditionally a state—indeed, a local—function: taking care of the medical needs of the poor. This history was told in Chapter 4 and is not repeated here.

Throughout its history of almost four decades, Medicaid has drifted—sometimes toward greater federal control, sometimes toward greater state autonomy. No state is compelled to participate in the Medicaid program, and even though most states quickly cashed in on the benefits Medicaid had to offer, Arizona resisted until 1982, when it was permitted to create a program to its own specifications under demonstration project waiver authority.[1] The lure of being able to attract to a state at least one federal dollar and potentially as many as four federal dollars for every state dollar spent on the Medicaid program has proved too much for the states to resist, and terminating Medicaid participation is not a realistic option for the states at this time.[2]

From the outset, Title XIX (the Medicaid statute) has imposed negative prohibitions and affirmative obligations on participating states. The program has always limited federal financial participation to coverage of certain categories of poor persons. For example, it has never permitted federal money to be used to cover working-age, nondisabled adults who do not have minor children, regardless of how poor they are.[3] Title XIX has also, from its adoption, required states that choose to participate in Medicaid to cover a set of "mandatory" categories of recipients, the "categorically needy." Originally this group included elderly and disabled persons and families of dependent children who were eligible for cash assistance.[4]

From the beginning, however, states have also been permitted a great deal of discretion as to the populations that they cover. The original Title XIX, for example, allowed the states to decide whether or not to cover the "medically needy"—those who were located within the categories covered by the cash-assistance programs (aged, disabled, and blind, as well as families of dependent children) but who had incomes that were both too high to allow them to qualify for cash assistance and too low to meet the costs of necessary medical care.[5] As time went on, more and more "optional" categories were added to the Medicaid menu, and the states became more and more disparate as to which of these groups they covered and which they did not.[6] A more important source of state discretion, however, has been the ability of the states to control financial eligibility levels for the cash-assistance programs to which Medicaid eligibility is tied. These have always varied significantly among the states, causing wide discrepancies as to the extent of Medicaid coverage.

The states also enjoy a great deal of latitude as to which benefits they cover. There are few services for which federal financial participation is not available. Although Title XIX purports to present a menu of covered services which the states may choose to cover, the final category, "any other medical care, and any other type of remedial care recognized under State law, specified by the Secretary," effectively makes federal Medicaid matching funds available for virtually any type of recognized medical care.[7] Federal financial participation is specifically not available, however, for some services. Most notably, it is not available for coverage of abortions that are not needed to save the life of the mother or in cases of rape or incest.[8] Title XIX also imposes several limitations on the states' ability to shift to the federal government the cost of services that historically were covered by the states. Thus, the Medicaid statute prohibits federal payments for services for prisoners or for persons under the age of 65 who are patients in mental hospitals.[9]

In contrast, the list of services that must be covered under federal law is fairly short and has grown relatively little over the years. States that participate in Medicaid must cover inpatient and outpatient hospital services; services in rural health clinics and federally qualified health centers; laboratory and X-ray services; skilled nursing facility services; early and periodic screening, diagnostic, and treatment services for children; family planning services; physician services; medical and surgical services furnished by dentists; home health services; medical transportation; and, to the extent permitted under state licensure laws, the services of nurse-midwives and nurse-practitioners for their categorically needy.[10] Even fewer services need to be made available to the medically needy, although the states are not permitted to limit benefits available to the medically needy to institutional care or care for the mentally ill or retarded.[11]

More burdensome to the states, however, have been regulatory requirements that pertain not to specific services but to the extent to which services must be provided if services are provided at all. The regulations require that "each service must be sufficient in amount, duration, and scope to reasonably achieve its purpose" and provide that "the Medicaid agency may not arbitrarily deny or reduce the amount, duration, or scope of a required service . . . solely because of the diagnosis, type of illness, or condition."[12] States must also offer to the categorically needy at least the services offered to the medically needy, and they cannot discriminate among groups of the categorically needy or the medically needy in the provision of services.[13]

Finally, Medicaid has all along imposed limits on the discretion of the states as to how to provide and pay for Medicaid services. The "statewideness" requirement of Title XIX, for example, limited the ability of the states to provide services through different approaches in different parts of the state.[14] The "free choice of provider" requirement precluded the states from requiring their recipients to receive care through a managed-care plan.[15] Title XIX also originally required the states to pay "reasonable cost" for inpatient hospital services—the Medicare standard of payment.[16] This requirement proved very costly for the states and significantly limited their ability to pay adequately for non-hospital and nursing home services.

Potentially, however, the most burdensome requirement imposed on the states by the original 1965 statute was the "comprehensiveness" requirement. Title XIX, as enacted, contemplated Medicaid as a program that would bring the deserving poor into the mainstream of American medical care within the foreseeable future. The original Medicaid statute, therefore, imposed on the states a requirement that they

[make] efforts in the direction of broadening the scope of care and services made available under the plan and in the direction of liberalizing the eligibility requirements for medical assistance, with a view toward furnishing by July 1, 1975, comprehensive care and services to substantially all individuals who meet the plan's eligibility standards with respect to income and resources, including services to enable such individuals to attain or retain independence and self-care.[17]

The implementation of this requirement was first delayed for two years in 1969, and then abandoned in 1972.[18] Nevertheless, it manifests an intention at the outset that Medicaid would achieve uniform coverage throughout the United States.

## Medicaid, 1965–1994: Expansion of Federal Control

During the early decades of the Medicaid program, there was a trend toward building a firmer federal floor under eligibility. The first major step in this direction took place in 1972, when the Aid to the Aged, Blind, and Disabled program was taken over by the federal government and renamed the Supplemental Security Income (SSI) program.[19] This new program substantially raised income eligibility levels in many states for the elderly, blind, and disabled, and thus it extended Medicaid eligibility significantly. In fact, the statute allowed states to exercise the "209(b)" option to retain more stringent eligibility levels in effect on January 1, 1972, but most states accepted the federal SSI income eligibility levels for their programs.[20] With SSI came also national standards for determining disability, which also made the state Medicaid programs more uniform (except in states that retained their own disability standards under the 209(b) option).

Over the decades, Congress has from time to time adopted additional eligibility mandates that have continued to expand and to encourage national uniformity of coverage among the elderly, blind, and disabled, including, for example, requirements for states to continue Medicaid coverage for persons who lost SSI or state supplement eligibility because of the 20% Social Security cost of living increase of 1972 or because of Social Security cost of living increases after 1977.[21] Under amendments adopted in the late 1980s and 1990s, state Medicaid programs are also required to cover the Medicare premiums and cost-sharing obligations for "Qualified Medicare Beneficiaries" (QMBs)—that is, those Medicare-eligible individuals whose income does not exceed 100% of the poverty level.[22] State Medicaid programs must also cover the Medicare Part B premiums for "Specified Low—Income Medicare Beneficiaries," or persons who would otherwise qualify as QMBs except that their income is between 100% and 120% of the federal poverty level;[23] and all or part of the Medicare Part A premiums of "Qualified Disabled and Working Individuals" (QDWIs), or persons who are disabled and employed with incomes below 200% of the poverty level.[24]

At the time the federal government took over the prior Aid to the Aged, Blind, and Disabled program in 1972, replacing it with the SSI program, it left control over Aid to Families with Dependent Children (AFDC) financial eligibility with the states. The states used this control quite effectively in the late 1970s and early 1980s, either to cut back AFDC eligibility levels or to leave eligibility levels unadjusted for inflation for long periods of time, particularly after the Reagan administration cut benefits in the early 1980s.[25] Between 1980 and 1992, AFDC eligibility levels (which also established eligibility for Medicaid) dropped more than 16%.[26] The AFDC population dropped by about 14.5% because of the 1981 Omnibus Budget Reconciliation Act (OBRA).[27] Between 1975 and 1985, the number of children receiving Medicaid actually declined.[28]

Beginning in 1984, however, a series of federal Social Security Act amendments began to federalize eligibility requirements for dependent children and pregnant women.[29] The Deficit Reduction Act of 1984 required states to cover all children born after September 30, 1983, and under the age of five living in families meeting AFDC income and resource requirements, regardless of whether the families had one or two parents. The following year eligibility for pregnancy-related services was extended to all pregnant women who met AFDC eligibility standards, regardless of family structure.[30] In 1986, eligibility for children and their families was first delinked from state AFDC eligibility standards by the OBRA of 1986, which gave states the option of covering pregnant women and children up to the age of five in families with incomes below 100% of the poverty line. A year later optional coverage was extended to pregnant women and children with incomes up to 185% of the poverty line and children below the age of five living below the poverty line. In 1988 states were for the first time required to cover pregnant women and infants under age of one with incomes below 100% of the poverty line.

The most revolutionary changes, however, occurred in 1989 and 1990, when omnibus budget reconciliation acts extended Medicaid eligibility first to all pregnant women and children up to age six in families with incomes below 133% of the poverty line,[31] and then to all children up to age 18 born after September 30, 1983, with incomes up to 100% of the poverty line.[32]

The effect of these statutes was to establish a federal floor undergirding Medicaid eligibility for SSI recipients in most states and for children in all. Only with respect to adult parents of dependent children did the states retain virtually unrestricted discretion over income limits. States could, of course, cover recipients with higher incomes (within limits) and expand coverage through adding optional categories, but by 1990 Congress had effectively established minimum federal financial eligibility standards for most of the populations that Medicaid covered.

There was also some movement between 1966 and 1990 toward greater uniformity with respect to services covered by Medicaid. The most important development here, no doubt, was the creation of the Early and Periodic Screening, Diagnosis, and Treatment (EPSDT) program, which became effective in 1969, and which obligated all states to screen children for medical problems and to provide treatment for problems identified.[33] But other services were also added to the list of federally required services over the decades. In 1980 Congress added a requirement for coverage of nurse-midwives, and a decade later, for nurse practitioner services.[34] States were required to cover family planning services in 1972 and services of federally qualified health centers in 1993. The 1989 OBRA responded to low participation rates in EPSDT by imposing high target participation rates on the states and by requiring the states to provide Medicaid services determined to be necessary under the EPSDT program, regardless of whether the service was otherwise available under the state program.[35] Although drugs remain an optional service under Medicaid, legislation adopted in 1990 establishing the Medicaid drug rebate program prohibited the states from refusing to cover medically necessary prescribed drugs manufactured by companies with a drug rebate agreement.[36] Finally, a number of courts during the 1970s and 1980s read the "amount, duration, and scope" and comparability requirements of the Medicaid statute and regulations liberally to broaden mandated coverage.[37]

Federal limits restricting the ability of the states to limit Medicaid payments also expanded during the 1970s and 1980s. In 1981 and 1982 Congress amended the Medicaid statute to give the states greater discretion in setting payment rates for hospitals and nursing homes than was available under the previous statute. The previous statute had tied Medicaid rates to Medicare rates, whereas the new "Boren Amendment" required states to pay an amount "reasonable and adequate to meet the costs that must be incurred by efficiently and economically operated institutions." The Boren Amendment was interpreted by the courts, however, as limiting the states' ability to manipulate payment rates.[38] The Supreme Court's *Wilder* decision in 1990, recognizing providers as having standing to enforce Medicaid requirements, further encouraged provider litigation to enforce these requirements.[39] Mandates imposed by Congress during the 1990s required the states to provide additional payments to disproportionate share hospitals and to increase their reimbursement for community health centers.[40] The 1989 OBRA also imposed a requirement on the states that Medicaid payment levels be "sufficient to enlist enough providers so that services . . . are available to . . . recipients at least to the extent that those services are available to the general population."[41]

These limits at their most ambitious only placed a federal floor under state eligibility, benefit, and payment levels, which continued to vary dramatically throughout the history of the program.[42] State Medicaid coverage of the non-elderly population varied from a low of 5.4% in Nevada to a high of 20.9% in Tennessee in 1996–1998.[43] Medicaid coverage of the non-elderly population with incomes below 200% of the poverty level varied from 14.2% in Nevada to 43.7% in Vermont over the same period.[44] In 1997, states ranged in their Medicaid costs per beneficiary from $1,048 (Virginia) to $2,507 (Alaska).[45] State Medicaid expenditures as a share of state budgets varied in 1994 from 5.3% (Alaska) to 29.2% (New York) of total state expenditures.[46] But for a time, the trend was toward greater national uniformity—not diversity—in the Medicaid program.

## The Tide Turns toward Greater State Discretion

In recent years, however, the movement toward greater federal control over the Medicaid program has reversed. Recent legislation and administrative actions have moved toward devolution of control over the Medicaid program to the states. In particular, a trend has occurred toward allowing states discretion to drop the floor, in addition to the discretion they have long enjoyed to raise the ceiling, of coverage.

To a considerable extent, this has been achieved though waivers of federal statutory requirements. In 1981, for example, Congress established the 1915(b) waiver program, which allowed the Department of Health and Human Services to waive specific requirements of the Social Security Act—most notably the freedom of choice requirement—and thus to permit states to adopt Medicaid managed-care programs that limit the freedom of choice of recipients.[47]

An even broader statutory avenue to devolution through waivers predated Medicaid. Section 1115 of the Social Security Act[48] had been adopted in 1962 and was extended to cover Medicaid at the time the program was created. Unlike § 1915(b), which only permitted waivers of specific sections of the Medicaid statute and for specified purposes, § 1115 permits waivers of virtually all provisions of the Medicaid program.[49] In 1981, § 1115 was used to allow Arizona to establish a Medicaid program based solely on managed care, an experiment that has continued now for over two decades.

In the mid-1990s, the "Contract with America" Congress attempted to end the Medicaid program, and to replace it with a block-granted "Medigrant" program, which would have devolved authority over the Medicaid program almost entirely to the states. The only remaining eligibility constraints would have been a requirement that states cover pregnant women and children under the age of 13 whose family income was below the poverty level and persons who were disabled under the state's definition of disability.[50] The only mandate that the statute imposed on the states as to services was that they had to cover immunizations for children and prepregnancy family planning services, and could not exclude preexisting conditions.[51] The legislation explicitly abolished the comparability; statewideness; amount, duration, and scope; and freedom of choice requirements of the Medicaid program.[52] It also would have capped the federal government's obligations on a year-to-year basis, thus ending Medicaid as a fiscal entitlement.[53] The only remedy available to individuals under the final Medigrant statute was a right to complain to the secretary, who, in turn, was to notify Congress and the state governor if the secretary found a pattern of complaints or an egregious finding of noncompliance against a state.[54] In short, the legislation would have ended Medicaid as an entitlement program.

President Clinton vetoed the Medigrant proposal. Legislation in the following two years, however, achieved many of its purposes. First, the 1996 Personal Responsibility and Work Opportunity Reconciliation Act (PRWORA) brought an end to the 60-year-old Aid to Families with Dependent Children program, putting in its place the Temporary Assistance to Needy Families (TANF) program.[55] This legislation essentially block-granted welfare for families, thus abolishing welfare for needy families as an entitlement and radically increasing the discretion of the states in governing family assistance programs. PRWORA was not supposed to significantly change the Medicaid program: families who had been eligible for Medicaid under the prior AFDC program remained eligible.[56] Indeed, PRWORA allowed the states to extend Medicaid coverage to families not previously covered.[57] In fact, however, hundreds of thousands of former Medicaid recipients were dropped from the rolls in the wake of PRWORA, some because they found employment with health insurance, but many others because they were either not told that they remained eligible for Medicaid when they lost cash assistance or because they were dissuaded from applying for Medicaid by aggressive tactics undertaken by the states to deter welfare applicants.[58] Indeed, coverage losses due to welfare reform largely reversed the gains accomplished through eligibility expansions in the 1980s and early 1990s for the poorest Medicaid recipients, leaving Medicaid enrollment in 1998 for families without income at levels comparable to coverage in 1980.[59] PRWORA also cut back dramatically on the eligibility expansions for disabled children.[60]

If the PRWORA had a profound effect on Medicaid eligibility, the Balanced Budget Act (BBA) of 1997 had an equally great effect on Medicaid services and payment.[61] First, a number of BBA provisions were directed at making it easier for the states to establish Medicaid managed-care programs. Perhaps the most important of these was a provision allowing the states to require recipients to enroll in managed-care plans; thus abolishing the free choice of provider requirement.[62] The BBA also permitted Medicaid to participate in Medicaid-only HMOs by repealing the prior requirement that at least one-quarter of HMO members had to be commercial (non-Medicare or -Medicaid) enrollees.[63] It further limited the right recipients had previously enjoyed to withdraw from a managed-care plan with one month's notice without cause, putting in its place a provision permitting recipients to terminate or change enrollment at any time for cause, but only within 90 days of enrollment or once a year thereafter without cause.[64] The BBA also allowed the implementation of mandatory primary care case-management programs (in which recipients are tied to a gatekeeper physician who must authorize all referrals) without an HHS waiver.[65] Medicaid managed care, which had previously only been possible with a waiver or on a voluntary basis, became an option universally available to the states.

The BBA also repealed or changed several payment requirements under the Medicaid statute. Most important, it repealed the Boren Amendment, replacing it with procedural provisions for hospital and nursing facility rate setting, which the courts quickly interpreted as not conferring substantive rights on providers.[66] The BBA also phased in a repeal of the requirement that states pay federally qualified health centers and rural health clinics 100% of their cost,[67] and limited the amount that states had to pay when they covered Medicare cost sharing to the rates their Medicaid programs paid for persons who were not Medicare beneficiaries.[68]

Yet another devolutionary feature of the BBA was the creation of the State Children's Health Insurance Program (SCHIP), an expansive program for providing health insurance coverage to poor children with family incomes from the Medicaid level up to 200% of poverty.[69] The SCHIP program was explicitly created as a nonentitlement program. The SCHIP statute states: "Nothing in this subchapter shall be construed as providing an individual with an entitlement to child health assistance under a State child health plan."[70] Indeed, the program can be understood as a choice by Congress to create a new nonentitlement program, having been blocked two years earlier in its attempt to end Medicaid itself as an entitlement program.[71] Significantly, none of the states that have created SCHIP programs independent of their Medicaid programs have recognized explicit state entitlements to SCHIP coverage, and 16 states expressly provide that SCHIP is not an entitlement—that is, that no individual has a right to SCHIP coverage.[72]

Finally, the Balanced Budget Act (BBA) also streamlined provisions for extending (for up to three years) § 1115 Medicaid waivers, facilitating the use of waiver authority as a means for creating alternative state approaches to the uniform national Medicaid program envisioned by Title XIX.[73] In fact, the Clinton administration had already, even before the BBA, moved ahead with aggressively granting waivers to the states. Prior to the Clinton administration, most § 1115 waivers had been granted for small-scale experiments (other than the Arizona program noted earlier).[74] President Clinton—who as a governor had pushed for increased flexibility for the states in the Medicaid program— placed much more emphasis on the waiver program. By the end of Clinton's second term, 18 states had implemented statewide comprehensive § 1115 demonstration projects—modifying their delivery systems, expanding coverage, or both—and $27 billion of federal Medicaid money, 20% of the total Medicaid budget, was being spent through waiver programs.[75] Several million Medicaid recipients were receiving services under waiver programs, and 2 million formerly uninsured persons were receiving Medicaid coverage under § 1115 programs.[76] Three states also received waivers in 2000 under the SCHIP program to cover parents of SCHIP recipients.[77]

With the George W. Bush administration, however, has come a change in emphasis in the § 1115 waiver program. On August 4, 2001, the Bush administration announced its Health Insurance Flexibility and Accountability Initiative (HIFA).[78] The primary focus of HIFA is to encourage comprehensive waiver programs to increase the number of insured individuals by using current Medicaid and SCHIP resources. Program expansions are to focus on individuals with incomes below 200% of the federal poverty level. In particular, the initiative contemplates cutting back on services or imposing additional cost-sharing obligations on optional Medicaid groups (who make up about 29% of current Medicaid recipients, including 56% of seniors and 43% of low-income parents).[79] The only limitations on services that must be provided to optional populations under HIFA are that the benefit package must be equivalent to a package permissible under SCHIP, and that cost-sharing obligations for children should not exceed 5% of family income. Benefits for the expanded populations need only cover "basic primary care," or nonspecialist physician services. Moreover, the states are strongly encouraged under the HIFA program to subsidize the purchase of private insurance, and they are not required to meet a specific cost-effectiveness test with respect to the purchase of private insurance, although aggregate costs of those enrolled in the private insurance premium assistance program are not supposed to be "significantly higher than costs would be under a direct coverage program."[80] The waiver program also does not impose any floor on benefits or ceiling on cost sharing on private plans, unlike current federal law.

Medicaid advocates have been highly critical of the HIFA program.[81] They point out that HIFA is likely to cut Medicaid benefits sharply for some of its most needy recipients, while providing inadequate benefits for newly covered populations and inefficient subsidies for private insurance. They note that the HIFA waiver template issued by the Center for Medicare and Medicaid Services, apparently contemplates enrollment caps, which currently are not permitted for Medicaid recipients. They argue that, in fact, the HIFA guidelines also do not require the states to reinvest their Medicaid and SCHIP savings in coverage expansions, as long as they do not impose additional costs on the federal government.

Perhaps the most serious complaint about the new guidelines, however, is that although they have the potential for radically changing the nature of the Medicaid program, they do so without congressional oversight. Indeed, the

.ver process does not seem to contemplate any public imput at the federal
/el, and CMS has refused to permit stakeholders to review waiver applications prior to approval.[82]

At the beginning of the twenty-first century, therefore, Medicaid is becoming a very different program—certainly different from what existed a decade
earlier, but even different from what was envisioned at the creation of Medicaid. While Medicaid has always been a federal/state cooperative program that
varied significantly among the states, it seemed for a time to be moving in the
direction of placing a more uniform federal floor under eligibility and benefits, and even under provider payments. Since the mid-1990s, however, the tide
has turned, and now devolution seems to be in full flood, leading to programs
that with federal acquiescence are becoming increasingly more disparate in
nature.

## Evaluating Devolution

Is devolution of the Medicaid program a good thing? It is not intuitively obvious that a person suffering from a serious illness and unable to afford medical
care should be able to receive that care at the expense of the American taxpayers in Minnesota, but not in Mississippi. Disparity in access to health care
is a problem in all nations, of course, no matter how committed the country is
to solidarity, and it continues to be a concern in the Medicare program, which
in theory provides the same benefits throughout the country.[83] But in most
public programs it is seen as a problem, not as a virtue to be celebrated.[84] Why,
therefore, are wide variations in the level of care provided by the Medicaid
program seen as a plus, while regional variations in the Medicare program are
seen as a serious deficiency?

The traditional argument for devolving power to the states is the idea of the
"laboratories of democracy": the states provide an opportunity to try out a range
of different experiments and thus, it is hoped, to come up with ideas for improving delivery of health care to the poor.[85] This is an idea with some appeal.
In fact, some state Medicaid programs have created innovative approaches that
have benefited the program more generally. Arizona, the first state to adopt a
statewide Medicaid managed-care program, illuminated the way for managed-
care programs subsequently adopted by other states across the country.[86] Tennessee and Oregon pioneered at piggy-backing expanded coverage for the poor
generally onto Medicaid through controlling the costs of the traditional Medicaid program, and over a dozen states now are attempting to expand health
insurance coverage through Medicaid waivers.[87]

However, the few states that have shown leadership in expanding coverage
are far outweighed by those that have limited eligibility expansions and tried

to manipulate the Medicaid system to maximize federal expenditures for minimal state effort. Two-thirds of the states still do not cover all parents of families with dependent children with incomes below the poverty level, even though they may do so under Medicaid law.[88]

Experiments with expanding coverage to new populations, or to providing care more efficiently, could be carried out, moreover, within a federal program. Even if Medicaid were totally operated by the federal government, any state that chose to could set up a state-funded program for populations not covered by the federal program, just as some do now. If the states no longer had to pay the billions of dollars that they must now contribute to the Medicaid program, moreover, they would have a great deal of money available to experiment with expanding coverage.

A second argument for devolution is that state government is closer to the people and more accurately reflects local tastes and desires, and thus authority for programs that do not need to be run at the national level should be devolved to the states. It is well known, however, that participation in national elections is much more widespread than in state elections and that people are more likely to follow national than state political news.[89] There is also evidence that state and local governments are more amenable to being dominated by interest groups and are particularly ill-suited for protecting the interests of the poor and of minority groups.[90]

Further, it is not obvious that reflection of local "taste" in programs for the poor is a good thing. The fact that poverty programs were left to the states when the United States embraced social insurance in the 1930s is explained to a considerable extent by the history of racism in the American South.[91] Southern congressmen and senators in the 1930s, largely Democrats and essential to Roosevelt's New Deal coalition, refused to cede to the national government control over programs for the poor that would have put poor African Americans on the same footing as the white poor in claiming benefits, and might also have dried up the pool of poor blacks that was essential for providing cheap agricultural and domestic labor.[92] For decades blacks were discriminated against in the federal/state cash-assistance programs, just as they were discriminated against in state and local public health programs.[93] Although explicit race discrimination has largely been eliminated in public programs, its legacy remains.

Indeed, the real explanations of why authority for running Medicaid is devolved to the states are largely historical and political.[94] As related in Chapter 4, there is a long tradition of dealing with the poor at the local, or at most, the state level, dating back at least to the Elizabethan poor laws. Even though middle-class social insurance programs—Social Security and Medicare—were taken over by the federal government in the 1930s and 1960s, programs for the poor, always suspect in American society, have by and large been left to the states, where intrusive administrators closer to the recipient can keep tighter control.[95] While the public is adverse to letting the poor die in the streets, it does not want them to become too comfortable, either. Thus programs for the poor are administered at lower levels of government, where those who administer the program can make life more intimately miserable for recipients.

For a time it was believed that this division of responsibility was required by the Constitution, though, as noted in Chapter 4, this notion has been rejected at least since the New Deal. Although in recent years the Supreme Court increasingly has returned to a recognition of state's rights, it has not questioned the authority of the federal government to care for the poor under the spending power, which is only limited by the Constitution to expenditures "in pursuit of the general welfare."[96] While history, therefore, may offer an explanation for devolution of power to the states, it does not offer a reason.

Moreover, there are good reasons why we may want to have a health-care program for the poor that is national in scope. First, there is oft-discussed problem of the "race to the bottom." One of the primary justifications for a federal system is that it creates a healthy competition among different jurisdictions, which, in turn, allows people to choose from among a variety of options the state that most closely matches their preferred level of publicly provided amenities and taxation.[97] While this competition may promote innovation and efficiency with respect to some government services, it has long been argued that it may result in a race to the bottom when redistributional programs, like Medicaid, are at issue.[98]

The argument is that any state offering more generous social programs risks, on the one hand, attracting recipients of the proffered benefit (who may move in from less generous jurisdictions) and, on the other, losing businesses or affluent taxpayers to jurisdictions that can afford to charge lower taxes because they offer less generous benefits. These forces result in a race to the bottom, as states restrict their benefits to an ever greater extent, or at least discourage any one state from getting too far out ahead of the others in generosity of its benefits.

The race to the bottom hypothesis has been extensively studied (or, at least, argued) in the cash-assistance context.[99] There is some evidence of its existence in that context, particularly among contiguous states, but other studies find that welfare recipients do not move often, and, when they do, they are more likely to move to find work or for family support rather than to obtain more generous benefits.[100] Given the fact that jurisdictions with more generous benefits tend to have higher living costs, a move rarely would result in a substantially improved economic situation in any event.[101]

The effect of Medicaid on the migration of potential recipients has not been well studied.[102] It seems quite conceivable, however, that people who need medical care and are not eligible for public health coverage in the jurisdiction in which they find themselves might move, at least to a neighboring jurisdiction, to obtain a more generous public health insurance program.[103] It seems even more likely, moreover, that businesses might move their operations from jurisdictions with high taxes and generous Medicaid programs to those with lower taxes.[104] But the key factor in the race to the bottom hypothesis is not whether recipients or businesses and taxpayers actually move, but whether politicians fear that they might.[105] As long as state politicians fear that generous public health insurance programs might make their state more attractive to indigents or less attractive to business, the states are not going to become too generous in providing health insurance for the poor. Thus, the possibility of a race to the bottom poses a real barrier to providing health-care coverage for the poor at the state level.

These considerations are much less of a factor at the national level. It is unlikely that people from other developed nations would move to the United States solely for medical benefits, as most of them already enjoy them, and people from developing nations already have ample economic incentives for moving here without regard to health care. By the same token, businesses and affluent taxpayers will find few developed countries with tax rates lower than the United States, and they already face economic incentives to move production to less-developed countries if it is otherwise possible or beneficial for them to do so. Thus the national government can raise taxes to cover health insurance programs without undue fear for its international competitive situation.

It is also likely that administration of a health insurance program for the poor at the federal rather than the state level would be more efficient. Although the states have traditionally lacked the administrative capacity of the federal government, and still vary considerably in their administrative expertise, some argue that state governments operate with greater efficiency than the national government.[106] It is difficult to believe, however, that running more than 50 different Medicaid programs, each with its own state bureaucracy (plus a federal bureaucracy to supervise them all)—and each with its own eligibility, benefit, and payment policies; information systems; and program operations—is efficient.

A clear example of the inefficiencies created by the current program is the gaming that has gone on for the past two decades as the states have tried to maximize their federal matching revenues. In the late 1980s and 1990s the primary scheme that was used to this end was to collect provider contributions and then match them with disproportionate share hospital payments.[107] The 1980 and 1981 OBRAs had created the disproportionate share hospital (DSH) program to permit states to make special payments to hospitals that provided high volumes of care to low-income or Medicaid patients. The provision saw little use initially, but several states (beginning with West Virginia) figured out

in the late 1980s that the DSH program could be combined with provider donations (permitted under a 1985 Health Care Financing Administration rule)
or provider taxes to obtain large sums of federal money. For example, a state
could collect $10 million from a hospital as a "provider donation," pay a $12
million DSH payment to the hospital, collect $6 million from the federal gov-
ernment at a 50% match rate, and pocket $4 million.[108] Once the states real-
ized this possibility, the DSH program grew dramatically—from $1.4 billion or
2% of Medicaid spending in 1990, to $17.5 billion or 15% of total Medicaid
spending by 1992.[109] By 1992, the DSH program accounted for 35% of New
Hampshire's spending and 43% of Louisiana's. DSH payments accounted for
much of the dramatic growth in the Medicaid program in the early 1990s.

Federal legislation in 1991, 1993, and 1997 stanched the worst abuses of the
DSH program by banning provider donations and limiting provider taxes and
DSH payments. In the late 1990s, however, the states discovered another
means of extracting money from the federal government without true state
matching contributions—"upper payment limit" (UPL) arrangements. Under
federal Medicaid regulations, states may not pay providers as a class more than
the amount Medicare would pay for the same service—the upper payment
level.[110] Prior to 2001, county and local facilities were grouped with private facilities in a "non-state owned" class. Where a gap existed between the amount
a state paid nonstate-owned providers and the UPL, the states could pay the
difference to local government-owned facilities as a supplemental payment.
Federal matching funds were then collected on this payment. The state finally
retrieved the money from local government through an intergovernmental
transfer, thus obtaining federal matching funds on money that was never really spent by the state. The federal cost of UPL financing grew from $313 mil-
lion in 1995 to $1.4 billion in 1998, to an estimated $3 billion in 2001, lifting
Pennsylvania's true federal matching rate from 54% to 65% and New Jersey's
from 50% to 60%.[111] In 2001, Medicaid created a new class for county and local providers, and in January 2002, CMS attempted to limit upper payment
limit abuses by restricting state payments to county and local hospitals to 100%
of Medicare payments following a transition period, but the rule was challenged
by litigation and delayed.

The larger point here is that as long as the Medicaid program is operated
by the states but funded in large part by the federal government, the states
face incentives to use the program to extract extra dollars out of the federal
government. Moreover, these funds may not always be used for the purposes
for which the funds were intended. In the past decade, tens of billions of dollars have been taken from the federal government in this way. These program
abuses have badly distorted the ongoing debate regarding funding health care
for the poor, as they have resulted in dramatic but artificial program cost increases and made the Medicaid program to appear to be more of a burden on

the states than in fact it is. It would be far more responsible for the federal government to spend its taxpayers' money directly for medical care for indigents, rather than to have to continually struggle with state manipulation of the system.

State attempts to maximize federal Medicaid matching funds, in contrast, are very understandable, given the fiscal situation of the American states. Medicaid spending, like spending on welfare programs generally, is countercyclical.[112] When the economy declines, Medicaid spending increases. This is obviously true because Medicaid eligibility is tied to income and employment, and as employment and income wane, more people become eligible for Medicaid. When the economy enters a recession, however, state revenues drop; thus, as the cost of Medicaid programs increases, the ability of states to pay for them diminishes.

When welfare expenses increase at the federal level, the federal government can simply borrow to get through the recession, or, if necessary, raise taxes. But 49 of the 50 states are not permitted to engage in deficit spending.[113] They must balance their books at the end of every year. Many states, moreover, have adopted constitutional amendments or other limitations that make raising taxes very difficult. Over half of the states have adopted tax and expenditure limits, which often require legislative supermajorities to raise taxes.[114] As Medicaid program costs are one of the biggest item in the budget of most states, about 20% of all state spending, the states face serious financial crises when recessions drive Medicaid costs up.[115] The mild recession of 2000 to 2002, for example, caused serious problems for Medicaid programs in most of the states.

In sum, although the trend has clearly been toward devolution of authority over the Medicaid program in the past decade (following modest earlier movements toward federalization of eligibility standards and, to a lesser extent, benefits and payment requirements), this should not be regarded as a salutary development. Even though there are historical, and political, explanations for why Medicaid is a joint federal and state program, administered at the state level, the problem it addresses is a national problem and demands a national solution.

This is not to say that there is no role for state or local government in an ideal health-care system. Throughout the world, nations that provide national health-care entitlements also provide a role for local or regional governments in health-care delivery, planning, and even financing. But entitlement to health-care services should not depend on the accident of where a person who needs medical care is located within the United States. A national floor over eligibility and benefits is needed.

Our national experience with Medicaid points to another important truth as well: entitlement for medical care should not depend on being poor, and in particular on fitting into a category of poor persons that can be categorized as "worthy." Our experience with Medicaid, as described in this chapter and in Chapter 5, has demonstrated that a program for the poor will always be politically vulnerable, underfunded, and generally inadequate. No other developed country covers only its poor with its health-care entitlement programs (though some provide extra benefits, such as the waiver of cost-sharing requirements to the poor). Only if the poor are included in a comprehensive program for the general population will they receive adequate and dignified health care. What such a system might look like is developed in Chapter 11.

# Notes

1. See Nelda McCall, "The Arizona Health Care Cost Containment System," in *Remaking Medicaid*, edited by Stephen M. Davidson and Stephen A. Somers (San Francisco: Jossey-Bass, 1998), 127.

2. The "federal medical assistance percentage," the percentage of Medicaid expenditures covered by the federal government, can (under 42 U.S.C. § 1396d(b)) amount to as much as 83% of state Medicaid expenditures; currently, the federal government covers no more than 77% of any state's expenditures, and about one-quarter of the states receive only 50%. See Department of Health and Human Services, "Federal Financial Participation in State Assistance Expenditures," *Federal Register* 66 (November 30, 2001): 59,790.

3. In 2001, however, seven states covered adults such as childless adults who were not otherwise eligible for Medicaid, under the § 1115 waiver authority discussed in this chapter. See Cindy Mann, *The New Medicaid and CHIP Waiver Initiatives* (Washington, D.C.: Kaiser Commission on Medicaid and the Uninsured, 2002), 15.

4. Social Security Amendments of 1965, Pub. L. 89-97. § 1902(a)(10). 79 Stat 286, 345 (1965).

5. Pub. L. 89-97, § 1902(a)(10)(B), 79 Stat. 286, 345 (1965).

6. The Commerce Clearing House (CCH) Medicare and Medicaid Guide currently lists 35 categories of persons that must be covered by state Medicaid programs and 23 optional coverage groups. One of the optional groups, however, the medically needy, is listed as including nine subgroups. See *Medicare and Medicaid Guide* (Chicago: CCH, 2002), ¶¶ 14,231, 14,251.

7. 42 U.S.C. § 1396d(a)(27).

8. The most recent prohibition on payment for abortions is found in the 1994 Hyde Amendment, Departments of Labor, Health and Human Services, and Education Appropriation Act of 1994, Pub. L. 103-112, § 509, 107 Stat. 1082, 1113 (1994). See 42 C.F.R. §§ 441.200–441.208.

9. 42 U.S.C. § 1396d(a). Before 1984, Medicaid payments were also limited for patients in tuberculosis sanitariums.

10. 42 U.S.C. § 1396a(a)(10)(A); 42 C.F.R. §§ 410.210 and 441.15.

11. See 42 C.F.R. § 440.220.

12. 42 C.F.R. §§ 440.230(b) and (c). The states are permitted to limit services based on medical necessity or utilization control purposes. 42 C.F.R. § 440.230(d).

13. 42 U.S.C. § 1396a(a)(10)(B); 42 C.F.R. § 440.240.

14. 42 U.S.C. § 1396a(a)(A)(1).

15. 42 U.S.C. § 1396a(a)(23).

16. Pub. L. 89-97, § 1902(a)(13); 79 Stat, 286, 345–346 (1965).

17. Pub. L. 89-97, § 1903(e); 79 Stat., 286, 350 (1965). The federal guidelines interpreting the statute stated that "comprehensive care includes all preventive, diagnostic, curative and rehabilitation services or goods furnished, prescribed, or ordered by a recognized practitioner of the healing arts within the scope of his practice." U.S. Department of Health, Education and Welfare, *Handbook of Public Assistance Administration*, Supplement D: *Medical Assistance Programs* D-5142 (1966), quoted in David F. Chavkin, "Medicaid and Viagra: Restoring Potency to an Old Program?" *Health Matrix* 11 (2001): 189, 190.

18. See Chavkin, "Medicaid and Viagra," 190–195.

19. The SSI program was created as Title XVI of the Social Security Program by section 301 of the Social Security Amendments of 1972. Michael S. Sparer, *Medicaid and the Limits of State Health Reform* (Philadelphia: Temple University Press, 1996), 33.

20. 42 U.S.C. §§ 1619(b) and 1396a(f). Twelve states continue to be "209(b)" states. CCH, *Medicare and Medicaid Guide*, 15,504.

21. 42 U.S.C. § 1396a(a); 42 C.F.R. §§ 435.134 and 435.135.

22. 42 U.S.C. § 1396d(p) (adopted in 1986).

23. 42 U.S.C. § 1396a(a)(10)(E)(iii).

24. 42 U.S.C. §§, 1396a(a)(10)(E)(ii) and 1396d(s).

25. See Michael B. Katz, *The Price of Citizenship: Redefining the American Welfare State* (New York: Metropolitan Books, 2001), 81–82; John K. Iglehart, "Federal Policies and the Poor," *New England Journal of Medicine*, 307 (1982): 836.

26. Sparer, *Medicaid and the Limits of State Health Reform*, 46.

27. Steven G. Craig, "Should States Be Responsible for New Directions in Health Provision? Lessons from Other Policy Areas," in *Health Policy, Federalism, and the American States*, edited by Robert F. Rich and William White (Washington, D.C.: Urban Institute, 1996), 221, 244.

28. Frank J. Thompson, "The Faces of Devolution," in *Medicaid and Devolution*, edited by Frank J. Thompson and John J. DiIulio (Washington, D.C.: Brookings Institute, 1998), 23.

29. See Karl Kronebusch, "Children's Medicaid Enrollment: The Impacts of Mandates, Welfare Reform, and Policy Delinking," *Journal of Health Politics, Policy, and Law* 26 (2001): 1223, 1228.

30. 42 U.S.C. § 1396a(a)(10)(A)(III and 1396d(n).

31. 42 U.S.C. §§ 1396a(a)(10)(A)(i)(IV) and (VII); 1396a(l)(1)(A),(B), and (C); and 1396a(l)(2)(A) and (B).

32. 42 U.S.C. § 1396a(a)(10)(A)(i)(VII); and 1396a(l)(1)(D) and (2)(C).

33. 42 U.S.C. §§ 1396d(a)(4)(B) and 1396d(r).

34. Sparer, *Medicaid and the Limits of State Health Reform*, 48.

35. 42 U.S.C. § 1396r(5).

36. 42 U.S.C. § 1396r-8(d)(4)(B); Chavkin, "Medicaid and Viagra," 206.

37. See Patricia A. Butler, "State Limits on the Amount, Scope, and Duration of Services under Medicaid," in *The Medicaid Experience*, edited by Allen D. Spiegel (Germantown, Md.: Aspen Systems, 1979), 35.

38. Thompson, "The Faces of Devolution," 31–34.

39. *Wilder v. Virginia Hosp. Ass'n.*, 496 U.S. 498 (1990).

40. Sparer, *Medicaid and the Limits of State Health Reform*, 49.

41. 42 U.S.C. 1396a(a)(30)(A).

42. See Sparer, *Medicaid and the Limits of State Health Reform*, 31–65.

43. Christopher Trenholm and Susanna Kung, *Disparities in State Health Coverage: A Matter of Policy or Fortune?* (Washington, D.C.: Academy for Health Services Research and Health Policy, 2000): 4–5.

44. Ibid.

45. Ibid., 9–10.

46. Steven D. Gold, "Health Care and the Fiscal Crisis of the States," in *Health Policy, Federalism, and the American States*, edited by Robert F. Rich and William D. White (Washington, D.C.: Urban Institute Press, 1996), 108–109.

47. 42 U.S.C. § 1396n(b), added by Pub. L. 97-35, Omnibus Budget Reconciliation Act of 1981, § 2175, 95 Stat 357, 808 (1981).

48. 42 U.S.C. § 1315.

49. Only a handful of requirements, such as the federal matching rate, cost-sharing requirements for some populations, and quality-assurance requirements cannot be waived.

50. Balanced Budget Act of 1995, 104 Cong., 1st Sess. H.R. 2491, § 2111.

51. Ibid., § 2111(c), (d) and (e). The act also required a maintenance of effort equal to 85% of prior Medicaid expenditures to cover low-income families and elderly and disabled persons. Ibid., § 2112.

52. Ibid., § 2116(a).

53. Ibid., § 2121(b).

54. Ibid., 2154(g).

55. Pub. L. 104-193, 110 Stat. 2105 (1996).

56. 42 U.S.C. § 1396u-1. Individuals whose TANF grants were terminated because they refused work could also be terminated from Medicaid, but their minor children could not be.

57. Ibid., § 1396u-1(b)(2)(B) and (C).

58. See Joel Ferber and Theresa Steed, "The Impact of Welfare Reform on Access to Medicaid: Curing Systemic Violations of Medicaid De-Linking Requirements," *St. Louis University Law Journal* 45 (2001): 145.

59. Kronebusch, "Children's Medicaid Enrollment," 1241.

60. Pub. L. 104-193, Title II, Subtitle B 110 Stat 2105-2188 (1996).

61. Balanced Budget Act of 1997, Pub. L. No. 105-33, 111 Stat. 251 (1997).

62. 42 U.S.C. § 1396u-2(a)(1)(A). Special rules prohibited the states from requiring certain high-needs children, Native Americans, or Medicare beneficiaries from enrolling in managed-care organizations and generally required states to permit recipients the choice of at least two managed-care entities. 42 U.S.C. § 1396u-2(a)(2) and (3).

63. Required under former 42 U.S.C. § 1396b(m)(2)(A).

64. 42 U.S.C. § 1396u-2(a)(4)(A).

65. 42 U.S.C. §§ 1396d(a)(25) and (t).

66. 42 U.S.C. § 1396a(a)(13)(A). See, e.g., *Evergreen Presbyterian Ministries, Inc. v. Hood*, 235 F. 3d 908 (5th Cir. 2000); *Indep. Acceptance Co. v. State of Cal.*, 204 F. 3d 1247 (9th Cir. 2000).

67. Pub. L. 105-33, § 4712.

68. 42 U.S.C. § 1396a(n)(2).

69. 42 U.S.C. §§ 1397aa et seq.

70. 42 U.S.C. § 1397bb(b)(4).

71. See Sara Rosenbaum and David Rousseau, "Medicaid at Thirty-Five," *St. Louis University Law Journal* 45 (2001): 7, 41–42.

72. Sara Rosenbaum et al., "Devolution of Authority and Public Health Insurance Design: National SCHIP Study Reveals an Impact on Low-Income Children," *Houston Journal of Health Law and Policy* 1 (2001): 33.

73. See 42 U.S.C. § 1315(e). The Medicare, Medicaid, and SCHIP Benefits Improvement and Protection Act of 2000 created an even more streamlined procedure for granting state waiver requests, as well as an automatic approval default where HHS does not respond to a state request within 45 days. See 42 U.S.C. § 1315(f).

74. See Jeanne Lambrew, *Section 1115 Waivers in Medicaid and the State Children's Health Insurance Program: An Overview* (Washington D.C.: Kaiser Commission on Medicaid and the Uninsured, 2001).

75. Ibid.

76. Ibid.

77. Ibid.

78. Health Care Financing Administration, "Guidelines for States Interested in Applying for a HIFA Demonstration," available at www.hcfa.gov/medicaid/hifa/hifagde. htm (cited June 11, 2002).

79. See Edwin Park and Leighton Ku, *Administration Medicaid and SCHIP Waiver Policy Encourages States to Scale Back Benefits Significantly and Increase Cost-Sharing for Low-Income Beneficiaries,* (Washington, D.C.: Center on Budget and Policy Priorities, 2001); Testimony by Ronald F. Pollack, Executive Director Families USA before the Senate Committee on Health, Education, Labor and Pensions, March 12, 2002, "HIFA: Will It Solve the Problem of the Uninsured?" available at http://www.familiesusa.org/finalsenateMarch2002.pdf (cited October 21, 2002).

80. Health Care Financing Administration, "Guidelines for States," 3.

81. See Park and Ku, *Administration Medicaid and SCHIP Waiver Policy*; Mann, *The New Medicaid and CHIP Waiver Initiatives*; Pollack, "HIFA: Will It Solve the Problem of the Uninsured?"

82. Pollack, "HIFA: Will It Solve the Problem of the Uninsured?" 4.

83. See, e.g., Eric C. Schneider et al., "Racial Disparities in the Quality of Care for Enrollees in Medicare Managed Care," *Journal of the American Medical Association* 287 (March 13, 2002): 1288–1294; Adam Wagstaff and Eddy van Doorslaer, "Equity in Health Care Finance and Delivery," in *Handbook of Health Economics*, edited by A. J. Culyer and J. P. Newhouse (Amsterdam: Elsevier, 2000), 1804.

84. John E. Wennberg, Elliott S. Fisher, and Jonathan S. Skinner, "Geography and the Debate over Medicare Reform," *Health Affairs Online* available from www.healthaffairs.org (cited 13 February 2002).

85. The bromide traces its origins to a quote from Justice Brandeis in *New State Ice Co. v. Liebmann*, 285 U.S. 262, 311 (1932): "It is one of the happy incidents of the federal system that a single courageous State may, if its citizens choose, serve as a laboratory; and try novel social and economic experiments without risk to the rest of the country."

86. Arguably, the disastrous attempt by California to move Medicaid recipients into HMOs in the early 1970s also demonstrated how not to go about implementing Medicaid managed care. See Carol N. D'Onofrio and Patricia Dolan Mullen, "Consumer Problems with Prepaid Health Plans in California: Implications for Serving Medicaid Recipients through Health Maintenance Organizations," in *The Medicaid Experience*, edited by Allen D. Spiegel (Germantown, Md.: Aspen Systems, 1979), 361–378.

87. See Jeanne Lambrew, *Section 115 Waivers.*

88. Families USA, *Disparities in Eligibility for Public Health Insurance: Children and*

*Adults in 2001* (Washington, D.C.: Families USA, 2002), available from http://www.familiesusa.org/media/pdf/disparities_in_eligibility.pdf (cited October 21, 2002).

89. Jerry L. Mashaw and Dylan S. Calsyn, "Block Grants, Entitlements, and Federalism: A Conceptual Map of Contested Terrain," *Yale Journal on Regulation* 14 (1996): 300, 310.

90. See Sheryll D. Cashin, "Federalism, Welfare Reform, and the Minority Poor: Accounting for the Tyranny of State Majorities," *Columbia Law Review* 99 (1999): 552, 596–599, 612–618.

91. See Robert C. Lieberman, *Shifting the Color Line: Race and the American Welfare State* (Cambridge, Mass.: Harvard University Press, 1998), 118–176; Jill Quadagno, "From Old-Age Assistance to Supplemental Security Income: The Political Economy of Relief in the South, 1935–1972," in *The Politics of Social Policy in the United States*, edited by Margaret Wier, Ann Shola Orloff, and Theda Skocpol (Princeton, N.J.: Princeton University Press, 1988), 235–263.

92. Leiberman, *Shifting the Color Line*.

93. See David Barton Smith, *Health Care Divided: Race and Healing a Nation* (Ann Arbor: University of Michigan Press, 1999).

94. See Stephen D. Surgarman, "Welfare Reform and the Cooperative Federalism of America's Public Income Transfer Programs," *Yale Law and Policy Review* 14 (1996): 123.

95. Ibid.

96. *South Dakota v. Dole*, 483 U.S. 203, 207 (1987). Indeed, the Supreme Court has questioned whether "general welfare" imposes any enforceable restrictions on the Congress. Ibid., n. 2, citing *Buckley v. Valeo*, 424 U.S. 1, 90–91 (1976). When Congress exercises the spending power through joint federal/state programs, like Medicaid, it also must make conditions imposed on the funding clear enough so that the states know the consequences of program participation, must impose only those conditions that are in some way related to the national purpose of the program, and must not otherwise invade the state's constitutional rights. *South Dakota v. Dole*, 209.

97. This is, of course, the Tiebout hypothesis, which stems from Charles Tiebout, "A Pure Theory of Local Expenditures," *Journal of Political Economy* 64 (1956). See also Thomas R. Dye, *American Federalism: Competition among Governments* (Lexington, Mass.: Lexington Books, 1990).

98. The leading advocate of this position is Paul E. Peterson, and its classic statement is found in Paul E. Peterson and Mark C. Rom, *Welfare Magnets: A New Case for a National Standard* (Washington, D.C.: Brookings Institute, 1990).

99. See Sanford F. Schram and Samuel H. Beer, eds., *Welfare Reform: A Race to the Bottom?* (Washington, D.C.: Woodrow Wilson Center Press, 1998), a compilation of recent research on the race to the bottom hypothesis.

100. Mark Carl Rom, Paul E. Peterson, and Kenneth F. Schreve Jr., "Interstate Competition and Welfare Policy," in *Welfare Reform: A Race to the Bottom?* edited by Sanford F. Schram and Samuel H. Beer (Washington, D.C.: Woodrow Wilson Center Press, 1998), 21 (confirming earlier research showing interstate competition to avoid attracting welfare recipients), and Sanford F. Schram and Joe Soss, "Making Something out of Nothing: Welfare Reform and a New Race to the Bottom," in ibid., 83, 94–95 (summarizing studies showing little evidence of migration).

101. Schramm and Soss, "Making Something out of Nothing," 96–98.

102. See Frank J. Thompson, "Federalism and the Medicaid Challenge," in *Medicaid and Devolution*, edited by Frank J. Thompson and John J. DiIulio (Washington,

D.C.: Brookings Institute, 1998), 273 (stating that a systematic literature search discovered only one publication on the subject that found some support for the hypothesis).

103. Some states that have established programs for the uninsured, such as Minnesota and Washington, have imposed residency requirements to avoid this problem. See Department of Health and Human Services, "Eligibility Criteria and the Verification Processes," available at http://aspe.hhs.gov/health/reports/resource/eligibility_criteria. htm (cited 6 June 2002).

104. Frances Fox Piven, "Comment on Interstate Competition and Welfare Policy," in *Welfare Reform: A Race to the Bottom?* edited by Sanford F. Schram and Samuel H. Beer (Washington, D.C.: Woodrow Wilson Center Press, 1998), 43; Daphne A. Kenyon, "Health Care Reform and Competition among the States," in *Health Policy, Federalism, and the American States*, edited by Robert F. Rich and William White (Washington, D.C.: Urban Institute, 1996), 253, 264–268.

105. Kenyon, "Health Care Reform and Competition among the States," 269.

106. See John D. Donahue, *Disunited States* (New York: Basic Books, 1997), 46–48; Thompson, "Federalism and the Medicaid Challenge," 264–268.

107. See Teresa A. Coughlin and David Liska, *The Medicaid Disproportionate Share Hospital Payment Program: Background and Issues* (Washington, D.C.: Kaiser Family Foundation, 1997): Teresa A. Coughlin and Stephen Zuckerman, *States' Use of Medicaid Maximization Strategies to Tap Federal Revenues: Program Implications and Consequences* (Washington, D.C.: Urban Institute, 2002).

108. Coughlin and Liska, *The Medicare Disproportionate Share Hospital Payment Program*, 2–3.

109. Ibid., 3.

110. Leighton Ku, *Limiting Abuses of Medicaid Financing: HCFA's Plan to Regulate the Medicaid Upper Payment Level* (Washington, D.C.: Center for Budget and Policy Priorities, 2000).

111. Ibid.

112. See Vernon Smith and Eileen Ellis, *Medicaid Budgets under Stress: Survey Finds for State Fiscal Year 2000, 2001, and 2002* (Washington, D.C.: Kaiser Commission on the Uninsured, 2001); Kaiser Commission on Medicaid and the Uninsured, *The Role of Medicaid in State Budgets* (Washington, D.C.: Kaiser Commission on Medicaid and the Uninsured, 2001).

113. All except Vermont

114. Thompson, "Federalism and the Medicaid Challenge," 270.

115. Smith and Ellis, *Medicaid Budgets under Stress*, 2–3.

# 8

# Tax Credits for
# Health Insurance:
# Disentitlement of
# America's Workers?

A MERICA'S third most costly health-care entitlement program is its most effective in terms of lives covered, but also one of its most maligned. For the past half century, most Americans with health insurance have been covered through their place of employment. A major factor in bolstering employment-related insurance has been the entitlement of employers who offer and employees who purchase employment-related health insurance to sizable tax subsidies. The payments that an employer makes to purchase employment-related group health insurance for its employees are considered to be business expenses of the employer and are thus not included in the employer's taxable income.[1] Moreover, § 106 of the Internal Revenue Code provides that employment-provided health insurance is also not taxable income to the employee, while § 105 excludes from employee income the value of medical benefits purchased with employment-related insurance.[2] When these provisions are read together, they totally exempt the value of employment-related health benefits from income taxation. The value of employer-provided insurance is also excluded from payroll taxes for Social Security and Medicare. Combined, these provisions afford a tax subsidy valued at $111.2 billion in 1998 to support employment-related health insurance.[3]

Moreover, employers are not limited to offering insured benefits to their employees, but are also permitted under the tax code to exclude the costs of self-insuring their employee's health-care costs. In 2001, about one-half of all employees worked for self-insured plans.[4] The Employee Retirement Income Security Act of 1974 (ERISA) offers special protections to self-insured plans, shielding them from state insurance regulation and premium taxes.[5] Employers large enough to self-insure, therefore, can save significant costs by avoiding state mandates and taxes. They are also largely free from liability in state court if their decisions regarding benefits harm their insureds.[6] Finally, self-insured companies are permitted to obtain reinsurance to cover their losses above a maximum amount without losing their self-insured ERISA status, thus allowing them to enjoy all of the benefits of self-insured status while controlling the risks.[7]

## Criticisms of Employment-Based Health Insurance Tax Subsidies

Although employment-related health insurance covers far more Americans than do all of America's public health-care entitlement programs combined, the tax subsidies that support this system are widely criticized.[8] Health economists and conservative critics condemn the tax subsidies as inefficient, claiming that they promote excess insurance coverage, which, in turn, encourages excess consumption of health-care services and drives up health-care costs.[9] They also claim that these tax subsidies are inequitable because tax exclusions provide larger subsidies for the wealthy (who are in higher tax brackets and thus benefit more from exclusions and deductibles), much lower subsidies for those with minimal income (who pay no income taxes),[10] and no subsidies at all for those who cannot obtain employment-related insurance and must purchase their insurance in the individual market.[11]

Some conservative critics also denounce employment-related insurance as inefficient because the employer (rather than the employee) chooses the insurer and the insurance policy, and thus insureds are not allowed to choose the coverage that best meets their needs and resources.[12] That is, employees may be forced by virtue of their being part of a group to purchase more insurance than they want, or be offered less than they need, or be deprived of access to the particular providers they would choose.[13] Indeed, the employer may choose a health plan or policy strictly on the basis of cost or to suit the needs of key employees, even though the plan or policy does not suit well the needs or desires of most employees.[14] Moreover, if (as often happens) an employer changes insurers or networks while an employee is employed the employee may have no choice but to switch doctors or providers, despite long-term relationships or on-going treatment.[15]

The fact that insurance in the United States is largely employment-related is further faulted for causing "job lock"—that is, for forcing employees to remain in jobs that do not fully use their potential talents or that they would not otherwise choose, because moving to more productive or satisfying jobs would mean sacrificing insurance benefits if the prospective new employer does not offer health insurance benefits or only offers insurance subject to waiting periods or preexisting conditions clauses.[16] Indeed, an employee may be deterred from changing jobs simply because the employee's current primary care physician or specialist is not part of the network offered through the health benefits program of a different prospective employer. The fact that health insurance depends on employment is also criticized for discouraging early retirement or moves to self-employment, and for forcing spouses, who would prefer to remain out of the workforce, to become or remain employed to provide coverage for their partners who do not have insurance available through their own work.[17]

The high and continually rising cost of employment-related health insurance is also widely regarded as playing a major role in dampening wage growth in recent years, and has been criticized for making American industry less competitive with foreign countries. Economists generally agree that the cost of employment-related insurance is ultimately borne by employees; although in some circumstances, the cost might be borne, at least in the short run, by employers or passed on to consumers.[18] Thus, the competitive position of American industry is probably not substantially affected by health-care costs. It appears very likely, however, that the rapid increase in the cost of fringe benefits in the United States in recent years, and of health insurance in particular, has sopped up most of the increased value of worker productivity and contributed to constraining wage growth. Between 1970 and 1991, the years of greatest growth in health-care costs, wages and salaries of American workers grew only four-tenths of 1% in inflation-adjusted dollars, while employer health expenditures grew 234.1%.[19]

Because most employees (and apparently most employers) do not perceive health insurance as an employee expense, however, and because health insurance is in any event purchased with tax-free dollars, it is widely believed that employees and their representatives have not been as aggressive in combating increases in health-care costs as they could be. Indeed, much of the backlash against managed care in recent years might have been avoided had employees understood that managed care was saving them, rather than their employers, billions of dollars.[20]

## Why Does Employment-Related Health Insurance Persist?

The persistent popularity of employment-related health insurance is grounded in the significant advantages that it offers over other forms of private insurance. Indeed, private employment-related group insurance is common in many countries throughout the world, even where public insurance is otherwise available and private insurance is not supported by tax subsidies.[21] The simple fact is that health insurance is more available and affordable to groups than to individuals, and common employment is the most natural basis on which to form insured groups.

Employment-related group health insurance is attractive to insurers because they face less danger from adverse selection when they sell coverage to employment-related groups than they do in individual markets.[22] Persons who obtain insurance through their job are less likely to be procuring insurance because they anticipate imminent health-care costs.[23] Those healthy enough to work, moreover, are better risks than persons who are retired or otherwise not employed. Also, in general, the larger a group, the more broadly risk is spread within it, so large employment groups offer safer risk pools to insurers.

Insurers also face lower administrative costs when dealing with employers than they do when contracting with individuals (and lower costs dealing with larger employers than with smaller employers), and thus they can sell policies with lower administrative cost "loadings."[24] Much of this difference is attributable to lower marketing costs. In the individual and small group market, insurance is marketed by agents who must be paid commissions, which can consume a substantial share of the premium. Insurers also have to spend more on mass advertising when they market to individuals. Insurers in the individual and small group markets must cover the cost of underwriting and of "risk premiums" for covering riskier individuals or groups.[25] Insurers that deal with groups can offload on the human resources divisions of employers some functions, like keeping track of employee enrollment and perhaps even carrying out certain claims processing functions, which would otherwise add to the costs paid by the insurer. Employment-related insurance is thus much less expensive for large employers and their employees than for small employers and their employees, while individual policies uniformly cost the most.

Employers can also purchase health insurance at lower costs than individuals because they have greater market power and can thus drive tougher bargains with insurers.[26] Employers are sophisticated repeat players in purchasing health insurance. Employers were the major factor driving the growth of managed care in the 1980s and 1990s, and some of the most advanced have been driving the movement toward quality purchasing as well.[27] The Leapfrog Group employer consortium, for example, has committed itself to purchasing services only from providers that take certain steps to improve patient safety and reduce errors.[28]

Although the interests of employers and employees do not fully coincide when employers offer health insurance to their employees, many employers, in fact, do a reasonably good job of looking after the interests of their employees.[29] Most employees who obtain employment-related group health insurance are offered a choice of at least two health benefit packages, and many are offered several options.[30] The human resources departments of employers often see themselves as employee advocates, and they spend a fair amount of their time fielding complaints from employees and arguing with insurers on behalf of employees.[31] Of course, there are limits to how forceful employers can be in representing employees in disputes with insurers—they are also interested in holding down costs—but it would be a mistake to see employers as being interested solely in insurance cost as opposed to employee satisfaction.

As noted, much of the popularity of employment-related insurance is also attributable to the fact that, even if the cost of employment-related health insurance is borne by employees, it is largely hidden from them.[32] Few employers offer employees a choice of taking either health insurance or an additional amount of income equal to the full cost of the health insurance. Even employers who would prefer to offer their employees this choice would have to pay the employer's share of payroll taxes on the cash compensation and thus could not offer the full value of the benefits (even before the employee paid income taxes) without incurring extra expense. Employers currently pay on average 85% of single coverage and 73% of family coverage premiums, and nearly all employers pay 50% or more of premiums.[33] Thus the full cost of health insurance is rarely immediately recapturable by the employee who declines coverage.

Although economists argue convincingly that employees will in most instances bear the cost of their health insurance in the end, this reality is not sufficiently immediate to most employees to convince them to forego health insurance now in hopes of eventually gaining higher wages. Moreover, even though elaborate economic studies purport to be able to detect the cost of employment-related insurance being passed back to employees, the simple fact is that in most employment markets, employers who offer health insurance benefits also offer higher wages than those who do not offer health insurance, in large part because they are competing for better qualified employees.[34] Thus prospective employees rarely face the choice between a job with health benefits on the one hand, and another job without benefits but with fully compensating higher wages on the other.

Some of the problems noted in the preceding discussion have also been addressed in recent years through federal and state legislation. The Health Insurance Portability and Accountability Act of 1996 (HIPAA)—the major federal law addressing these problems—contained several provisions directed at increasing the portability of employment-related coverage and also at improving the functioning of the small group market, the most problematic part of the employment-related insurance market.[35] It limited the scope and duration of preexisting condition exclusions and restricted their application when an already insured employee simply moves from one employer to another, thus loosening job lock.[36] HIPAA prohibited discriminatory underwriting or differential premiums within groups and required insurers who write in the small group market to offer and guarantee renewal to any small group in the market.[37] It also required insurers in states that do not have an alternative program for insuring uninsured individuals to offer individual coverage to individuals who have previously been insured by a group insurer for at least 18 months, again reducing job lock.[38] Most states have also adopted insurance reforms in the small group market, such as requiring guaranteed offer or renewability of insurance to small groups and limiting rate differentiation, to try to make small group coverage more affordable to employers.[39]

To date, these reforms have not dramatically changed the nature of employment-related health insurance.[40] The federal reforms do not touch on the most fundamental problem with small group markets—affordability. It is one thing to require insurers to offer insurance to small groups, quite another to assure offers at an affordable price. Prohibiting preexisting condition clauses has no doubt facilitated some employment moves, but it does not help those employers who would like to move to a job that simply does not offer insurance, or those who would prefer to leave an insured employer and strike out on their own. But the federal and state reforms do make employment-related insurance, already a superior alternative to individual insurance, an even better deal for some who might not otherwise have been able to afford it or who might have otherwise been locked into a particular job because of the prospect of preexisting condition exclusions.

## The Most Significant Problem with Employment-Related Insurance

In the end, the greatest limitation of the employment-related insurance tax preference entitlement is that it does not afford Americans a right to health insurance by virtue of their citizenship or residency in the United States, but rather provides an entitlement to a tax subsidy (the value of which varies depending on the extent of the insured's tax exposure), which only benefits employees who (1) work for employers that offer health insurance benefits and (2) choose to accept those benefits (and to pay the employee's share of health insurance premiums).

Approximately 41 million Americans are currently uninsured.[41] This figure masks a much more dynamic picture however: while 44 million were uninsured at any particular point in time in 1998, and 43 million in 1997, half of those persons uninsured in 1998 were insured in 1997 and visa versa.[42] Though as many as 55 million persons lack insurance at some point or another during any given year, only 40% of the uninsured go without coverage for 18 months or more.[43] Some of the uninsured are at any one moment temporarily between insured jobs, and thus may only be uninsured for short periods of time.[44] These persons are often eligible for continuation coverage under provisions of the federal Consolidated Omnibus Budget Reconciliation Act of 1985 (COBRA) or under state law, but COBRA coverage is quite expensive, and many choose to forego it.[45] For a young person in good health with limited means, this may be a reasonable judgment. But if that person has an accident or becomes seriously ill while uninsured, the results can be financial disaster. Some 65% of the uninsured earn less than 200% of the federal poverty level, and thus they have little ability to pay should they need expensive care while uninsured.[46]

Many of the uninsured who are not employed are not likely to be employed any time soon, and their uninsured status is not likely to be temporary. Many are nearing retirement age without significant marketable skills.[47] About 37% are in poor, fair, or good health.[48] The uninsured who are of advanced age or who have chronic medical conditions not only face difficulty finding work but also with locating affordable insurance coverage (or any insurance) in the individual insurance market.[49] Figures 8–1 and 8–2 provide a summary of uninsured in the United States in March 2001.

Most of the uninsured, however—about 80%—are in families with at least one employed worker.[50] About one-quarter are in families with workers who were offered insurance by their employers, but decline it.[51] Many of those who decline insurance offered by their employers, almost two-thirds, have coverage from another source, usually through a spouse or parent but sometimes through a public program.[52] Some who refuse employer-provided insurance may also be young and healthy, and able to purchase insurance in the individual market for less than the premium share that would have to be paid to obtain employment-related coverage.[53]

Many persons who are eligible for employment-related insurance decline it without having any other source of coverage. Very few of these do so because they do not value insurance: 9% of those who declined offered coverage were otherwise uninsured, according to one recent study.[54] By contrast, about one-half of the uninsured who were offered insurance but declined coverage did so because of cost.[55] This problem is exacerbated because firms employing low-wage employees require higher employee contributions for health insurance coverage on average than do firms with higher wage employees.[56] Those who decline insurance while in poor health are left to the mercies of safety-net providers or the bankruptcy courts.[57]

Most of the uninsured, about 60%, are in families that do not have the option of obtaining employment-related insurance, however, and thus are denied the benefit of the health insurance tax preference entitlement.[58] Many of these workers are employed by firms that do not offer insurance to their employees. This is particularly true of workers employed by very small businesses. Small

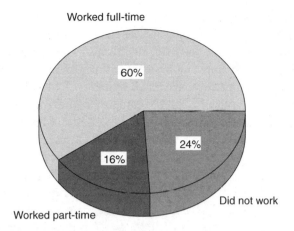

**FIGURE 8–1.** Employment status of the uninsured for entire year, 2000. *Source:* U.S. Census Bureau, Current Population Survey, March 2001.

employers face much higher insurance costs than do large employers because they cannot offer large risk pools to insurers and cannot obtain the benefits of lower insurer administrative costs available to large employers. But a more important factor may be that small employers are often found in low-skill/low-wage industries where insurance benefits are not necessary to attract qualified employees and where minimum wage laws may diminish the ability of employers to pass the costs of insurance back to employees.[59] The combined result of these factors is that the employees of small businesses often miss out on the benefits of employment-related insurance.

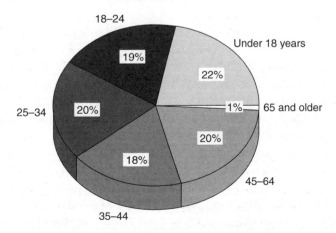

**FIGURE 8–2.** Age of the uninsured for entire year, 2000. *Source:* U.S. Census Bureau, Current Population Survey, March 2001.

Many of the working uninsured are also employed part-time or are in temporary employment arrangements, and they are not offered the insurance that is available to full-time employees.[60] Health insurance does not cost the employer any less for part-time employees than for full-time, and employers who may be forced by competitive labor market forces or by federal laws that prohibit discrimination in favor of highly compensated employees to offer insurance coverage to all full-time employees are often not required to offer it to part-time employees. Part-time and temporary employees, moreover, are often low-skill/low-wage employees who will work whether or not they have health insurance, thus competitive pressures do not force employers to cover these employees. Only 27% of employees who work fewer than 21 hours a week and 50% of those who work 21 to 34 hours a week are offered insurance by American employers, compared to 85% of full-time workers.[61]

If persons who are not offered employment-related insurance do not qualify for a public health insurance entitlement, as will likely be true for most adults, their only option will be to purchase health insurance in the individual insurance market. For those who are young and healthy and reasonably well off, this may be a realistic option. For those who are older and who have chronic medical conditions, it will only be an option if they have sufficient income to pay the high rates charged in that market. Individual insurers are quite adept at screening out high-risk applicants, and to date, state reforms have not been very effective in keeping them from doing so.[62] They also commonly engage in the practice of "reunderwriting," regularly reviewing the health of individual insureds and dropping or raising the premiums of those whose health status changes.[63] In fact, a recent Institute of Medicine report noted that one-half of all currently uninsured persons had previously had individual insurance, but had presumably lost it because it had become unaffordable or because the insurer refused to renew the policy.[64]

Although a study published in 2001 showed that individual nongroup coverage was much higher among the near-elderly than among younger groups, it also showed a recent dramatic drop in the proportion of the near-elderly moving to individual coverage upon retirement, a trend that is likely attributable to increasing premiums.[65] Another study found that 21% of individually-insured individuals aged 50 to 64 spent 10% or more of their family income on medical expenses, and almost 50% reported spending $3,500 or more each year.[66] The same study found that annual premium costs for individual policies in states that did not require community rating were twice as high for 50-year-olds as for 25-year-olds, and three to four times as high for 60-year-olds. Other studies, on the other hand, have found that many of the uninsured do have sufficient income to purchase individual insurance, and that many persons with chronic medical conditions are able to find insurance in the individual market,[67] but all studies agree that many uninsured persons cannot afford individual insurance, and that persons with serious health problems face difficulties in finding individual insurance. A person aged 60 with income at 150% of the poverty level would have to spend one-third of his income for a $1,000 deductible health insurance policy and one-half for a $250 deductible policy.[68] Thus, our nation's dependence on employment-related insurance, and the lack of viable alternatives for many uninsured, leaves us with far more persons without health insurance, and often without medical care, than are found in other nations.

## The Individual Tax Credit Solution

One much-touted approach to addressing the problems posed by employment-related insurance is to alter the nature of our tax subsidies while improving the functioning of the individual insurance market. As noted at the outset, the tax exclusions and deductions that currently undergird employment-related health insurance have received harsh criticism from health economists and from conservative health policy analysts. The alternative to the current tax preferences most frequently championed by these critics is a tax credit that could be used by individuals to purchase individual health insurance.[69]

On its face, a tax credit for the purchase of nongroup insurance would address many of the problems found in the current system. First, receipt of the tax credit would not need to be tied to employment. Thus the insured would neither be locked into a particular job nor bound by a particular employer's choice of insurers. Individuals could freely move between jobs—or even withdraw from the employment market or become self-employed—without losing health insurance coverage. The credit would allow beneficiaries to pursue their own insurance preferences. Insureds could (in theory, at least) purchase as much or as little insurance as they desired and choose the managed-care organization or insurer that best met their needs.

It is also argued that a tax credit regime would ameliorate (at least to some extent) the equity problems that attend employment-related insurance. Everyone (or everyone whose income was below a certain maximum level, depending on the proposal), would be entitled to a tax preference, not merely those who were employed by an employer who offered health insurance.[70] Moreover, the credit would either have the same nominal value to its holder regardless of income level, or it would decline in value as income increased, in contrast to the current deduction, which is more valuable to higher-income individuals.

Since the proposed credit, unlike the current deduction, would be limited in amount, recipients of the credit would be fully responsible for any amount they chose to spend above the value of the credit. Supporters of tax credits argue that this would limit the extent of overinsurance, and thus of overconsumption of health care services.[71] This would in turn, it is argued, help to contain rising health-care costs.

Tax credit proposals are another manifestation of the trends toward devolution and individualization noted elsewhere in this book. These proposals call for the devolving of health insurance purchasing from employers to individuals. They advocate the breaking down of group solidarity—even the limited solidarity currently found within our employment-related health insurance system—in favor of autonomous individual insurance coverage. While addressing some of the problems presented by employment-related insurance, they present serious new problems of their own.

First, tax credits will be of little value to most of the uninsured unless they are both fully refundable (i.e., they would have to be available whether or not the recipient actually owes taxes, like the current earned income tax credit) and advanceable (they would have to be available when premiums were due rather than at the end of the tax year as a refund). Some 45% of the uninsured do not pay any taxes against which a credit could be applied.[72] If tax credits were only available to those who otherwise paid taxes, therefore, they would do little to help the uninsured. The uninsured would also benefit little if they had to wait until the end of the tax year to collect their credits. It will be necessary for credits to be advanced throughout the tax year, either as direct payments to insurers or through diminished withholding of income and payroll taxes, to low-income beneficiaries. However, this will necessitate reconciliation between projected and actual taxes at the end of the tax year, and it might require repayment of credits. Many of the uninsured lack insurance precisely because their employment and income is continually in flux. Making stable determinations of eligibility will be difficult.[73] It is because of this uncertainty, and of the fear of having to give money back to the government, that 99% of recipients of the earned income tax credit wait until the end of the year to collect their credit rather than collecting it on a regular basis throughout the year, as they are entitled to do.[74] But if beneficiaries of the tax credit underestimate their income, and thus receive excessive credit prepayments, recouping overpayments at the end of the tax year from these beneficiaries, whose income and resources are marginal at best, will be difficult and unpopular. This problem could, in turn, be avoided by basing tax credits on income from prior years, but variability of income from year to year for many of the uninsured would make this solution also problematic.[75]

Second, even refundable and advanceable credits will be of modest value in the current individual insurance market. As noted, individual insurance policies are attended by high administrative expenses, and they cost on average far more than group policies for equivalent benefits. Insurers selling in the individual market also risk-underwrite, and individual insurance is much more expensive for older persons or persons with chronic diseases than for younger and healthier individuals. Recent studies indicate that tax credits at the levels currently being discussed would not begin to cover the cost of health insurance for any but the lowest-risk uninsureds, and that higher-risk individuals would have to spend unrealistic proportions of their family incomes to secure insurance.

One study, for example, concluded that a family with income of $30,000 would have to spend 10% to 15% of its income to purchase an average group family insurance policy if the family were given tax credits in the $2,000 to $2,500 range found in most tax credit proposals.[76] Another found that a healthy 55-year-old male earning 200% of the poverty level would have to spend 17% of his income for premiums and out-of-pocket expenses to obtain coverage with a $1,000 credit.[77] Yet another study, examining the insurance that could be bought for a $1,000 tax credit, found that a healthy nonsmoking 55-year-old woman would not be able to find a $1,000 policy in 24 of 26 of the states studied, and in the 2 states where plans were available, she would only be able to find policies with $5,000 deductibles.[78]

Third and finally, tax credits would be of value only to those persons who in fact collect and use them. The fact that nearly one-quarter of uninsured adults and two-thirds of uninsured children are currently eligible for public coverage (Medicaid or SCHIP), but have not gone to the (often considerable) effort required to apply, bodes ill for a high take-up rate for tax credits.[79] In fact, only one-quarter of those eligible for the supplemental health insurance tax credit available briefly in the early 1990s as part of the earned income tax credit actually took advantage of it.[80] Extensive—and expensive—marketing of both the tax credit program and the policies to be purchased by it, would be necessary to assure reasonable take-up.[81]

Some advocates of the tax credit approach minimize these problems, believing that associations will naturally emerge to aggregate purchasing power and risk in a manner that basically mirrors employment-related groups, or that direct marketing approaches will emerge that will reduce marketing and underwriting costs. Although association plans already exist, to date they have behaved like traditional insurers, finding it more profitable to pick off favorable risks through biased selection than to control costs.[82] Current proposals for association plans, free from regulation at the state level, also closely resemble unregulated multiple employer welfare arrangements, which engaged in extensive fraud in the 1980s until congressional hearings into abuses led to changes in Department of Labor policy and greater state regulation.[83] Association plans are likely to attract good risks away from traditional plans, causing traditional coverage rates to go up and providing little new coverage for the uninsured.[84]

Direct marketing is beginning to emerge over the Internet, but costs for many potential insureds are still high. In fact, the studies described here that found individual policies to be unaffordable generally located policies over the Internet.

Some tax credit advocates also advocate "bare-bones" policies, often with high deductibles and cost sharing. These policies might be more affordable to the uninsured than traditional insurance, but they also have very little value, and where they have been offered they have had few takers.[85] Health care for expensive conditions is already available to the uninsured through public safety-net providers or is received by the uninsured from private providers and written off as bad debt. If a "bare-bones" policy does nothing more than cover catastrophic care, it offers the poorest uninsured little that they do not already have, and it is unlikely to be worth even its modest cost.

Other tax credit advocates would couple tax credits with a highly regulated market for individual insurance, usually in some form of managed competition.[86] They would attempt to organize the market for individual insurance, perhaps requiring guaranteed issue or guaranteed renewal, or community rating, or purchasing cooperatives. This could make insurance somewhat more affordable or available, but experience with similar reforms to date has not been encouraging, and, in the end, these efforts are likely to be of marginal value.[87] Purchasing cooperatives in the small group market, for example, have broadened choice but not generally brought down prices.[88]

One of the most serious problems with proposals to support the individual market through tax credits, moreover, has yet to be mentioned—"crowd out." While tax credits are likely to make insurance affordable to some of the uninsured, they are also likely to encourage some employers to drop coverage they currently offer, and to cause some low-risk persons currently covered through their employers to drop their employer-based coverage, seeking coverage instead in the individual market. One study calculates that a program offering refundable tax credits of $1,000 for individuals and $2,000 for families would be taken up by 18.4 million Americans, but that the number of uninsured would fall by only about 4 million, as many of those who took up the credits would be those already currently insured, while others currently insured would lose insurance altogether as their employers dropped health insurance.[89] People with incomes under 100% of poverty level make up 45% of the uninsured, but only 1.3 million of these would take up the tax credits at the levels studied, and those under the poverty level would benefit from only 26% of the net spending on credits.[90] More generous individual tax credit proposals might extend coverage to 9 to 13 million currently uninsured persons, but would do so at a cost of $2,500 to $3,100 per year per newly insured person.[91] Those left behind in employment-based insurance in the wake of individual tax credits are likely to be those whose care is the most expensive, which will further undermine the viability of the employment-based insurance market.

There are ways of dealing with the crowd-out issue. For example, tax credits could be targeted only to those who are currently uninsured. Implementing such a scheme would be difficult, however, because there is so much mobility presently between insured and uninsured status. Denying credits to those already insured would also reward employees and employers who had not previously attempted to secure insurance and punish those who had. Moreover, a program to identify those who dropped insurance (or were dropped from insurance) simply to qualify for the credit would be costly and difficult to administer, and it would discourage participation in the new plan even by those who could qualify for it.[92] Alternatively, the tax credit could be made available to also cover those who receive insurance through their employer.[93] This strategy may be the most promising, as it would take advantage of the economies inherent in the group market, and would be more equitable than the current deduction. It has garnered considerable interest from more liberal members of Congress in the recent past.[94] Any tax credit program that covers significant numbers of those currently uninsured, however, is going to cost a great deal in terms of additional lives insured.

If one builds sufficiently intricate tax and regulatory programs, it might be possible that some additional uninsured persons might procure valuable insurance coverage at an affordable cost through the use of tax credits. But what would be the cost in terms of damage to our existing system (which, in the end, covers most of our population reasonably well)? And how much would the new system increase administrative costs (which make no additional health care available)?[95] And do we really want to turn over the administration of our nations' health insurance system to the Internal Revenue Service, the most likely candidate to oversee the tax credit system?

## Conclusion

Although the United States has never developed a system of universal health coverage for all of its residents, it has developed a system of tax subsidies that covers most of its working age residents and their families through employment-related insurance. Because this system encourages group solidarity at the employer level, it deals reasonably effectively with the problems of biased selection that bedevil individual health insurance markets. It is a system with many faults, but its great virtue is that it has extended insurance to 172 million Americans, far more than have been reached by the individual insurance market, and even more than are covered by public insurance.

Our current employment-based health insurance system is plagued by many problems. Most of these—inequity of distribution of benefits, job lock, and dampening effects on wage growth—would be solved if we embraced a social insurance or national health insurance system. In no other country, for example, is job lock a major concern; nor do the wealthy receive more public subsidies for their health insurance than the poor. In most countries, financing of health insurance is progressive, not regressive as in the United States. Yet the proposals currently being debated for devolution and individualization head in the wrong direction. They would only modestly expand coverage at best, would do little for the sick and elderly uninsured (those most in need of coverage), and might well destroy a system that currently works reasonably well. What we need, rather, is a program that will build on, not tear down, what we already have.

Fortunately, in designing such a system, we are not alone. We can look to over a century of experience that other countries have had in designing and operating health-care systems based on entitlements. To see what we can learn, we now turn to the two major models of health-care finance that have emerged for doing this: national health service models, exemplified by the British National Health Service; and social insurance models, exemplified by the German social health insurance system.

# Notes

1. 26 U.S.C. § 162(a); 26 C.F.R. § 1.162-10.(a).

2. While 26 U.S.C. § 105(a) in fact states that payments from health insurance are included in gross income, § 105(b) excludes from gross income insurance payments for medical expenses of the taxpayer and the taxpayer's spouse, children, or other dependents.

3. John Sheils and Paul Hogan, "Cost of Tax-Exempt Health Benefits in 1998," *Health Affairs* 18, no. 2 (March/April 1999): 176–181. A more recent estimate puts the cost at $140 billion; see Stuart M. Butler, "Right Diagnosis, Wrong Prescription," *Health Affairs* 21, no 4 (July/August 2002): 101–102. While this chapter focuses on the federal tax subsidy, most states that have income taxes base their income taxation on federal taxable income or federal adjusted gross income and would, therefore, also exclude from income taxation employer payments for health insurance. State tax expenditures for employment-related health insurance amounted to $13.6 billion in 1998. Ibid.

4. Kaiser Family Foundation and Health Research and Education Trust (HRET), *Employer Health Benefits, 2001 Survey* (Washington, D.C.: Kaiser Family Foundation, 2001), 130.

5. See 29 U.S.C. § 1104(a); Barry Furrow et al., *Health Law*, 2nd ed. (St. Paul, Minn.: West Group, 2000), §§ 8-3–8-4.

6. Furrow et al, *Health Law*, § 8-5.

7. Ibid., § 8-3(b).

8. See, e.g., Grace-Marie Arnett, ed., *Empowering Health Care Consumers through Tax Reform* (Ann Arbor: University of Michigan Press, 1999); Stuart M. Butler and Edmund F. Haislmaier, *A National Health System for America* (Washington, D.C.: Heritage Foundation, 1989).

9. See Michael Tanner, "What's Wrong with the Present System?" in *Empowering Health Care Consumers through Tax Reform*, 27–34. The classic statement of the the-

sis that excessive insurance causes welfare loss is found in Mark V. Pauly, "The Economics of Moral Hazard: Comment," *American Economic Review* 58, no. 40 (1968): 531–537.

10. In 1998 the health insurance tax exclusions resulted in annual tax expenditures of $2,357 for a family earning $100,000 or more and $71 for a family earning less than $15,000. The nation spent $26.2 billion in tax expenditures for families earning $100,000 or more and $1.4 billion for families earning less than $15,000. Sheils and Hogan, "Cost of Tax-Exempt Health Benefits in 1998," 180.

11. Two exceptions to this general statement are the self-employed, who may from 2003 deduct the cost of health insurance from their income, subject to certain limits, under 26 U.S.C. § 162(1); and those whose medical expenses, including insurance premiums, exceed 7.5% of their adjusted gross income, who may deduct medical costs above that amount under 26 U.S.C. § 213.

12. See Mark Pauly, Allison Percy, and Bradley Herring, "Individual versus Job-Based Health Insurance: Weighing the Pros and Cons," *Health Affairs* 18 (1999): 28–34.

13. David Hyman and Mark Hall, "Two Cheers for Employment-Based Insurance," *Yale Journal of Health Policy, Law, and Ethics* 2 (2001): 27–57.

14. See, exploring the "reverse agency" problem of employer purchase of employee insurance, Dayna B. Matthew, "Controlling the Reverse Agency Costs of Employment-Based Health Insurance: Of Markets, Courts, and a Regulatory Quagmire," *Wake Forest Law Review* 31 (1996): 1037.

15. See Thomas Bodenheimer and Kip Sullivan, "How Large Employers Are Shaping the Health Care Marketplace—Part I," *New England Journal of Medicine* 338 (1998): 1003–1007.

16. See Jonathan Gruber and Brigitte C. Mandrian, *Health Insurance, Labor Supply, and Job Mobility: A Critical Review of the Literature* (Washington, D.C.: National Bureau of Economic Research, 2002); Jonathan Gruber, *Health Insurance and the Labor Market* (Washington, D.C.: National Bureau of Economic Research, 1998).

17. Gruber and Mandrian, *Health Insurance, Labor Supply, and Job Mobility*, 8–15, 19–22.

18. Mark V. Pauly, *Health Benefits at Work: An Economic and Political Analysis of Employment-Based Health Insurance* (Ann Arbor: University of Michigan Press, 1997); Alan B. Krueger and Uwe E. Reinhardt, "The Economics of Employer versus Individual Mandates," *Health Affairs* 13 (spring 1994): 34–53.

19. Cathy A. Cowan and Patricia A. McDonnell, "Business, Households and Government Spending, 1991," *Health Care Financing Review* 14, no. 3 (spring 1993): 238.

20. Hyman and Hall, "Two Cheers for Employment-Based Insurance," 28.

21. Employer-related group private insurance is common, for example, in France, where it insures cost-sharing obligations imposed under the social insurance scheme; in the United Kingdom, where it permits insurers to avoid the National Health Service queues; and in Canada, where it covers services not covered by the national health scheme. See Timothy Stoltzfus Jost, "Private or Public Approaches to Insuring the Uninsured: Lessons from International Experience with Private Insurance," *New York University Law Review* 76 (2001): 419.

22. See Hyman and Hall, "Two Cheers for Employment-Based Insurance," 31–33; Uwe E. Reinhardt, "Employer-Based Health Insurance: A Balance Sheet," *Health Affairs* 18 (November/December 1999): 125–126. The advantages with respect to risk pooling that groups, and in particular small groups, afford over nongroup policies may be exaggerated in most accounts. See Mary Pauly and Bradley Herring, *Pooling Health Insurance Risks* (Washington, D.C.: American Enterprise Institute Press, 1999).

23. Insurers can protect themselves further against adverse selection in the group market by requiring that a certain percentage of employees be enrolled or by only allowing new enrollment during specified open enrollment periods, as well as through the use of waiting periods and preexisting condition clauses also used in the individual market.

24. Pauly et al., "Job-Based Health," 33–35; Institute of Medicine, *Employment and Health Benefits: A Connection at Risk* (Washington, D.C.: National Academy Press, 1993), 108–111; Hyman and Hall, "Two Cheers for Employment-Based Insurance," 31.

25. Mark A. Hall, *Reforming Private Health Insurance* (Washington, D.C.: American Enterprise Institute Press, 1994), 6.

26. See James Maxwell and Peter Temin, "Managed Competition versus Industrial Purchasing of Health Care among the Fortune 500," *Journal of Health Politics, Policy, and Law* 27 (2002): 5–30 (documenting that large American businesses use their market power to purchase health insurance like other resources).

27. See William S. Custer, Charles N. Kahn III, and Thomas F. Wildsmith IV, "Why We Should Keep the Employment-Based Health Insurance System," *Health Affairs* 18 (November/December 1999): 119; Hyman and Hall,"Two Cheers for Employment-Based Insurance," 34–35.

28. See the Leapfrog Group, *Patient Safety*, available at http://www.leapfrog-group.org/safety1.htm (cited 19 June 2002).

29. See Pamela B. Peele, Judity R. Lave, Jeanne T. Black, and John H. Evans III, "Employer Sponsored Health Insurance: Are Employers Good Agents for Their Employees?" *Milbank Quarterly* 78 (2000): 5–21.

30. In 2001, 60% of employees had a choice of two or more plans available. Thomas Rice et al., "Workers and Their Health Plans: Free to Choose?" *Health Affairs* 21 (2002): 184.

31. Institute of Medicine, *Employment and Health Benefits*, 146–147; Judith R. Lave et al., "Changing the Employer-Sponsored Health Plan System: The View of Employees of Large Firms," *Health Affairs* 18 (2001): 114–115.

32. See Pauly, *Health Benefits at Work*.

33. Kaiser Family Foundation and HRET, *Employer Health Benefits, 2001 Survey*, 84.

34. This fact is reflected in studies that show that the demand of employers for health insurance is more related to worker characteristics, especially income, than to insurance price. M. Susan Marquis and Stephen H. Long, "To Offer or Not to Offer: The Role of Price in Employer's Health Insurance Decisions," *Health Services Research* 36, no. 5 (October 2001): 935–958.

35. See Furrow et al., *Health Law*, § 9-7.

36. 29 U.S.C. § 1181(a); 42 U.S.C. § 300gg-41(a).

37. 29 U.S.C. § 1182(a)–(b); 42 U.S.C. § 300gg-11(a)(1).

38. 42 U.S.C. §§ 300gg-41(a), (b), and (c) and 300gg-44.

39. See Jost, "Private or Public Approaches," 465–466.

40. See M. Susan Marquis and Stephen H. Long, "Effects of 'Second Generation' Small Group Health Insurance Reforms, 1993 to 1997," *Inquiry* 38 (2001/2002): 365–380; Mark A. Hall, "The Competitive Impact of Small Group Health Insurance Reforms," *University of Michigan Journal of Law Reform* 32 (1999): 685.

41. Department of Commerce, "Numbers of Americans with or without Health Insurance Rise, Census Bureau Reports," available at http://www.census.gov/Press-Release/www/2002/C602-127.html (cited October 16, 2002.)

42. Sherry A. Glied, "Challenge and Options for Increasing the Number of Americans with Health Insurance," *Inquiry* 38 (summer 2001): 92.

43. Ibid.

44. See Katherine Swartz, "Dynamics of People without Health Insurance," *Journal of American Medical Association* 271, no. 1 (1994): 64–66.

45. COBRA recipients must pay a premium equal to 102% of the total premium, including the employer's share, that would have been paid to the insurer for the recipient's insurance prior to the losing coverage (or of a self-insured employer's cost for insuring the recipient). This would often be far more than the employee was in fact paying prior to losing coverage. See 42 U.S.C. §§ 1162(3) and 1164. COBRA also only covers employers who employ 20 or more employees on a typical business day and have a group health plan.

46. Institute of Medicine, *Coverage Matters: Insurance and Health Care* (Washington, D.C.: National Academy Press, 2001), 62–63.

47. Glied, "Challenge and Options," 93. See also Marie C. Reed and Ha T. Tu, "Triple Jeopardy: Low Income, Chronically Ill and Uninsured in America," in Center for Studying Health System Change, available at www.hschange.org/CONTENT/411 (cited February 2002).

48. Glied, "Challenge and Options," 92.

49. See Jon Gabel et al, "Individual Insurance: How Much Financial Protection Does It Provide?" *Health Affairs Web Exclusive*, available at http://www.healthaffairs.org/WebExclusives/Gabel_Web_Excl_041702.htm (cited June 24, 2001); Families USA, "A 10-Foot Rope for a 40-Foot Hole," *Families USA* (Washington, D.C.: Families USA, 2002); Elisabeth Simantov, Cathy Schoen, and Stephanie Bruegman, "Market Failure: Individual Insurance Markets for Older Americans," *Health Affairs* 20 (July/August 2001): 139–148.

50. Glied, "Challenge and Options," 91.

51. Ibid.

52. Some 63% those who decline employer-offered insurance have employer-sponsored insurance through another source. Linda J. Blumberg and Len M. Nichols, "The Health Status of Workers Who Decline Employer-Sponsored Insurance," *Health Affairs* 20 (November/December 2001): 181.

53. About 2% of those who decline insurance receive "private, nongroup" coverage, and 55% of those who decline coverage are under the age of 34. Ibid., 182.

54. E. Richard Brown et al., *The State of Health Insurance in California* (Los Angeles: UCLA Center for Health Policy Research, 2002), 40.

55. Ibid. Others turned it down because they preferred to take higher pay instead, because they did not like the plan offered by their employer, because of concerns about immigration status, or for other reasons.

56. Kaiser Family Foundation and HRET, *Employer Health Benefits, 2001 Survey*, 93.

57. Approximately one-quarter of families filing for bankruptcy identify illness or injury as a reason for filing. Melissa B. Jacoby, Teresa A. Sullivan, and Elizabeth Warren, "Rethinking the Debates over Health Care Financing: Evidence from the Bankruptcy Courts," *New York University Law Review* 76 (2001): 387.

58. Glied, "Challenge and Options," 91.

59. Institute of Medicine, *Coverage Matters: Insurance and Health Care*, 97; Pauly, *Health Benefits at Work*, 100–104.

60. Institute of Medicine, *Coverage Matters: Insurance and Health Care*, 61.

61. Paul Fronstin, "Trends in Health Insurance Coverage: A Look at Early 2001 Data," *Health Affairs* 21 (January/February 2002): 191.

62. Katherine Schwartz, "Markets for Individual Health Insurance: Can We Make Them Work with Incentives to Purchase Insurance?" *Inquiry* 38 (2001): 133–145.

63. See "National Insurance Group Criticizes Reunderwriting Practice," *Kaiser Daily Health Policy Report*, June 12, 2002.

64. Institute of Medicine, *Coverage Matters: Insurance and Health Care*, 49.

65. Michael A. Morrisey and Gail A. Jensen, "The Near-Elderly, Early Retirees, and Managed Care," *Health Affairs* 20 (November/December 2001): 197–206.

66. Simantov et al., "Market Failure," 144.

67. Ibid., 146.

68. See M. Kate Bundorf and Mark V. Pauly, *Is Health Insurance Affordable for the Uninsured?* (Cambridge, Mass: National Bureau of Economic Research, 2002); Mark V. Pauly and Len M. Nichols, "The Nongroup Health Insurance Market: Short on Facts, Long on Opinions and Policy Disputes," *Health Affairs* Web Exclusive, http://www.healthaffairs.org/WebExclusives/Nongrp_TOC.htm (Cited October 24, 2002).

69. See, for a small sampling of recent proposals for tax credits, Lawrence Zelenak, "A Health Insurance Tax Credit for Uninsured Workers," *Inquiry* 38 (2001): 106–120; Arnett, *Empowering Health Care Consumers through Tax Reform*; National Association of Health Underwriters, Health Credit *One-Page Summary*, available at www.nahu.org/government/issues/tax_credits/summary.htm (cited June 6, 2002); Stuart M. Butler, "Reforming the Tax Treatment of Health Care to Achieve Universal Coverage," in *Covering America: Real Remedies for the Uninsured*, edited by Jack Meyer and Elliott Wicks (Washington, D.C.: Economic and Social Research Institute, 2001): 23–71; Mark V. Pauly, "An Adaptive Credit Plan for Covering the Uninsured," in ibid., 137–152; Lynn Etheredge, "A Flexible Benefits Tax Credit for Health Insurance and More," *Health Affairs* 20, no. 3 (2002): 8. See also Jost, "Private or Public Approaches," 420–421; William J. Scanlon, *Health Insurance: Proposals for Expanding Private and Public Coverage*, GAO-01-481T (Washington, D.C.: General Accounting Office (describing other proposals). Although proposals for replacing tax deductions with tax credits have not found general legislative support, tax credit proposals for dealing with specific groups have made some progress. H.R. 3009, which reestablished fast-track trade negotiating authority in the summer of 2002, for example, included tax credits for covering up to 65% of the cost of COBRA continuation coverage or the cost of state-sponsored high-risk pool or purchasing pool coverage for displaced workers.

70. Proposals often provide for a phase-out once income exceeds a certain level, usually pegged to some percentage (e.g. 200%) of the poverty level. See Lawrence Zelenak, "A Health Insurance Credit for Uninsured Workers," *Inquiry* 38 (summer 2001): 109. This is similar to the current earned income tax credit.

71. C. Eugene Steuerle and Gordon B. T. Mermin, "A Better Subsidy for Health Insurance," in *Empowering Health Care Consumers through Tax Reform*, edited by Grace-Marie Arnett (Ann Arbor: University of Michigan Press, 1999), 81.

72. Jonathan Gruber and Larry Levitt, "Tax Subsidies for Health Insurance: Costs and Benefits," *Health Affairs* 19 (2000): 73.

73. See Linda Blumberg, *Health Insurance Tax Credits: Potential for Expanding Coverage* (Washington, D.C.: Urban Institute, 2001): 4; Zelenak, "A Health Insurance Credit for Uninsured Workers," 110–111.

74. Scanlon, "Health Insurance," 8.

75. This idea has been proposed by the Bush Administration. See, Robert Cunningham, "Joint Custody: Bipartisan Interest Expands Scope Of Tax-Credit Proposals" *Health Affairs*, Web Exclusive, available at http://www.healthaffairs.org/WebExclusives/Cunningham_Web_Excl_091802.htm (cited October 24, 2002): w292.

76. Iris J. Lav and Joel Friedman, *Tax Credits for Individuals to Buy Health Insurance Won't Help Many Uninsured Families* (Washington, D.C.: Center for Budget and Policy Priorities, 2001).

77. Gabel et al., "Individual Insurance," W179.

78. Families USA, "A 10-Foot Rope for a 40-Foot Hole," 81.

79. Glied, "Challenge and Options," 93.

80. Zelenak, "A Health Insurance Credit for Uninsured Workers," 107.

81. Glied, "Challenge and Options," 99.

82. Mark A Hall, Elliot K. Wicks, and Janice S. Lawlor, "HealthMarts, HIPCs, MEWAs, and AHPs: A Guide for the Perplexed," *Health Affairs* 20 (January/February 2001): 142–152.

83. Eleanor Hill and Anne Schott, "Association Health Plan Provisions of H.R. 2990: Preemption of State Oversight Would Place Consumers and Small Employers at Risk," available at http://bcbshealthissues.com/relatives/19504.pdf (cited June 24, 2002).

84. James R. Baumgardner and Stuart A. Hagan, "Predicting Response to Regulatory Change in Small Group Health Insurance Market: The Case of Association Health Plans and Health Marts," *Inquiry* 38 (winter 2001–2002): 351–364.

85. Sherry Glied, Cathi Callahan, James Mays, and Jennifer N. Edwards, *Bare-Bones Health Plans: Are They Worth the Money?* (Washington, D.C.: Commonwealth Fund, 2002).

86. This model has traditionally been associated with Alain Enthoven. For a recent version of his approach, see Sara J. Singer, Alan M. Garber, and Alain C. Enthoven, "Near-Universal Coverage through Health Plan Competition," in *Covering America: Real Remedies for the Uninsured*, edited by Jack Meyer and Elliott Wicks (Washington, D.C.: Economic and Social Research Institute, 2001), 155–171.

87. See Elliot K. Wicks, Mark A. Hall, and Jack A. Meyer, "Barriers to Small-Group Purchasing Cooperatives" (Washington, D.C.: Economic and Social Research Institute, 2000); Stephen H. Long and M. Susan Marquis, "Have Small-Group Health Insurance Purchasing Alliances Increased Coverage?" *Health Affairs* 20 (October 2001): 154–160.

88. Long and Marquis, "Have Small-Group Health Insurance Purchasing Alliances Increased Coverage?"

89. Jonathan Gruber and Larry Levitt, "Tax Subsidies for Health Insurance: Costs and Benefits," *Health Affairs* 19, no. 1 (2001): 75–76.

90. Ibid., 77

91. See Glied, "Challenge and Options," 99.

92. Ibid., 96.

93. See, e.g., Jack A. Meyer and Elliot K. Wicks, "A Federal Tax Credit to Encourage Employers to Offer Health Coverage," *Inquiry* 38, no. 2 (2001): 202–213.

94. Cunningham, "Joint Custody."

95. See Jack A. Meyer, Sharon Silow-Carroll, and Elliot K. Wicks, *Tax Reform to Expand Health Coverage: Administrative Issues and Challenges* (Washington, D.C.: Kaiser Family Foundation, 2000) (describing administrative issues).

# 9

# The British National
# Health Service:
# The General
# Revenue-Financed
# Model of Health-Care
# Entitlements

THE British National Health Service (NHS) is generally regarded as the archetypical example of the national health service, general revenue financed, model of health-care financing and provision.[1] The hallmarks of the British "Beveridge model" are payment for health-care services from general taxes and direct government provision of health care. Neither of these characteristics exists purely in the British system. Although the health-care system is funded primarily through general revenue funding, about 12% of funding comes from national insurance contributions, a payroll tax that is a holdover from the pre-NHS days that funds various social security programs, and 6.3% is funded by user charges.[2] Also, most British general practitioners (GPs) are not government employees, but own their own practices as individuals or groups and provide services to the NHS on a contracted basis.[3] The NHS, moreover, has increasingly turned to private ownership of NHS hospitals as a means of financing new construction, and has begun to purchase services from private hospitals as well.[4] In general, however, the British system represents this model of health service provision, with its strong and weak points.

The British NHS was not the world's first public health service. Public ownership and provision of health-care services had developed in U.S.S.R. during the Communist period, and national health services were established in Costa Rica, New Zealand, and Mexico in the late 1930s and early 1940s.[5] The U.K., however, became the primary leader and example in a series of national transitions from social insurance to national health service funding of health services that continued for much of the second half of the twentieth century. Canada established its national health insurance program in 1968, Sweden in 1969, Denmark in 1973, Australia in 1975 and again in 1983, Italy in 1978, Portugal in 1979, Greece in 1983, and Spain in 1986.

We can learn much from the positive features of the British system in our study of entitlements. Britain has been very effective in holding down healthcare costs. It has also achieved much more equitable access to health care than has the United States. In turn, its emphasis on care of populations has facilitated an emphasis on primary care and coordination of care. It has also maintained a level of clinical freedom that has all but disappeared in the United States. Finally, its centralized organization allows it to attack systemwide problems in a more rapid and coordinated fashion than is possible in less centralized systems. But the British NHS also has its problems—in particular, the prevalence of waiting lists and the absence of the most modern technology. The system also exhausts considerable energy in continuous reorganization. After examining the history and structure of the NHS, I will turn to these issues.

## A Brief History of the NHS

Public provision of health care in England dates back to the 1834 poor laws, which required the appointment of a parish medical officer to look after the needs of the sick poor.[6] The poor laws also provided for the care of the sick in workhouses, some of which evolved into municipal hospitals.[7] The Local Government Act of 1929, which repealed the poor laws, authorized the establishment of municipal hospitals, which thereafter appeared in some localities. More common were voluntary hospitals, some of which dated back to the twelfth century.[8] The most prestigious voluntary hospitals were established by eminent patrons or charitable or religious societies to serve indigents and were staffed by consultants (specialist physicians) on a voluntary basis.[9] Although the consultants were usually not paid for their work in the hospitals, consultant status was highly beneficial in securing private business. Primary care was provided by general practitioners in the community, who would refer difficult cases to specialists.[10] Until medical registration reforms of 1858, the public also had access to a wide variety of alternative healers of varying persuasions and reputations.[11]

The British established a social insurance program in 1911 to insure workers for sick pay and general medical services.[12] It was a very limited and on the whole unsatisfactory program. It initially only covered 27% of the population, increasing to 43% by 1938.[13] It did not cover hospital or specialist services or the families and dependents of workers.[14] More affluent British workers had been covered since the nineteenth century by mutual insurance through the Friendly Societies.[15] But by the end of the war, there was a general understanding that more was needed, a belief promoted by the prestigious 1943 report of Lord Beveridge.[16]

Several developments came together at the end of the war that created a propitious environment for the founding of an NHS.[17] First, the British healthcare system entering the war was outdated, poorly organized, and totally inadequate in its provision for the poor, and it suffered further destruction during the war.[18] Second, Britain had in general a high degree of confidence in the national government coming out of World War II, and in particular had been impressed with the functioning of the Emergency Medical Service during the war.[19] Third, the Labor Party won an overwhelming and decisive electoral victory in the summer of 1945, affording it the power to create a national health service of its own design with minimal need to compromise.[20] The new Labor government struck out on a bold new path to create a socialized health service run from the center, though it did concede to some of the demands of the doctors, including independent contractor status for GPs and continuation of a right to private practice for specialists.[21] Finally, the postwar Labor Minister of Health, Aneurin Bevan, was a dynamic, forceful, and persistent leader, who was able to stamp on the NHS his own vision of a comprehensive national health service that persisted for much of the next half century.[22] The NHS came into existence in 1948.

## Organization of the NHS

The British National Health Service is one of the largest employers in the world, with around one million employees.[23] It spends over £60 billion a year. It is in a continual state of reorganization, an issue that will be addressed later in this chapter. The NHS is overseen by the Department of Health, which, in turn, is headed by the Secretary of State for Health.[24] The NHS executive has offices in Leeds and London and in eight regional offices throughout the country. These eight regional offices are being combined into four under the most recent reorganization as of this writing.[25] The Department of Health develops an annual budget for the NHS and distributes these funds throughout the NHS. It sets policy and practices for the NHS, provides guidance and support to the health authorities, and monitors performance.[26]

At the local level, the English NHS has always been directed by local health authorities, which were responsible for identifying and planning for the health needs of local residents and for making arrangements for services to be provided by NHS hospitals, primary care providers, and other agencies.[27] In Scotland this role has been carried out by health boards and in Northern Ireland by health and social services boards. In the 1990s, Margaret Thatcher's reorganization of the health service attempted to create an internal market by identifying the health authorities as "purchasers" and separating off the hospitals into separate provider organizations as NHS trusts.[28] With Labor's return to power in 1997, the notion of an internal market fell out of favor, even though the separation of purchaser and provider functions continued.

Under the government's most recent plan for NHS reorganization (as of this writing), England's 95 health authorities are to be combined into 28 "strategic health authorities."[29] The task of the strategic health authorities is to "lead the strategic development of the local health service and performance manage PCTs [primary care trusts] and NHS Trusts on the basis of local accountability agreements."[30] The strategic health authorities are responsible for establishing performance agreements with local PCTs and NHS trusts, and for monitoring compliance with these agreements.[31] The authorities are also responsible for allocating discretionary capital investment funds for future development of services.[32]

NHS trusts were established during the Thatcher reforms as self-governing hospitals. Although they are answerable to the Secretary of State for Health, they are essentially semi-autonomous, nongovernmental organizations.[33] While their primary task is running hospitals, they can also provide services in the community through health centers or clinics or in people's homes.[34] In Great Britain, unlike the United States or Germany, specialists are found almost exclusively within hospitals. GPs in the community serve a gatekeeper function, seeing patients initially and referring them to hospitals for outpatient specialists consultations, or perhaps for inpatient admission, as needed.

Primary care trusts are a creation of the government of Tony Blair, and are based essentially on a reconceptualization of Thatcher's internal market. Under the most recent reorganization, PCTs will be the "most local NHS organization" and will be "led by clinicians and local people."[35] They will control three-quarters of NHS funding and will be responsible for "commissioning" (that is, purchasing) services for their constituents from primary care providers (GPs, pharmacists, dentists, and optometrists), from community care providers, and from the NHS trusts.[36] They are also responsible for integrating health and social care.[37]

Over 99% of the U.K. population is registered with a GP.[38] GPs are responsible for about 90% of the contacts between patients and the NHS.[39] Community nurses, health visitors, dentists, opticians, pharmacists, and specialist therapists also work in the community, sometimes in teams together with GPs.[40] The NHS has also recently launched NHS Direct, which provides advice and referral over the telephone.

## The Nature of the NHS Entitlement

The NHS was founded on a vision of providing a comprehensive, publicly funded services, free at point-of-service delivery:

> Every man and woman and child can rely on getting all the advice and treatment and care which they need in matters of personal health; that what they get shall be the best . . . ; that their getting these shall not depend on whether than can pay for them, or any other factor irrelevant to the real need. . . . The service must be "comprehensive" in two senses—first, that it is available to all people and second, that it covers all necessary forms of health care.[41]

Section 1(1) of the National Health Service Act of 1946 and 1977 imposes on the Secretary of State (for Health), a duty

> to continue the promotion in England and Wales of a comprehensive health service, designed to secure improvement (a) in the physical and mental health of the people of those countries, and (b) in the prevention, diagnosis and treatment of illness, and for that purpose to propose to provide or secure the effective provision of services in accordance with this Act.

Section 3 continues:

> it is the Secretary of State's duty to provide . . . to such extent as he considers necessary to meet all reasonable requirements: (a) hospital accommodation; (b) other accommodation for the purpose of any service specified under this Act; (c) medical, dental, nursing and ambulance services; (d) such other facilities for the care of expectant and nursing mothers and young children as he considers are appropriate as part of the health service; (e) such facilities for the prevention of illness, the care of persons suffering from illness and the after-care of persons who have suffered from illness as he considers appropriate as part of the health service; [and](f) such other services as are required for the diagnosis and treatment of illness.

Although the National Health Service Act articulates aspirations and imposes obligations, it does not confer individual entitlements. No British man or woman is entitled to any particular service at the hands of the National Health Service.[42] In the words of an eminent group of British health policy analysts:

> One of the defining characteristics of the NHS—in contrast to many other health care systems—remains its repudiation of any notion of entitlements. Patients may have a right of access to health care, but, once access has been achieved, it is for providers to decide what treatment (if any) to offer within the constraints of the available resources.[43]

Tellingly, the Labor government has replaced the Patient's Charter, initiated in 1995 by the Thatcher government as a national patient "bill of rights," with a brochure that describes what patients can expect from the NHS.[44] But even the Patient's Charter was more a list of aspirations than a guarantee of rights.

Although NHS patients do not have a legal entitlement, the NHS, or more precisely the Department of Health and the Secretary of State who heads it, have a political obligation to fulfill the vision of the NHS. This obligation, as a political obligation, is taken very seriously by the British public. The public has a sense of ownership of the NHS that is quite different from the relationship that Americans have to their health-care system. During the year 2000, some 18,154 items (articles, letters, and editorials) mentioning the NHS appeared in the three dozen British papers that make up the British Westnews database, an average of more than one article per day per paper. These items represent a broad range of opinion and cover a wide variety of topics, but they uniformly show a concern about the operation and future of the NHS. In general, they recognize that there are limits to what the NHS can do—that it has limited resources and cannot give everybody every possible service. However, commentary on the NHS also evidences irritation, disappointment, even disillusionment with its many deficiencies.

Just because no individual has entitlement claims against the NHS does not mean that the law plays no role in NHS governance. In fact, the NHS is subject to a variety of legal constraints and is periodically called to account in the courts.

Basically, the NHS is a government agency and is thus subject to administrative law. Under British administrative law, a government agency must act legally, rationally, and in accordance with proper procedures.[45] These standards, however, are not unduly difficult to meet.

As has already been noted, the DOH is obligated to fund and to provide through the NHS "a comprehensive health service." It is conceivable, therefore, that the failure of the NHS to provide a particular service to a particular patient could be found to violate these statutory obligations. The statutes, however, are quite vague in the obligations they create, and the courts have traditionally declined the invitation to make them more specific.[46]

For example, the Court of Appeals stated in a recent case examining the duty established by § 3 of the National Health Act:

> the Secretary of State's section 3 duty is subject to two different qualifications. First of all there is the initial qualification that his obligation is limited to providing the services identified to the extent that he considers that they are necessary to meet all reasonable requirements. In addition there is a qualification in that he has to consider whether they are appropriate to be provided as part of the health service.

The first qualification placed on the duty contained in section 3 makes it clear that there is scope for the Secretary of State to exercise a degree of judgment as to the circumstances in which he will provide the services. . . . When exercising his judgment he has to bear in mind the comprehensive service which he is under a duty to promote as set out in section 1. However, as long as he pays due regard to that duty, the fact that the service will not be comprehensive does not mean that he is necessarily contravening either section 1 or section 3 . . . [A] comprehensive health service may never, for human, financial, or other resource reasons, be achievable. . . .

In exercising his judgment, the Secretary of State is entitled to take into account the resources available to him and the demands on those resources.[47]

The British courts have also not been particularly demanding when reviewing NHS decisions from the standpoint of rationality. The British standard of irrationality—*Wednesbury* unreasonableness[48]—is much like our own standard of arbitrary and capricious action. Lord Diplock defined it as follows:

It applies to a decision which is so outrageous in its defiance of logic or of acceptable moral standards that no sensible person who had applied his mind to the question to be decided could have arrived at it.[49]

In early cases, the courts demonstrated extraordinary deference in applying this standard to the NHS. In one of the most notorious cases, *R v. Central Birmingham Health Authority, ex parte Collier*, the Court of Appeal was asked to order the Health Authority to perform an operation on a four-year-old boy with a hole in his heart, whose surgery had been scheduled and canceled three times, and whose physician testified that "he desperately needed open heart surgery." In declining to intervene, the Court stated:

Even assuming that [the evidence] does establish that there is immediate danger to health . . . this court is in no position to judge the allocation of resources by this particular health authority. . . . There is no suggestion here that the health authority has behaved in a way which is deserving of condemnation or criticism. What is suggested is that somehow more resources should be made available to enable the hospital authorities to ensure that the treatment is immediately given.[50]

The court declined, moreover, to even ask the Health Authority why the surgeries had been canceled or to suggest consideration of other alternatives like transferring the case to a different hospital.

*Ex parte Collier* may well be no longer good law. In more recent cases the courts have begun to ask health authorities to give reasons for their decisions beyond the simple excuse that resources are short and that difficult decisions must be made. For example, a court observed the following in a recent case challenging a health authority's denial of payment for transsexual surgery:

In establishing priorities—comparing ten respective needs of patients suffering from different illnesses and determining ten respective strengths of their claims to treatment—it is vital: for (1) an authority accurately to assess the nature and seriousness of each type of illness, (2) to determine the effectiveness of various forms of treatment for it, and (3) to give proper effect to that assessment and that determination in the application of its policy.[51]

The courts in these cases did not order the health authority to provide the service, however, but just remanded the matter to the authority for further consideration.

Finally, recent cases have begun to recognize a duty on the part of health authorities to comply with legal procedural requirements in their actions, specifically to consult with community health councils when required to do so by regulation or statute.[52] This entitlement, however, is procedural, not substantive.

While the extent of discretion afforded the NHS and its health authorities in the allocation of resources excludes a claim of absolute entitlement to hospital services, a claim of entitlement to GP services may be stronger. The NHS (General Medical Services) Regulations of 1992,[53] paragraph 12, provides that "a doctor shall render to his patients all necessary and appropriate personal medical services of the type usually provided by general practitioners." Paragraph 43 requires that "a doctor shall order any drugs or appliances which are needed for the treatment of any patient to whom he is providing treatment under these terms of service by issuing to that patient a prescription form."

These duties, which have existed from the creation of the NHS in 1948, appear to be mandatory, devoid of the discretionary language found in the provisions of the NHS act dealing with the health authorities. In the recent case of *R. v. Secretary of State for Health, ex parte Pfizer*—a challenge brought by Pfizer against a Health Service circular urging GPs not to prescribe Viagra except in exceptional circumstances—the court held the circular to be unlawful.[54] Justice Collings observed that doctors are obligated to prescribe any treatments that they in their professional judgment deem to be necessary for their patients. In caring for their patients, "the GPs clinical judgment is supreme" and can only be overridden by an act of Parliament, not by mere executive order.[55] In other words, it may be that the British are entitled to primary care services, even though they may not be entitled to any particular secondary and tertiary care services.

New avenues have also opened up in the recent past for asserting an entitlement to health services as a matter of human rights law. In 1998, the British Parliament adopted the Human Rights Act, which went into effect in October 2000. The act incorporates into domestic law the 1951 European Convention of Human Rights.[56] It allows victims of human rights abuses to bring proceedings against civil authorities to enforce their rights in British courts.[57] The act does not allow the British courts to set aside acts of Parliament as violative of human rights, but does require the courts to interpret legislation in a manner that is consistent with human rights.[58] If this is not possible, the higher courts are enabled to issue a formal declaration that legislation is incompatible with the convention, though it remains enforceable.[59]

The convention has been invoked several times in cases challenging the decisions of NHS health authorities, but generally without success. In one case, *R. v. North and East Devon Health Authority, ex parte Coughlan,*[60] the court sustained a challenge to a health authority's attempt to move a patient whom it had promised a placement in an institution for the long-term disabled for life, relying in part on Article 8(1), "Everyone has the right to respect for . . . his home." In subsequent cases, however, the same argument has been given short shrift.

In *The Queen on Application of C v. Lincolnshire Health Authority,*[61] the High Court rejected another challenge based in part on article 8 of the European Convention of Human Rights to an NHS action closing a facility and moving a resident, deferring instead to the health authorities considered judgment as to how best to handle the resident's case. In another hospital closing case, the court dismissed a challenge based on article 8 of the European Convention on Human Rights as not having "any substance whatever."[62]

In the end, however, European Union (EU) law may have a greater influence on the NHS than European human rights law will have. In *ex parte Pfizer,* mentioned above, for example, the court also ruled against the Department of Health for failing to publish and communicate prospectively its criteria for deciding to exclude medicinal products from NHS coverage and, more specifically, for failing to communicate to Pfizer the objective reasons for excluding Viagra from NHS coverage.[63] Because the Viagra in question originated in another EU state (France, not surprisingly), the action of the NHS was in violation of EU law, which prohibits restrictions on the free flow of goods and services.[64]

A more recent case, not explicitly involving the NHS, may have far greater ramifications. In the *Smits–Peerbooms* case involving Dutch nationals who had sought medical care in Germany, the European Court of Justice held that, under articles 49 and 50 (ex articles 59 and 60) of the European Community Treaty, which prohibit barriers to the free movement of services, a national of one EU country can only be denied payment for treatment in another EU country "if equally effective treatment can be obtained without undue delay at an establishment having a contractual arrangement with the insured person's sickness insurance fund."[65] The court also held that if a prior authorization is necessary for treatment under national law, prior authorization decisions must be made on "objective, non discriminatory criteria which are known in advance, in such a way as to circumscribe the exercise of the national authorities' discretion, so that it is not used arbitrarily."[66] Authorization decisions also must be made within "a reasonable time" and "be capable of being challenged in judicial or quasi-judicial proceedings."[67]

As discussed later in this chapter, wait lists in the United Kingdom are legendary, while excess capacity for providing health services exists in some other European countries. There is the potential, therefore, that NHS patients could demand care in other countries with payment from the NHS. Nevertheless, the case is unclear as to what constitutes "undue" delay, and if and when the NHS moves to implement the decision, it is unlikely that a high proportion of those on the waiting lists will choose to travel to elsewhere in Europe for surgery.[68]

Rregardless of whether NHS patients are "entitled" to particular treatments from the NHS, they do have rights within the NHS. First, they have the right to complain. Any patient dissatisfied with care in the NHS may complain to the relevant NHS trust, health authority, GP, dentist, optician, or pharmacist.[69] If the complaint is not resolved satisfactorily, the complainant can request an independent review from the local health authority.[70] If the complainant is dissatisfied with the independent review, he or she may refer the matter to the Health Service Commissioner.[71]

During 1999–2000, some 86,536 complaints were received by the English NHS concerning the hospital and community health services.[72] In 2,061 of these cases, the complainant requested an independent review; of these, 296 reviews were granted. Also, 39,725 complaints were received regarding general medical and dental services; in 1,396 such cases, the complainant requested an independent review, and in 341 an independent review was granted. Between April 1, 2000, and March 31, 2001, some 2,595 complaints were filed with the Health Service Commissioner; of these, 241 were accepted for investigation. Four-fifths of the investigations involved clinical care.[73]

The current NHS complaint procedure was established in 1996. A recent review found widespread dissatisfaction, with a majority of those surveyed expressing dissatisfaction with the procedure, a majority considering the current procedure to be unfair or biased, and no more than 20% to 30% being satisfied with the time it takes to get the complaint resolved.[74] The most pervasive complaint about the complaint procedure was that NHS staff had a poor attitude regarding complainants, including "lack of respect, lack of sympathy and understanding; patronizing, aggressive and arrogant attitudes."[75] The few complainants who proceeded to the independent review process were even less satisfied with the process and result.[76]

Both the existence of a national complaint process and dissatisfaction with that process are characteristics of a national health service. Neither the United States nor Germany has a centralized process through which one can complain to the government about health-care services. A patient may complain to a licensure board about a particular type of professional, or an insured may submit a complaint to a state external review procedure in the United States or to the social courts in Germany, but, because the health-care delivery system is decentralized, there is no central complaint procedure.

In England (and in some other countries with national health services) a centralized complaint process exists. Because the English populace feels an ownership of the NHS, they consider themselves entitled to be treated decently by it. Thus, tens of thousands of patients complain every year. Because the NHS has very limited resources, however, and because patients are in fact not entitled to all of the services they desire, dissatisfaction with the process is rife.

Patients who are actually injured by inadequate medical care are not limited to the complaints procedure, moreover; they may also sue for medical negligence. This is true in instances of ordinary negligence, of course, although the English courts have historically been very deferential to the medical profession in these cases. But in some cases the real problem has been more systemic and resource based. In *Bull v. Devon Health Authority*,[77] for example, a baby suffered brain damage at birth because the NHS hospital took an hour rather than the standard 20 minutes to produce a physician when one was needed. The health authority was held liable for failure to provide the plaintiff with treatment that met the standard of care. In sum, while the NHS patient may not be entitled to the provision of a particular service, if the services that are provided (or withheld from) the patient breach the standard of care for the profession, the patient may be able to recover for consequent injuries in negligence.

## Benefits of National Health Service Model

### Equitable Access to Health Care

The British media, like their American counterparts, tend to focus on the negative aspects of the British National Health Service. But the NHS has much to commend it. The greatest strong point of the British system is that health care is available to all; indeed, it is more or less equitably available.

In fact, every British citizen has an equal right to free health care from the NHS. Where patient charges exist, they are generally waived for welfare recipients, children, and the elderly. Eliminating geographic disparities in the distribution of health-care professionals and facilities has been a conscious policy of the NHS since its inception, and geographic disparities had been significantly eliminated by the 1980s.[78] There is some evidence that manual and semiskilled workers use more GP services than skilled and professional workers, though there is also evidence that NHS expenditures are higher for higher social groups.[79]

Comparative measures of equity of reported access to health care by survey respondents clearly favor the United Kingdom over the United States. Table 9–1 reports the results of a recent study comparing access to health care for the United States and the United Kingdom (and for a third country with a national health service, Canada). The statistics shown in this table, however, represent access to health care for the total population. More telling are statistics comparing access for residents with below or above-average income. Only 4% of U.K. residents with below-average income surveyed in 2001 reported

TABLE 9–1. Citizens' Views of Access to and Quality of Care, Three Countries, 2001 (Percent of Respondents)

| | CANADA | UNITED KINGDOM | UNITED STATES |
|---|---|---|---|
| **Access** | | | |
| Very or extremely difficult to see a specialist | 16 | 13 | 17 |
| Somewhat difficult to see a specialist | 28 | 22 | 22 |
| Not too or not at all difficult to see a specialist | 51 | 53 | 59 |
| Somewhat or very difficult to get care on nights or weekends | 41 | 33 | 41 |
| Did not fill a prescription due to cost | 13 | 7 | 26 |
| Did not get medical care due to cost | 5 | 3 | 24 |
| Did not get test, treatment, or follow-up due to cost | 6 | 2 | 22 |
| Did not get dental care due to cost | 26 | 19 | 35 |
| Problems paying medical bills | 7 | 3 | 21 |
| **Quality** | | | |
| Rated overall medical care received by family in last 12 months as | | | |
| Excellent | 20 | 21 | 22 |
| Very good | 34 | 32 | 35 |
| Good | 32 | 30 | 28 |
| Fair | 9 | 13 | 10 |
| Poor | 3 | 2 | 3 |
| Rating of physician responsiveness as excellent or very good | | | |
| Treating you with dignity and respect | 79 | 73 | 72 |
| Listening carefully to your health concerns | 74 | 67 | 65 |
| Providing all the information you want | 67 | 58 | 63 |
| Spending enough time | 62 | 54 | 58 |
| Being accessible by phone or in person | 55 | 48 | 52 |

Source: Adapted from Robert J. Blendon, "Inequities in Health Care: A Five-Country Survey," Health Affairs 21 (May/June 2002), 182, 183, based on the 2001, Commonwealth Fund/Harvard/Harris 2001 International Health Policy Survey.

problems paying their medical bills in the preceding year, compared to 35% of Americans of below-average income.[80] Only 16% of British respondents of below-average income in a recently published survey reported that it was "extremely or very difficult to see a specialist," compared to 30% of lower-income respondents from the United States.[81] By contrast, 9% of above-average-wealth Britons reported difficulties in getting access to specialists, compared to 8% of above-average-wealth Americans. And 7% of Britons of below-average wealth reported not filling a prescription during the preceding year due to cost, compared to 39% of below-average-wealth Americans.[82] A total of 56% of Britons of below-average income rated as excellent or very good medical care they had received during the preceding year, while 15% rated it as fair or poor medical, compared to 45% of below-average-income Americans who rated the care they had received as excellent or very good, and 20% who rated it as fair or poor.[83] In sum, although inequities still exist in health status between the wealthy and the poor in the United Kingdom, differences in access to health care are far less than in the United States, and a conscious and continual effort is being made to provide health care more equitably.

## Effective Cost Control

A second virtue of the British health-care system is that it is very cheap. In 2000, the United Kingdom spent 7.3% of its gross domestic product on health care, about $1,763 (purchase parity adjusted) per capita, the least of any Group of 7 country, and less than the OECD average.[84] By comparison, Germany spent 10.6% of GDP, or $2,748 per capita, and the United States spent 13% of its GDP, or $4,631 per capita (nearly three times as much as the British). Indeed, the United Kingdom is one of the few countries in the world that is consciously trying to increase its expenditures on health care, with a current target of increasing its expenditures to the level of the European Union (EU) median.[85]

Not only are overall expenditures lower in the United Kingdom, however, but sector by sector the United Kingdom spends less as well. The United Kingdom spent $320 per day per patient in hospital costs in 1996, as compared to $1,128 in the United States and $489 in Canada.[86] Although spending on prescription drugs has risen steeply in the United Kingdom as in every other developed country, only about $229 per capita was spent on prescription drugs in 1997, which is about one-half the U.S. level of $451 and less than the German level of $283.[87] Physicians also earn less in the United Kingdom—the ratio of average physician income to average employee income was 1.4:1, compared to 3.4:1 in Germany and 5.5:1 in the United States.[88]

A primary reason for the United Kingdom's low expenditure levels would seem to be that the vast majority of expenditures flow from a single source, the national treasury.[89] The NHS budget must compete with other public priorities (including, often most importantly, holding down the level of taxation), in the annual budget process.[90] Because the NHS is an institution of the national government, moreover, all funding comes from the center, without contributions from local or regional governments.[91] Thus fiscal discipline imposed by the central government is not dissipated by local or regional spending.

Another key factor in maintaining fiscal discipline is the limited role of private spending in the United Kingdom. Private spending on health care makes up only 1% of the British GDP, compared to 2.4% of GDP in Germany, 2.5% in France, 2.8% in Canada, and 7.4% in the United States.[92] Only about 15% of health care in the United Kingdom is paid for by private funds.[93]

As in other countries, private spending takes the form of either private insurance or out-of-pocket spending. Approximately 7 million people in the United Kingdom (about one-eighth of the total population) have private insurance.[94] About 60% of these receive private insurance through their employment, 30% have individual policies, and 10% receive insurance through professional associations or trade unions.[95] After growing in the 1980s, when it was encouraged by tax incentives from the Thatcher government, the private insurance industry stagnated in the 1990s, with tax incentives being revoked by Labor in 1997.[96]

Private insurance is primarily relied on for faster and more convenient access to hospital care, particularly for elective procedures.[97] The privately insured still rely primarily on the NHS for primary care, where satisfaction levels are high, although private GP services that are conveniently located for busy working people and offering immediate consultations for a standard fee are beginning to appear.[98] Private health insurance tends, rather, to be used to purchase hospital care in private facilities, though some private pay beds have always been available within the NHS, and many NHS specialists carry on a private practice on the side.[99] The primary value of private insurance is that it enables insureds to jump the queue and get access to health care more quickly. The most common surgeries done in the private sector, therefore, tend to be those for which waits are long in the public sector, including cataract removals, hernia repairs, hip replacements, and stripping of varicose veins.[100]

Private expenditures also include out-of-pocket payments. These take two forms. First, some U.K. residents pay for private care out of pocket. Because essential medical care is covered by the NHS, it is quite possible to forego private insurance but to purchase private care when faster or more convenient care is desired. Approximately 20% of treatment in private health-care facilities is purchased out of pocket rather than through insurance.[101] The most commonly performed procedure in English private hospitals is abortion, and while some abortions are covered by insurance, others are paid for out of pocket.

Out-of-pocket payments also cover patient cost-sharing obligations in the NHS. While the founding principle of the NHS was that services would be free, as early as 1949 the government decided to impose a copayment for pharmaceuticals (not actually imposed until 1951), causing Anuerin Bevan, the founder of the National Health Service to resign.[102] Prescription charges have grown steadily since then, though 84% of all NHS prescriptions are exempt from prescription charges because their recipients are children, the elderly, those needing long-term medication, and those who receive income support.[103] Cost-sharing charges are also imposed for optical care—the NHS does not pay for spectacle frames and only partially subsidizes the cost of lenses, though the elderly and children are covered.[104] Dental charges are also substantial, and many dentists now practice outside of the NHS.[105] Long-term care and abortion services are also largely financed through the private sector.[106] In total, however, only about 6% of NHS income is from patient charges, and many of the most needy receive care free from cost sharing.

The availability of private health insurance to those who are relatively well to do has the potential for undermining support for the NHS, but most U.K. citizens still rely primarily on the NHS for care. Employment-related health insurance has not become the norm, even though it has become more common for higher-income members of society, and private expenditures have not become a significant source of health-care finance. Although private insurance and private health care offer a safety valve for persons who are not satisfied with NHS care, health-care expenditures remain largely under government control. The government has exercised this control quite forcefully, and thus health-care expenditures in the United Kingdom are among the lowest found in developed nations.

## Emphasis on Primary Care

A third strong suit of the British health-care system is its emphasis on primary care. Virtually every person in the United Kingdom is registered with a general practitioner. These tend to be long-term relationships, making health education, prevention, and management of care more possible.[107] British GPs are broadly trained in primary care and manage most health-care services for their patients.[108] About one-half of GP compensation is paid on a capitated basis, with additional allowances for practice maintenance, health-promotion payments for running health-promotion and chronic disease-management programs and for achieving target levels of childhood immunization and cytology screening, and fee-for-service payments for certain services like contraception.[109] GPs also get extra compensation based on the proportion of their patients who live in deprived or rural areas, recognizing the greater health needs of these populations.[110]

Access to specialists and to hospital care is available only through general practitioners. Unlike gatekeeper physicians in U.S. managed-care plans, however, the role of the British GP is not to discourage access to specialists and hospital care but to manage effectively the patient's care and to seek consultations when necessary.[111] The most recent reorganization of the health service has been directed toward increasing the power of general practitioners within the service, assigning to primary care trusts the task of commissioning services from the hospitals and other health service providers.

General practitioners tend to practice in small groups, with one or two part-timers or trainees attached to the practice. About 30% of GPs, however, still practice on their own, and larger groups (of six or more doctors) are becoming more common.[112] Practices may also include a district nurse (who is trained for work in the community and sometimes paid by the local NHS trust) and health visitors—specialist nurses who work with children, mothers, and the elderly—as well as practice nurses who assist the physician within the practice.[113]

Most practices now work on an appointment system, and appointments are generally available reasonably quickly. A recent survey of general practice found that 29% of respondents had to wait two to three days for an appointment; only 25% had to wait four or more days. Some 80% of respondents reported that they received an appointment as soon as necessary; 84% of those with appointments were seen within half an hour of arriving at the doctor's office.[114] Also, 87% of those surveyed were satisfied with the length of their consultation with their GPs, 87% reported that they were given enough information about their treatment by their GP, 84% felt they were listened to, and 78% reported that their opinions were taken seriously. British GPs also continue to make house calls, unlike their American counterparts. In the same survey 14% of those registered with a GP had made after-hours phone calls to reach their GP, and 43% of those received a visit from their own GP or a locum tenens. In sum, the British have achieved to a considerable degree a cost-effective and well-accepted primary care–led health service.

The British emphasis on primary care has led to a relatively strong emphasis on public health and prevention. The British health service, like health-care systems throughout the developed world, is focused primarily on sickness, not on wellness. But the NHS does have more of an emphasis on preventive care and health promotion than is found in the United States and other countries where health-care systems are organized on a more individualistic basis. Maintenance of health was a fundamental principle of the NHS Act, and successive governments have affirmed a commitment to disease prevention.[115] GPs are also responsible for maintaining registers of patients with specified chronic diseases; monitoring diet, physical activity, and smoking habits; providing annual health checks for persons over 75; and carrying out breast and cervical cancer screening.[116] District nurses and health visitors assigned to general practices are also responsible for public health responsibilities.[117]

The performance of the United Kingdom in preventive health care is relatively strong. Some 92% of children are immunized for diphtheria, pertussis, and tetanus by 12 months of age, compared to 84% in the United States.[118] A comparative study of health system performance found that the United Kingdom provided more cost-effective diabetes care than the United States did, achieving outcomes that were one-third better with one-third lower costs.[119] The study attributed the U.K.'s superior performance to better triaging of cases and use of a team approach—that is, better coordination of care.[120]

## Clinical Freedom

Another positive characteristic of the NHS is its preservation of clinical freedom, both in running the NHS and in serving patients. With the rise of managed care in the United States, there has been an increasing tendency for treatment decisions to be made by insurers rather than by doctors: in general, managed-care companies are run by lay leadership. By contrast, professional autonomy had been one of the founding principles of the NHS.[121] During most of the first four decades of the NHS, doctors and, somewhat later, nurses played a major role in running the service. Consultants played a major role in resource allocation within the hospitals, while "matrons," or nurse administrators, played a major role in hospital administration.[122] GPs and other health-care professionals ran the primary care services.

Beginning in the mid-1980s, a series of reforms have emphasized the importance of management in the NHS and built up the power of professional managers.[123] The internal market reforms of the 1990s went even further in enhancing the power of managers, both within the health authorities and within the NHS trusts. The managers have never been more than moderately successful, however, in wresting control of the health service from the clinicians. Utilization review, as it is found in the United States or even in Germany, does not exist in the United Kingdom.[124] Consultants still largely control their patient lists and play a major role in resource allocation within hospitals.[125] Under the current government health plan, GPs will gain control over health-care resources and will control purchasing of services within health authorities.[126] In sum, physicians have considerably more power in the United Kingdom than in many other countries to make decisions on behalf of their patients.

## Central Coordination and Direction

The Institute of Medicine's 2000 report, *To Err Is Human*, brought into sharp focus the problems of medical error and poor-quality medical care in the United States.[127] The report revealed medical error to be the eighth most significant cause of death in the United States and disclosed a host of quality deficiencies in America's health-care system. The report concluded:

> The decentralized and fragmented nature of the health care delivery system (some would say "nonsystem")[of the United States] also contributes to unsafe conditions for patients, and serves as an impediment to efforts to improve safety. . . . For example, when patients see multiple providers in different settings, none of whom have access to complete information, it is easier for something to go wrong than when care is better coordinated. At the same time, the provision of care to patients by a collection of loosely affiliated organizations and providers makes it difficult to implement improved clinical information systems capable of providing timely access to complete patient information. Unsafe care is one of the prices we pay for not having organized systems of care with clear lines of accountability.[128]

Indeed, the diffuse responsibilities of state licensing boards, the federal Medicare program, the federal and state Medicaid program, private accreditation and certification agencies, private payers, public health insurance programs, and private and public providers makes any kind of coordinated approach to the problems of error and poor quality in the United States hopeless.

England, confronted with a similar awakening to the problem of quality in the late 1990s, adopted a coordinated, nationwide approach to the problems, which continues to unfold. First, it established the National Service Frameworks (NSF) to establish national standards of care for specific conditions and the National Institute for Clinical Excellence (NICE) to evaluate and provide guidance for the use of new technologies.[129] Second, it established instruments to monitor compliance with the emerging standards and guidelines and to collect data on performance: the Commission for Health Improvement (CHI) to inspect NHS organizations; the Performance Assessment Framework of performance indicators to assemble data on performance; and the National Patient Safety Agency to collect and analyze information on adverse events.[130] It also created a Council for the Regulation of Healthcare Professionals to address problems in its professional regulatory process identified in an investigation into deaths in the pediatric heart surgery unit in Bristol; and the National Clinical Assessment Authority to assist health authorities dealing with particular problem doctors.[131] Finally, it established incentives to encourage and reward improvement: a special performance fund to fund progress toward goals; a system of earned autonomy to reward institutions that do well; and a star rating system to both reward good performers and shame poor performers.[132] It is still too early to evaluate the success of the British approach, and it is possible that it will simply result in more bureaucracy, but it is moving ahead and seems reasonably coherent and well thought out.

Moreover, there is evidence of the possibilities of centralized approaches to other problems. Breast cancer has been targeted as a particular concern and focus of investment, leading to a dramatic increase in breast cancer screening and treatment and decline in mortality rates and waits for treatment.[133] The important point, however, may be simply that the British system makes a coherent and coordinated approach to problems like quality possible, a possibility that is sorely lacking in our own nonsystem.

## Problems with the NHS System

### Lack of Resources, Prevalence of Wait Lists

Despite all of its strong points, the NHS also faces serious problems that gives one pause in putting it forward as a model for emulation. First, and foremost, the NHS is underresourced. This fact is evidenced in the condition of U.K. health-care facilities. Of the current NHS properties, 29% predate 1948.[134] NHS hospitals are often crowded, with most rooms having four to six beds, and some older hospitals still having large open wards with 24 or more beds.[135] As the most recent government NHS plan acknowledges, food has been poor in quality, and cleanliness has left much to wish for.[136] Many facilities just appear generally shabby.

Lack of resources has long been most publicly evident in the persistence of waiting lists for surgery and inpatient treatment. The NHS was formed through a simple nationalization of the existing British health-care system. The British hospitals had suffered through the depression and the war, and many were outdated and dilapidated at the time they were taken over.[137] The founders of the NHS badly underestimated the resources that would be necessary to operate the service, and some had wrongly believed that as health care was extended throughout the British population, improved health would lead to a decline in expenditures.[138] After three years of serious cost overruns, the government put a clamp on further expenditure growth in the NHS, and health expenditures did not rise significantly again until the mid-1960s.[139] Though NHS expenditures have risen slowly over the decades—and at certain periods such as the early 1970s, the early 1990s, and the early 2000s, resources have risen dramatically—the NHS has always been underfunded.[140]

Throughout the history of the NHS, waiting lists have been a problem, particularly for elective surgery.[141] Wait lists have grown and sometimes diminished over the history of the service, but they have always been there. Time and again, the government in power has adopted programs to reduce the size of the lists and the length of time that those on the lists have to wait. But each time, waiting list size and duration have risen again as the new program lost its potency, or waiting lists have been simply reconfigured to conform to the precise requirements of the government program.[142] Waiting times for emergency treatment have also become an issue leading to horror stories of hours, even days, spent waiting to be seen in emergency room corridors.[143] As of this writing in the spring of 2002, the NHS claims that progress is being made on wait times: that the number of English residents waiting more than one year for treatment was 48.3% lower than a year earlier, and that waits of over 15 months had been virtually eliminated.[144]

Any economist can explain that if the supply of a good or service is limited by the state while demand is not constrained by price (because the care is free to the consumer), demand will exceed supply, and the available supply will need to be rationed.[145] One reasonable response to limited supply is certainly to ration by queue. While this economic explanation is helpful in understanding the problem faced by the NHS, it is not wholly adequate. The problem is more complicated than a simple shortfall of supply in the face of demand.

First, waiting lists have existed historically primarily for a relatively short list of conditions, which still account for a large proportion of the patients on the list. These conditions include varicose veins, hernias, painful or immobile joints, cataracts, enlarged tonsils, and women awaiting sterilization.[146] They have a number of characteristics in common: they are not generally life threatening, they are predominantly problems of older persons, and they are routine. They are also not inherently interesting conditions, about which articles are published and on the basis of which reputations are made.[147] They are, most importantly, conditions that doctors who are being paid on a salary rather than a fee-for-service basis would prefer not to spend their days dealing with.

Second, queues are the visible result of a complex interplay of resource shortages, some of which may be as attributable to inadequate planning or allocation rather than to an absolute lack of resources. A current problem, for example, is "bed blocking"—hospital beds occupied by elderly patients well enough to be discharged to the community but remaining in the hospital because of lack of after-care resources. A recent report found that 10% or more of hospital beds were blocked, resulting in the cancellation of nearly 5,000 surgeries in the first quarter of 2001.[148] Another problem is lack of staff. The NHS is experiencing a serious shortage of health-care practitioners, particularly doctors and nurses. One study estimates that there was a shortfall of 22,000 unfilled vacancies for nurses in 2000, while another survey found 1,214 vacancies for GPs.[149] The Labor government has committed itself to increasing NHS staff, but training new health-care professionals takes time, as well as resources.

Third, the length of the NHS waiting lists cannot be taken simply at face value. Statistics both under- and overrepresent the true nature of the problem. In fact, NHS patients wait in line at least twice before they are operated on in NHS hospitals.[150] First, they wait for an outpatient appointment to be seen by a specialist after they have been referred by their GP. If the specialist believes that the patient needs surgery or other inpatient treatment, the patient will be placed on a second list to receive the actual operation. It is the second, waiting for a surgery, list that is usually the focus of wait list discussions. Some doctors prefer to keep their inpatient surgery lists short, and thus they delay outpatient consultations until their surgical calendar clears up. Others believe that they should see their patients as soon as possible to determine the severity of the problem and then operate as conditions warrant. Patients with less severe conditions tend to wait while more severe conditions are addressed, but from time to time when the government demands action on the lists the more severe cases must wait while those patients who have been waiting a long time with less severe conditions are cleared from the list. Waiting lists are not necessarily kept current and may be redundant between hospitals and specialists. A considerable number of patients found on waiting lists, from 10% to 30%, in fact no longer require surgery, either because their condition has cleared up spontaneously or because they have already been operated on elsewhere.[151]

Another important point to note about the U.K. waiting list process, moreover, is that, in the end, the lists are not solely a matter of consumer demand but rather of professional judgment. A GP must first decide that a patient needs to see a specialist before the patient can get a consultation. A consultant must next decide that the patient needs surgery before the patient progresses to the hospital waiting list. Waiting lists exist, therefore, not simply because of a gap between supply and demand, but rather because of a gap between supply and need, as professionally determined.

It is very possible, however, that gaps between need and supply also exist in other countries, including the United States. One attempt to quantify the shortfall in the United States between need and supply with respect to denial of treatment of the uninsured and underinsured, found that implicit waiting lists in the United States were worse than the explicit lists in the United Kingdom.[152] Supporting this hypothesis, doctors from the United States report much more often when surveyed that their patients have difficulty affording the care they need, while U.K. doctors are more likely to report shortages of resources such as the latest medical or diagnostic equipment or hospital beds.[153]

Nor is greater availability of private access to physicians necessarily an answer to the problem of queues. In theory, the availability of private treatment alternatives should relieve the problem of lists and take pressure off the NHS. In fact, it is believed that NHS consultants who also practice privately encourage their patients to "go private," and the specialties with the longest waiting lists are those specialties that have the highest private incomes.[154] It may also be true that longer waiting lists are due in part to the amount of time NHS doctors spend in private practice.[155] Therefore, maintaining a list may be to the economic benefit of consultants who are also allowed private practice. Although long lists could be evidence of a hospital's inefficiency, they are also used to argue for additional resources, sometimes quite successfully.[156] Hospitals that keep their lists down can appear to be hospitals that are coping fine without additional resources.

## Lack of Access to Technology

However serious our problems of undertreatment may be in the United States currently, one can imagine how much more serious they would be if we cut our health-care expenditures by two-thirds to reach British levels. Low health-care spending is also apparent in the relative lack of expensive health-care technology in Great Britain. The United Kingdom had only 3.4 magnetic resonance imagers per million persons in 1998, compared to 7.6 in the United States.[157] In 1997 only 41 coronary bypass procedures were performed per 100,000 population in the United Kingdom, compared to 223 in the United States.[158] Only 27 patients per 100,000 were undergoing dialysis in the United Kingdom in 1998, compared to 74 in the United States.[159] One recent report claimed that among the 15 European Union nations, only the Greeks had to wait longer than Britons for new cancer treatments, which might take three years longer to arrive in Britain than in Sweden, with much of the delay attributable to government objections that the drugs were not "cost effective."[160]

One can argue, of course, that high-technology equipment and procedures are too available in the United States, but outcomes data comparing the United States and the United Kingdom are more persuasive. Breast cancer mortality in the United Kingdom, for example, is 34 per 100,000 women per year compared to 28 in the United States.[161] Breast cancer five-year survival rates are 67% in the United Kingdom, compared to 83% in the United States and 73% for the EU average. In the United Kingdom fewer than 4% of male lung cancer patients survive for more than five years, compared to 12% in the United States, while 60% of colon cancer patients survive at least five years in the United States compared to 34% in the United Kingdom.[162] Life expectancy at age 80 is 9 years for females and 7.5 years for males in the United States; it is 8.5 years for females and 6.7 years for males in the United Kingdom.[163]

This is also not to say that the United Kingdom is technologically primitive. Despite the very limited resources that it dedicates to health service provision, the United Kingdom continues to have a significant role in health-care research and innovation. Some of the world's most prestigious hospitals and medical centers are found in the United Kingdom. NHS doctors developed the technique on which the modern approach to hip replacement is based, as well as cataract surgery.[164] The favorable attitude of the United Kingdom to stem cell research promises to make it a leader in this developing technology. But technology is not as readily available and does not diffuse as rapidly in the United Kingdom as in the United States or in other European nations.

## The Continuous Reorganization

Another great weakness of the NHS is its chronic and continuous attempts at reorganization. For three decades the British governments in power have labored under the illusion that somehow reorganizing the National Health Service will solve its problems. The first reorganization in 1974 introduced district health authorities and consensus management.[165] The Griffiths reforms of 1994, led by a supermarket magnate, created general managers.[166] Margaret Thatcher's radical market reforms, initiated in 1991, attempted to split the purchaser/provider functions within the NHS to create an internal market.[167] While this change created a whole new administrative level and a great many more management jobs in the NHS—and added considerably to the complexity and information demands of the system—there is little evidence that it improved the system's quality or responsiveness.[168] When Labor returned to power in 1997, it had the good sense not to put the NHS through another total upheaval by dismantling all of the structures that the Conservatives had created, but it did eliminate some of the structures the Conservatives had put in place, such as GP fundholding, and created some of its own, such as primary care trusts. Its latest aspirations are reflected in the Wanless Report, which calls for dramatic expansion of expenditures, capacity, and quality in the NHS by 2022.[169]

With these changes have come frequent reconfigurations of the NHS organizational chart.[170] Regional health authorities were reduced in number and became regional NHS offices; then, in turn, these were reduced in number again. Local health authorities became local health purchasing authorities and are now being reduced in number to become strategic health authorities, with unclear responsibilities. GPs contracted initially with executive councils, next with family practitioner committees, then with family health services authorities, while now the GPs must form primary care trusts.[171]

All of this has taken place in the context of an endless series of green papers, white papers, legislation, regulations, and NHS plans, which have created a sizeable bureaucracy and high transactions costs. The NHS is one of the biggest businesses in the world, and it is understandable that governments, which are accountable for the NHS, would try to find some way to manage it. It is also understandable that when governments come to power with a different ideological orientation than their predecessors, they would try to shape the service to fit their ideals.

One must also appreciate the complexity of the NHS: the government is not only responsible to its patients as patients, but also to its (often unionized) employees as an employer; to its doctors and nurses in their capacity as professionals; and to the private sector, which serves as a potential source of capital and partner in the provision of health-care services. It is unrealistic to hope that the government could ever devise the perfect organization for the NHS, and thereafter leave it alone to do its job. But the political nature of the NHS at times does get in the way of its role as a health-care provider.[172]

## Conclusion

What can we learn, then, from the experience of the NHS? Perhaps the most important lesson of the British experience for our purposes is the importance of legal health-care entitlements. The fact that a British citizen cannot successfully sue the NHS for denied services goes far to explain why services are often not available. If only populations, and not individuals, are eligible for health, then governments are free to make health-care services available at any level they choose. Entitlements are vital if health care is in fact to be available to all. The NHS experience also illustrates the danger of depending on a single source of funding for health care, particularly public funding. If a health service is to be publicly funded, funding should come from several sources—both general revenues and hypothecated taxes, for example—or from both national and regional governments. Finally, the British experience illustrates the problems of excessive political entanglement that can accompany a centralized health service.

The British experience also has positive lessons to teach us, however. It is possible to control health-care costs very effectively in a public system: we need not fear the doomsday scenarios of the privatizers. Public health-care systems, moreover, make possible much more equitable access to health care and can facilitate primary and coordinated care. They also can allow professionals the freedom to use their own judgment in serving their patients. Although the British NHS system is flawed, in sum, we should still attend to it in considering the redesign of our own badly flawed system.

## Notes

1. The discussion in this chapter refers primarily to the English National Health Service. The Scottish Health Service has always been somewhat independent of the English system, and with devolution the Welsh and Northern Irish systems are differentiating themselves somewhat more as well.

2. European Observatory on Health Care Systems, *Health Care Systems in Transition: United Kingdom* (Copenhagen: European Observatory of Health Care Systems, 1999): 33.

3. Ibid., 54.

4. Ruth Levitt, Andrew Wall, and John Appleby, *The Reorganized National Health Service*, 6th ed. (Chelthenham: Stanley Thornes Publishers, 1999), 100–101; Allyson M. Pollock, Jean Shaoul, and Neil Vickers, "Private Finance and 'Value for Money' in NHS Hospitals: A Policy in Search of a Rationale?" *British Medical Journal* 224 (May 18, 2002): 1205–1209; Rebecca Paveley, "NHS Buys 100,000 Private Operations to Cut Waiting Lists," *Daily Mail* (26 October 2001), 15.

5. World Health Organization (WHO), *World Health Report, 2000* (Geneva: WHO, 2000), 12–13.

6. Judith Allsop, *Health Policy and the NHS: Towards 2000*, 2nd ed. (London: Longman, 1995), 16–18.

7. Levitt et al., *The Reorganized National Health Service*, 9.

8. Ibid., 7–9; Geoffrey Rivett, *From Cradle to Grave: Fifty Years of the NHS* (London: King's Fund, 1998), 4.

9. Rivett, *From Cradle to Grave*, 7–8; Rob Baggott, *Health and Health Care in Britain* (Houndsmills: Macmillan Press, 1998), 86–87.

10. Allsop, *Health Policy and the NHS*, 18–19.

11. Ibid., 17.

12. Ibid., 20–22.

13. Ibid., 22–23.

14. Ibid.

15. Baggott, *Health and Health Care in Britain*, 87; Lawrence R. Jacobs, *The Health of Nations* (Ithaca, NY: Cornell University Press, 1993), 44–45.

16. Charles Webster, *The National Health Service: A Political History* (Oxford: Oxford University Press, 1998), 6–15.

17. See, generally, Jacobs, *The Health of Nations*.

18. Webster, *The National Health Service*, 3–5.

19. Ibid., 6–7; Jacobs, *The Health of Nations*, 112–116.

20. Webster, *The National Health Service*, 12–13.

21. Jacobs, *The Health of Nations*, 178–180.

22. Ibid., 13–15.

23. "The NHS Explained: What is the NHS," in *National Health Service Online*, available at www.nhs.uk/thenhsexplained/what_is_nhs.asp (cited June 4, 2002).

24. European Observatory on Health Care Systems, *Health Care Systems in Transition*, 13.

25. "Shifting the Balance of Power within the NHS, Securing Delivery," available at www.doh.gov/uk/shiftingthebalance/execsum.htm (cited July 27, 2001).

26. "Shifting the Balance of Power," available at www.doh.gov.uk/shiftingthebalance/shifting1.htm (cited July 27, 2001).

27. Levitt et al., *The Reorganized National Health Service*, 40–50. These were called "area health authorities" from 1974 to 1986, and "district health authorities" from 1982 to 2001, though their function changed in 1991.

28. Ibid., 42–46.

29. "New Health Authorities Boundaries: Shifting the Balance of Power in the NHS to Patients and FrontLine Staff," in NHS, available at www.doh.gov.uk.shiftingthebalance/press18dec2001.htm (cited May 20, 2002).

30. "Shifting the Balance of Power within NHS." Available at www.doh.gov.uk/shiftingthebalance/execsum.htm (cited July 27, 2001).

31. *Shifting the Balance of Power*, in NHS, available at www.doh.gov.uk/shiftingthebalance/shifting1.htm (cited July 27, 2001).

32. Ibid.

33. Levitt et al., *The Reorganized National Health Service*, 53.

34. Ibid.

35. "Shifting the Balance of Power within the NHS," available at www.gov.doh.uk/shiftingthebalance/shifting1.htm (cited July 27, 2001).

36. Ibid.

37. Ibid.

38. European Observatory on Health Care Systems, *Health Care Systems in Transition*, 53.

39. Ibid.

40. Ibid., 54–56.

41. *A National Health Service*, CMD 6502 (1944) 5, 9.

42. Rudolf Klein, Patricia Day, and Sharon Redmayne, *Managing Scarcity: Priority Setting and Rationing in the National Health Service* (Buckingham: Open University Press, 1996).

43. Ibid., 39–40.

44. "Your Guide to the NHS," available at http://www.nhs.uk/nhsguide/home.htm (cited June 27, 2002).

45. Christopher Newdick, "Judicial Supervision of Health Resource Allocation: The U.K. Experience," in *Readings in Comparative Health Law and Bioethics*, edited by Timothy Stoltzfus Jost (Durham, N.C.: Carolina Academic Press, 2000), 61.

46. Diane Longley, *Public Law and Health Service Accountability* (Buckingham: Open University Press, 1993), 79–82; Christopher Newdick, *Who Shall We Treat? Law Patients and Resources in the NHS* (Oxford: Clarendon Press, 1995).

47. *R v. North and East Devon Health Authority, ex parte Coughlan* [1999] Lloyds Rep. Med. 306, 314 per Sedley L.J.

48. Lloyds Rep. Med. 306, 314 per Sedley L.J., from *Associated Provincial Picture House Ltd. v Wednesbury Corporation* [1948] 1 K.B. 223 (which established the doctrine).

49. *Council of Civil Service Unions and Others v. Minister for the Civil Service* [1985] A.C. 374, 410.

50. Unreported, quoted in Newdick, *Who Shall we Treat?* 66–67.

51. *R. v. N.W. Lancashire HA, ex parte A, D & G* [1999] 1999 WL 1142599 (July 29, 1999).

52. *R. v. N.W. Thames RHA ex parte Daniels* [1999] Lloyd's Rep. Med. 306.

53. SI 1992/6354, sched 2.

54. [1999] 3 C.M.L.R. 875.

55. *R. v. Secretary of State for Health, ex parte Pfizer Ltd.* (1999) 3 C.M.L.R. 875 (Q.B. 1999).

56. Human Rights Act of 1998, 1999 Chap. 42, § 5(1).

57. Ibid., § 7(1).

58. Ibid., § 3.

59. Ibid., § 4.

60. 2 WLR 622 [2000].

61. *The Queen on Application of C v. Lincolnshire Health* (QBD Administration Court, September 6, 2001).

62. *The Queen on the Application of P v. Surrey Oakland NHS Trust*, 2001 WL 824999 (QBD Administrative Court, June 12, 2001). See also *Queen v. Brent, Kensington, and Chelsea and Westminster Mental Health NHS Trust*, 2002 WL 45361 (QBD Administrative Court, February 13, 2002), distinguishing *Coughlan* on its facts.

63. *R. v. Secretary of State for Health ex parte Pfizer Ltd.*, 875.

64. Specifically, the NHS violated Directive 89/105, articles 6 and 7, implementing articles 28 and 30 of the European Community Treaty, as amended.

65. European Court of Justice (ECJ) (2001), July 12, 2001, *Smits–Peerbooms*, C-157/99. In another case decided the same day, the ECJ held that when payment for services in another European country is required under this standard, payment must be made on the basis of the payment schedules of the treating, not the paying, country. ECJ (2001), July 12, 2001, *Vanbraekel*, C-368/98.

66. *Smits–Peerbooms*, ¶ 90.

67. Ibid. See, discussing these cases, Elias Mossialos et al., *The Influence of EU Law on the Social Character of Health Care Systems in the European Union*, Report Submitted to the Belgian Presidency of the European Union (November 19, 2001).

68. See Tessa Reilly, "Preparing for Patient Export," *Online BMAnews* (October 25, 2001).

69. "Local Resolution of Complaints," in *National Health Service: Patients Voice*, available at www.nhs.uk/patientsvoice/local_resolution.asp (cited June 3, 2002).

70. "Independent Review of Complaints," in *National Health Service: Patients Voice*, available at www.nhs.uk/patientsvoice/independent_review.asp (cited June 3, 2002).

71. "Health Service Commissioner," in *National Health Service: Patients Voice*, available at www.nhs.uk/patientsvoice/health_service_review.asp (cited June 3, 2002).

72. Department of Health, Statistical Press Notice, *Handling Complaints: Monitoring the NHS Complaints Procedure, England, 1999–2000*, (Washington, D.C.: U.S. Department of Health, 2001).

73. "Complaints Rise," in *NHS Magazine Online*, available at www.nhs.uk/nhs-magazine/story398.htm (cited June 3, 2002).

74. "System Three Social Research, *NHS Complaints Procedure: National Evaluation* (March 2001), available at http://www.doh.gov.uk/nhscomplaintsreform/evaluation.htm (cited June 27, 2002).

75. Ibid., 23.

76. Ibid., 25.

77. *Bull v. Devon Health Authority*, [p1993] 4 Med. L. R. 117 (decided in 1989), discussed in Newdick, *Who Shall We Treat?* 97–98, 111–112.

78. Allsop, *Health Policy and the NHS*, 133–134.

79. Ibid., 134–136.

80. Robert J. Blendon et al., "Inequities in Health Care: A Five-Country Survey," *Health Affairs* 21 (May/June 2002): 182–191.

81. Ibid., 184.

82. Ibid., 185.

83. Ibid., 189. About 45% of above-average-wealth Britons reported care that they had received as excellent or very good, and 16% as fair or poor, compared to 65% of above-average income Americans who rated the care they had received as excellent or very good, and 9% as fair or poor.

84. The Group of 7 consists of the United States, Britain, Italy, France, Germany, Japan and Canada. *Organization of Economic Corporation and Development (OECD) Health Data, 2002* (Paris: OECD, 2002).

85. Nicholas Timmins, "A Time for Change in the British NHS: An Interview with Alan Milburn," *Health Affairs* 21 (May/June 2002): 134. The government's intention to increase funding is a very popular policy, supported by 72% of the population, including 54% of the members of the opposition, Conservative, party. Peter Riddell, "Tories Suffer as Public Approves Health Budget," *Times* (London) (April 24, 2002), 14.

86. The Commonwealth Fund, *International Health Policy*, "Multinational Comparisons of Health Systems," (visited 27 June 2002). available at www.cmwf.org/programs/international/comp_chartbook_431.asp (cited June 27, 2002).

87. OECD Data, U.S. Data from 1998. (Paris: OECD).

88. Uwe Reinhardt, Peter S. Hussey, and Gerard Anderson, "Cross-National Comparisons of Health Systems Using OECD Data, 1999," *Health Affairs* (May/June 2002): 169–181.

89. Richard Freeman, *The Politics of Health in Europe* (Manchester: Manchester University Press, 2000), 44–45.

90. Donald Light, "Policy Lessons from the British Health Care System," in *Health Care Systems in Transition: An International Perspective*, edited by Francis D. Powell and Albert F. Wesson (Thousand Oaks, Calif.: Sage, 1999), 327, 329–330. See, describing the budget process, Giovanni Fattore, "Cost Containment and Health Care Reforms in the British NHS," in *Health Care Cost Containment in the European Union*, edited by Elias Mossialos and Julian Le Grand (Brookefield, Vt.: Ashgate, 1999), 733, 735–740.

91. Local government pays for social care, which is closely related to health care, however.

92. Carl Emmerson, Christine Frayne, and Alissa Goodman, *Pressures in U.K. Health Care: Challenges for the NHS* (London: Institute of Fiscal Studies, 2000), 14.

93. Ibid., 24

94. Ibid.

95. European Observatory on Health Care Systems, *Health Care Systems in Transition*, 43.

96. Baggott, *Health and Health Care in Britain*, 165.

97. European Observatory on Health Care Systems, *Health Care Systems in Transition*, 44–45.

98. Ibid., 55.

99. Baggott, *Health and Health Care in Britain*, 166; Levitt et al., *The Reorganized National Health Service*, 105–106.

100. European Observatory on Health Care Systems, *Health Care Systems in Transition*, 67–68.

101. Emmerson et al., *Pressures in U.K. Health Care*, 24.

102. Baggott, *Health and Health Care in Britain*, 107.

103. Ibid.

104. Levitt et al., *The Reorganized National Health Service*, 72.

105. Ibid., 70.

106. Baggott, *Health and Health Care in Britain*, 168.

107. Light, "Policy Lessons from the British Health Care System," 335.

108. Ibid.

109. European Observatory on Health Care Systems, *Health Care Systems in Transition*, 91.

110. Light, "Policy Lessons from the British Health Care System," 338–339.

111. Ibid., 336.

112. Levitt et al., *The Reorganized National Health Service*, 67.

113. Baggott, *Health and Health Care in Britain*, 68.

114. NHS Executive, *National Surveys of NHS Patients: General Practice 1998, Summary of Key Findings* (London: NHS Executive, 1999).

115. Levitt et al., *The Reorganized National Health Service*, 121.

116. European Observatory on Health Care Systems, *Health Care Systems in Transition*, 59.

117. Ibid., 54–55.

118. The Commonwealth Fund, "Multinational Comparisons" chart II-2.

119. Martin Neil Baily and Alan M. Garber, "Health Care Productivity," Brookings Papers on Economic Activity: *Microeconomics* (Washington, D.C.: Brookings Institution, 1997): 143, 158.

120. In the other conditions and procedures considered by this study—cholelithiasis (gallstones), breast cancer, and lung cancer—the United States performed as efficiently or more efficiently than the United Kingdom, largely because of use of more effective technologies and shorter hospital stays. Despite the fact that the United States used fewer resources for treatment of these conditions, however, it paid much more for the resources it used and had higher administrative costs. Ibid.

121. Allsop, *Health Policy and the NHS*, 29–30.

122. Ibid., 44–45; Rivett, *From Cradle to Grave*, 109, 179–180, 190–191, 333.

123. Webster, *The National Health Service*, 162–174.

124. There is a primarily informational review of prescribing practices for GPs; see Levitt et al., *The Reorganized National Health Service*, 71.

125. Robert West, "Joining the Queue: Demand and Decision-Making," in *Rationing and Rationality in The National Health Service: The Persistence of Waiting Lists*, edited by Stephen Frankel and Robert West (Houndsmills: Macmillan, 1993), 42, 58–59; Klein et al., *Managing Scarcity*, 83.

126. "Shifting the Balance of Power." Available at www.doh.gov.uk/shiftingthebalance/shifting1.htm (cited July 27, 2001).

127. Institute of Medicine, *To Err Is Human: Building a Safer Health Care System* (Washington D.C.: National Academy Press, 2000).

128. Ibid., 3. See also Institute of Medicine, *Crossing the Quality Chasm: A New Health Care System for the 21st Century* (Washington, D.C.: National Academy Press, 2001).

129. Peter C. Smith, "Performance Management in British Health Care: Will It Deliver?" *Health Affairs* (May/June 2002): 103–115. See also Julian Le Grand, "Further Tales from the British National Health Service," *Health Affairs* 21 (May/June 2002), 116, 118–119; Derek Wanless, *Securing Our Future Health: Taking a Long-Term View, Final Report* (London: HM Treasury, 2002), 21–27.

130. Smith, "Performance Management," 107–108; Kieran Walshe, "The Rise of Regulation in the NHS," *British Medical Journal* 324 (April 20, 2002): 967.

131. Department of Health, "Press Release: Better Protection for the Patient" (March 5, 2002).

132. Ibid., 108–110.

133. Department of Health, "Press Release: Further Progress in the Battle against Breast Cancer" (March 15, 2002); Reinhard Busse, *The British and German Health Care Systems* (London, Anglo-German Foundation, 2002), 44.

134. Wanless, *Securing Our Future Health: Taking the Long View, Interim Report* (London HM Treasury, 2001), 122.

135. Peter R. Hatcher, "United Kingdom," in *Health Care and Reform in Industrialized Countries*, edited by Marshall W. Raffel (University Park: Pennsylvania State University Press, 1997), 232.

136. Secretary of State for Health, *The NHS Plan* (London: NHS, 2000), 46–47. The NHS spends currently about £2.50 per day for food, compared to £4.10 per day in Germany. Wanless, *Securing Our Future Health, Final Report*, 31.

137. Rivett, *From Cradle to Grave*, 5.

138. Ibid, 110.

139. Webster, *The National Health Service*, 30–38.

140. Klein et al., *Managing Scarcity*, 37–48; Emmerson et al., *Pressures in U.K. Health Care*, 4–6.

141. John Cullis, "Waiting Lists and Health Policy," in *Rationing and Rationality in the National Health Service*, Stephen Frankel and Robert West, eds. (London, MacMillan, 1993) 15,19; Emmerson et al., *Pressures in U.K. Health Care*, 34.

142. See, e.g., Levitt et al., *The Reorganized National Health Service*, 130, 252; Baggott, *Health and Health Care in Britain*, 260–261.

143. Jenny Hope, "Crisis in Casualty? It's Pretty Disappointing says Milburn," *Daily Mail* (October 26, 2001), 15; Audit Commission, "Acute Hospital Portfolio: Review of National Findings—Accident and Emergency," available at http://www.audit-commission.gov.uk/reports/AC-REPORT.asp?CatID=?ProdID=037F9E79-DF51-4823-96B9-E87DF4B58EB9 (cited October 21, 2002).

144. Department of Health, "Friday, May 10, 2002, Statistical Press Release Notice: NHS Waiting List Figures,: available at http://tap.ukwebhost.eds.com/doh/intpress.nsf/page/2002-0224?OpenDocument (cited June 25, 2002).

145. Cullis, "Waiting Lists and Health Policy," 14–17.

146. Stephen Frankel, "The Origins of Waiting Lists," in *Rationing and Rationality in the National Health Service*, edited by Stephen Frankel and Robert West (London: Macmillan, 1993), 6.

147. Ibid., 11.

148. Beezy Marsh, "'Bed Blocking' Is 100 Times Worse, Admits Whitehall," *Daily Mail* (October 15, 2001), 17.

149. "Search for Staff to Fulfill Health Pledges," *The Guardian*, 2001 WL 21558767 (May 23, 2001), .

150. See Stephen Farrow and David Jewell, "Opening the Gate: Referrals from Primary to Secondary Care," in *Rationing and Rationality in the National Health Service*, 63; Stephen Frankel and Margaret Robbins, "Entering the Lobby: Access to Outpatient Assessment," in ibid., 80; Ian Harvey, "And So to Bed: Access to Inpatient Services," in ibid., 96.

151. Harvey, "And So to Bed," 103–104.

152. Cullis, "Waiting Lists and Health Policy," 23–37.

153. Robert Blendon et al., "Physicians' Views on Quality of Care: A Five-Country Comparison," *Health Affairs* 20 (May/June 2001): 233.

154. Le Grand, "Further Tales," 126. The latest NHS consultant contract attempts to control, but does not eliminate, the private practice of consultants. NHS update, "NHS Consultant Contract Puts Patients First" (June 25, 2002).

155. See Harvey, "And So to Bed," 105.

156. Secretary of State, *The NHS Plan*, 2000 (Norwich, England: HMSO, 2000), 28.

157. Gerard Anderson and Peter Sotir Hussey, "Comparing Health System Performance in OECD Countries," *Health Affairs* 20 (May/June 2001): 225.

158. Ibid.

159. Ibid.

160. Rachel Ellis, "Britons Are Last to Receive Latest Anticancer Drugs: NHS patients Years Behind Most of Europe, Says Survey," *Mail on Sunday* (June 24, 2001), 44.

161. The Commonwealth Fund, "Multinational Comparisons," chart V-2.

162. Edward Heathcoat Amory, "By Any Audit, the NHS Has Declined," *Daily Mail* (June 1, 2001) 6; Wanless, Securing Our Future Interim Report, 122.

163. The Commonwealth Fund, "Multinational Comparisons," chart IV-5.

164. Secretary of State, *The NHS Plan*, 22.

165. Levitt et al., *The Reorganized National Health Service*, 15–18.

166. Ibid., 17–18.

167. Secretary of State for Health, *Working for Patients* (London: HMSO, 1990); Levitt et al., *The Reorganized National Health Service*, 18–23.

168. Julian Le Grand, *Evaluating the National Health Service Reforms*, edited by Ray Robinson and Julian Le Grand (New Brunswick, N.J.: Transaction Books, 1994), 246–253.

169. Wanless, *Securing Our Future Health Final Report*.

170. Examples can be found in Levitt et al., *The Reorganized National Health Service*.

171. See Webster, *The National Health Service*, 20, 109, 179.

172. See Rivett, *From Cradle to Grave*, 482–483; Richard Smith, "Oh NHS, Thou Art Sick," *British Medical Journal* 324 (January 19, 2002): 127.

# 10

# The German
# Health-Care System:
# The Social Insurance
# Model of Health-Care
# Entitlements

═══════════════

THE German public health-care system is the world's oldest public health-care financing system—and one of the most successful. Initiated by Otto von Bismarck in 1883, the German social health insurance system served as the model for public health insurance systems throughout the world through the middle of the twentieth century, and it continues to exemplify one of the primary approaches to public health-care financing. Although the German system is relatively expensive by international standards, it is less so than our own American system, and it makes available to Germans universal access to sophisticated and up-to-date health care with minimal rationing of services. It is useful to study, therefore, as a model for health-care entitlements.

In fact, the German system can assist our consideration of entitlements in four important respects.

1. The model of social insurance, created in Germany and followed in the design of our own Medicare system, has proved adept at developing both a psychological expectation of and cultural commitment to health-care entitlements, which, in turn, have led to a high level of societal commitment to the sharing of health-care risk.
2. The German approach of affording statutory—indeed, constitutional—guarantees of health care on the one hand but operationalizing them

through quasi-public, self-governing, corporatist insurance and provider institutions on the other hand, creates a system in which political, professional, and market forces all play a part. At its best, this system draws on professional expertise, democratic governance, and legal oversight to offer a reasonably effective, responsible, and accountable system of health-care provision and coverage.

3. The German system of negotiated, fixed sectoral budgets affords a greater capacity for exerting fiscal discipline than the U.S.'s open-ended budgetary entitlements, but at the same time it provides greater flexibility than the more constrained British National Health Service.

4. The German social court system, as it operates in the context of the health-care system, provides a useful model of how courts can protect entitlements while still observing budget controls.

In this chapter I explore these aspects of the German system. I further examine how they are operationalized in two particular contexts: making coverage decisions with respect to new or unconventional medical treatments and payment for physician's services. Finally, I conclude by noting several emerging problems with the German system.

## The Social Insurance Approach to Entitlements

The German system of social health insurance offers an alternative to both socialized medicine and private insurance. Because Germany's social insurance system is created and directed by public law and based on the principle of social solidarity, coverage is free from the capricious inequity of markets, with their tendency to offer generous protection to the healthy and wealthy and little to the sick and the poor. Because it is a contributory insurance system, however, it affords entitlements that are relatively protected from the political vicissitudes of public budgets.

The German social insurance system was originated by Bismarck in an effort to offer increased security to the working class, thus enhancing their allegiance to the Prussian state and diminishing the attractiveness of socialism.[1] Originally the system only included workers in designated industries, and only those whose income was below 2,000 Marks a year.[2] Over the decades, however, the system has expanded to cover other occupational groups—transport and office workers in 1901, unemployed persons in 1918, seamen in 1927, dependents of fund members in 1930, pensioners in 1941, farmworkers in 1966, and students and disabled persons in 1975—while the income coverage level has also gradually increased.[3] Coverage is still far from universal, however. Only 74% of the population are mandatory members of the social health insurance funds or dependents of members.[4] Civil servants and persons whose incomes do not exceed a level of 3,375 euros monthly (in 2002) are not required to participate, though they are permitted to do so, and about three-fifths do. This brings the total proportion of the population covered by statutory health insurance to about 88%.[5] Many of those who are not required to purchase public insurance, however, purchase private insurance instead—about 9% of the total population—while another 2% are police officers or those in military or civilian service and are entitled to free government care. About 9% of the population also carry supplementary private insurance, in addition to social insurance coverage, to cover items and services not covered by the compulsory insurance, such as crowns and dentures.[6] Although those not bound by the social insurance obligation may also go without insurance, only about one-tenth of 1% do so.[7]

The German social health insurance system is not a welfare program. It is means-tested, but the income limits (there are no asset limits) cap the obligation—not the entitlement—to participate. That is, the income limits are intended to excuse the wealthy from participating if they choose not to, not to limit the program to covering indigents, excluding all others. These income limits, therefore are set high enough so that a broad cross-section of respectable, comfortably well off, citizens participate. While there may be a certain cachet in being privately insured, there is no shame in being publicly insured.[8]

The fact that a broad cross-section of German society participates in the social health insurance system means that the system has become a part of the German culture. One recent poll, for example, found that 84% of insureds surveyed agreed with the solidarity principle, under which younger insureds supported older, and healthy support sick.[9] Only 6.3% disagreed. Support was largely independent of age, income group, and party affiliation. Another poll found that 80% of Germans surveyed rejected the position that those who were often sick should pay higher premiums for insurance, but 51% supported the position that those who smoked, participated in extreme sports, or otherwise followed unhealthy life styles should pay higher premiums.[10] Finally, another poll found that 60% of Germans support bringing civil servants and the self-employed into the social insurance system, including a majority of the members of each of those groups who were surveyed.[11]

In turn, this popular support has translated into strong political support. As is the case with our own social insurance program, Medicare (and unlike our welfare program, Medicaid), politicians treat the program with considerable respect. The system has survived and grown through the end of the monarchy, the Weimer republic, the Nazi period, and several changes of the party in power since World War II. Even though social insurance was maintained in form only in the East during the Communist period, traditional social insurance was restored immediately as soon as the Berlin Wall fell.[12] In recent years conserva-

tive governments have laid more emphasis on patient cost sharing, while socialist governments have emphasized placing the responsibility on providers for
constraining costs, but all major parties in Germany favor a strong social health
insurance system.[13] The health insurance entitlement, therefore, is based on a
solid political consensus.

The German health-care system is financed through "contributions" from
employers and employees based on income, essentially a payroll tax, which vary
by insurance fund, but currently average about 14% of wages.[14] The employer
and employee each contribute half of this amount.[15]

This nexus between the employee's contribution and insurance coverage
means that there is a settled expectation of health insurance in Germany. The
worker who has contributed all of his working life, month in and month out,
to a health insurance fund considers himself simply to be receiving that which
he is owed when he goes to the doctor, the hospital, or even the spa. The relationship between the worker, the insurance fund, and the doctor is not formally one of contract, nevertheless it is an exchange relationship.

This attitude of entitlement is reflected in the resistance of Germans to rationing. Recent surveys, for example, have found that 60% of Germans reject
a reduction in services covered by the social insurance funds as an approach
to cost control, 73% oppose the use of financial incentives to encourage cost
consciousness on the part of doctors, and 79% oppose reducing the utilization
of expensive, but medically indicated, treatments.[16] Of those surveyed, 89%
take the position that savings should come from other state expenditures rather
than from the health-care system.[17] Over half of those questioned in another
poll agreed with the proposition that "health services should receive unlimited
funding, which means that all types of treatment are given equal priority," and
only 30% supported some form of prioritization.[18]

In this respect, the psychology of social insurance systems is markedly different from that of national health services. As noted in Chapter 9, there is
clearly a sense of ownership in national health services, which are publicly financed and publicly owned. Recipients expect a certain level of service and
feel aggrieved when this level of service is not realized. Yet the understanding
is that the entitlement is collective rather than individual.[19] No one individual
member of society can expect the national health service to satisfy all individual needs. Rather, the expectation is one of fair and equitable treatment as a
member of the collective that has a claim on the health-care system.

Insureds in a social insurance system have a more individualized claim. They
contribute as individuals, are members of a social health insurance fund as individuals, have an individual relationship with fund doctors, and expect services as individuals.[20] This individual expectation of entitlement has contributed
to a demand for a high level of service in the German health-care system and
a comparatively high level of technical sophistication.

## A Legal Entitlement in a Corporatist Environment

Although not all Germans are required to participate in the social health insurance system, for those subject to the insurance obligation, social health insurance is both a legal obligation and a legal entitlement. The health-care legal entitlement is deeply grounded. Indeed, the German Constitution itself protects a bounded right to health insurance. Section 1 of Article 20 of the German Constitution states: "The German Republic is a democratic and a social federal state." Article 20 is one of the two sections of the Constitution that cannot ever be amended;[21] it is one of the foundational "eternal principles" of the German state.

The Constitution does not further elaborate on what it means for Germany to be a "social state," but this concept clearly encompasses a commitment to social justice, social equality, and social protection against the vicissitudes of life.[22] The social state principle is limited in its scope, however; it must be reconciled with the principle of freedom, recognized by article 1 of the Constitution, which has been interpreted as including the concepts of self-responsibility and self-help.[23] That is to say, in German constitutional law the principle of solidarity exists in tension with the principle of subsidiarity.[24] Therefore, while the provision of social health insurance has been recognized as a basic obligation of the state, those with sufficient means to insure themselves are free to decline participation in the social health insurance system and can choose, rather, to purchase private insurance (or to go without).

For those Germans required to participate in the program, or who do so voluntarily, social health insurance is a statutory entitlement. The German social insurance system is established by the Social Code.[25] Section one of the First Book of the Social Code (which establishes general provisions for the social insurance system) sets out the task of the Social Code as realizing the constitutional goal of creating a social state:

> The rights granted under the Social Code shall serve in the realization of the goals of social justice and social security, including social and educational services. To these ends it should also: insure an existence compatible with human dignity, provide equal opportunity for the free development of personality, particularly for young persons, protect and promote the family, make it possible to earn a living through a freely chosen occupation, and assist the prevention or overcoming of particular burdens of life, including assistance with self-help.

The Fifth Book of the Social Code specifically establishes the German social health insurance system.[26] Section five of the Fifth Book of the Social Code creates a duty to be covered by the health insurance and specifies those whom it binds, including, among others, workers, employees, apprentices, the unemployed, farmers, artists and publicists, the handicapped, students, and retired, and the families of insured persons.

The social health insurance system is managed through the social health insurance funds. These funds, of which there are currently about 400,[27] evolved out of the older guild and fraternal society funds.[28] Historically, fund membership was determined by type of employment (with special funds for sailors, miners, and farmers and for certain crafts); or by employer (with many larger businesses having their own funds). Blue-collar workers who did not fit into a particular employment-related fund belonged to a local fund.[29] White-collar workers could choose among a number of "substitute" funds, which grew out of the survivors of the mutual funds which antedated the statutory system.[30] Although the vast majority of funds (318 in 2001) are company funds, most Germans currently belong to the local or substitute funds.

Since 1996, most Germans have been able to choose freely among the local or substitute funds and among the company funds and guild funds that choose to open themselves to the public. This freedom of choice was established by the 1993 Health Care Reform Act in the hopes of holding down health-care costs by encouraging competition among funds.[31] The insureds can change whenever they choose, but must remain with the new fund for at least 18 months.[32] Only the farmers', miners', and sailors' funds, as well as company and guild funds that choose to, remain legally closed.[33]

Historically, premium costs were lower for the company and substitute funds, which covered younger and healthier workers, and higher for the local and occupation-related funds, which had older and sicker members. At the same time, as free choice of funds was instituted in 1996, a risk-equalization scheme was implemented, which moves money from funds with higher contribution rates and more favorable risk structures (measured in terms of age and sex of members) to those with less favorable characteristics.[34] Beginning in 1999, the system also began moving revenue from the funds in the former West Germany to funds in the former East Germany.[35] Amendments to the risk-structure adjustment laws in 2002 introduced a national risk pool to cover 60% of costs of individuals with annual expenditures above 20,000 euros and provision for extra compensation for individuals enrolled in disease-management programs; they also endorsed the creation of a morbidity-based risk-adjustment system by 2007.[36] By 2000, 9.6% of total fund expenditures moved through the risk-adjustment system, while the percentage of fund members who paid a contribution rate varying more than 1% from the average premium dropped from 27% in 1994 to 7% in 1999.[37] While the risk-structure equalization program has led to more equity in contributions for social health insurance, it also has created a situation in which the continued existence of separate funds, with the heightened administrative expenses they bring, makes less and less sense.

Those whom the law requires to participate in the social health insurance system are entitled by statute to receive the services specified in the third chapter of the Fifth Social Code Book, including services necessary for the prevention, early diagnosis, and treatment of diseases, as well as family planning and rehabilitation services.[38] Services must be provided "adequately, effectively, and economically," and only to the extent necessary.[39] Services are generally provided in kind rather than in cash.[40] Historically, however, the most important benefit of the social health insurance funds was sick pay, which was provided directly, and which still makes up about 5% of health insurance expenditures.[41]

Members of the health insurance funds are entitled to receive goods and services from any doctor, hospital, pharmacy, or other provider or professional that participates in the health insurance program. Since virtually all professionals and providers do participate, Germans have much greater freedom of choice of provider than do most Americans.

The insured's entitlement to health care in Germany is realized within the context of the three-cornered relationship that exists among the insured/ patient, the health insurance fund, and the health-care providers and their institutions.[42] First, the insured has a direct relationship with his or her insurance fund, both as an insured participant and as a member. As a participant, the insured is entitled to a rather comprehensive list of benefits, including physicians service, hospital care, some dental care, drugs, and the services of various therapists.[43] The participant may also be entitled to supplemental health-promotion benefits provided under the regulations of the insurance fund.[44] If the participant has a family, they also are entitled to receive services as beneficiaries of the fund, without extra charge.[45]

Insureds are also members of their funds, which are self-governed, nonprofit corporations.[46] In most funds, the day-to-day administration of the fund is managed by an executive board. This board is elected by a governing assembly half of which is elected by the fund members and the other half of which is elected by the employers for the blue-collar funds, and all of which is elected by the members for the white-collar funds. This assembly adopts the bylaws and regulations of the funds, establishes its budget, sets its contribution rate, and elects the governing board.[47] Elections for the assembly are held every six years.[48]

The insured also has a relationship, of course, with his or her health-care provider. Private insurance in Germany reimburses insureds on an indemnity basis for services they purchase from providers. Social insurance participants, on the other hand, receive services directly from their providers, who, in turn, look to the insurance funds for payment. Doctors and dentists are paid through the providers' corporate organizations.[49] Participants may freely choose among doctors or dentists in private practice who treat social insurance patients.[50] Once a patient chooses a family doctor, however, the patient is expected to remain with that doctor for at least a quarter of a year and cannot change unless he or she has a sufficient reason.[51] In the German system, however, the doctor does not function as a gatekeeper—the patient may self-refer to specialists.[52] Specialists of virtually all kinds, including those who use expensive and highly sophisticated equipment, have office-based practices; indeed, only 40% of doctors in office-based practices are general practitioners.[53] Patients, therefore, have direct access to a wide range of services.[54]

Insureds relate to health-care providers as patients. The doctor–patient relationship is a contractual relationship under the civil law, and under the terms of the Social Code, providers owe to their patients the same duty of care as is imposed under the civil contract law.[55] This is a duty to provide diagnosis and treatment in accordance with the standard of the profession, to refer the patient to a specialist or hospital or to seek a consult regarding the patient where necessary, and to inform the patient about the disease and its treatment.[56] To complete the triangle, providers also have contractual relationships with the social health insurance funds. For doctors and dentists, this relationship is mediated through corporate institutions.

In general, the German economy and society are organized on a corporatist basis—that is, individuals are organized into corporate institutions based on their interests and positions in society and in the economy.[57] These institutions, in turn, relate to each other and to the state in furtherance of the interests of their members. Doctors who serve publicly insured patients are members of their state or region's Kassenärztliche Vereinigung, or association of insurance doctors.[58] Dentists are members of their Kassenzahnärztliche Vereinigung. These associations negotiate agreements with the corresponding state's health insurance fund associations.[59] The funds are obligated to pay doctors in accordance with the requirements of the law and the terms of these agreements. The doctors, in contrast, are corporately obligated to make certain that health-care services are adequately available to the members of the health funds.[60] This obligation exists even if the payment that the funds offer for any particular service does not cover the doctor's costs of providing that service.[61]

Although hospitals are also members of corporate institutions, they negotiate with the social health insurance funds directly rather than through these institutions. Increasingly, however, hospitals are paid on the basis of case- and procedure-specific payments, which are established on a corporatist basis. Under recently adopted legislation, reimbursement will move to a complete diagnosis-related group prospective payment system by 2004.[62] The social health insurance funds, however, only cover the operating costs of hospitals; capital costs are still covered by the states and allocated according to state capital development plans.[63]

In sum, in contrast to the United States, where health-care entitlements commonly exist in bilateral relationships between the insured, beneficiary, or recipient, on the one hand, and the insurer or government health-care program, on the other, German entitlements arise in a much more complex environment. The German participant in the social health insurance system has a legal entitlement to the provision of health-care goods and services. An obligation to fulfill the patient's entitlement rests on the insurer, but also on the doctor or other relevant provider and on the corporate organizations representing doctors or other providers. Even though the health insurance fund bears the ultimate legal obligation to satisfy this requirement, the entitlement is usually not asserted directly by the insured against the insurer. Rather, the insured looks to the doctor, the dentist, the hospital, or the pharmacist for services. These persons and entities then look to the insurance funds for reimbursement once services have been provided.

Only in a few circumstances are insurers faced with individual claims.[64] Requests for exotic forms of durable medical equipment, experimental treatments, or alternative medicine seem to be the only claims for health-care services that regularly result in disputes between the social insurance funds and their members.[65] Indeed, the claims of doctors and dentists are normally processed by the corporate institutions rather than by the insurers, as will be explained more fully later in this chapter. In turn, the insurers only pay over lump sums based on negotiated budgets to the corporatist institutions. Even these corporate institutions rarely review individual claims, however, choosing rather to focus on aggregate prescribing or treatment patterns, as explained later in this chapter.

This system affords considerable discretion to health-care providers to care for their patients according to their own medical judgment based on the medical needs of the patient. The patient's legal entitlement in Germany rarely leads to a legal conflict. Conflict (more often economic or political than legal) takes place within and between the corporatist institutions and does not directly involve the individual patient. The direct conflicts often found in the United States (between the needs and desires of the patient for medical treatment, the professional judgment of the doctor as to what services are medically appropriate, the hope of the doctor paid on a capitated basis to make a profit, and the incentives of the insurer or managed-care organization to hold down expenditures to increase profits) have until now been less starkly apparent in the German social health insurance setting.

## Health-Care Budgets

German providers are in most instances paid on a fee-for-service basis, and the inflationary tendencies of fee-for-service payment systems have long been clear. Fee-for-service creates strong incentives for noneconomical overprovision of services. In Germany, fee-for-service reimbursement has had to be tempered with other measures to control the cost of services and, more specifically, to control utilization. The most important of these measures is the application of health-care budgets.

Sectoral health-care budgets in Germany are made possible by the fact that participants and beneficiaries of the German social insurance funds receive in-kind services from providers rather than indemnity payments from the funds. For the major sectors of health care—ambulatory physician care, hospital care, and dental care—resources are allocated through budgets negotiated between representatives of the health insurance funds and representatives of the providers or of their corporatist institutions.[66] Pharmaceutical expenditures have also been budgeted from time to time.

For example, for the past two and a half decades, the regional unions of insurance doctors have annually negotiated budgets with the social health insurance funds for funding all physicians' services within the region. At first these budgets were voluntary, but since 1989 they have been mandatory.[67] The budgets are negotiated with reference to the principle of premium stability: health insurance premiums must not grow at a rate greater than the rate of inflation generally.[68] They are negotiated within guidelines established by the Concerted Action in Health Care organization, which represents all of the major interest groups in health care and which was established in part to guide these negotiations.[69] Though § 72 of the Social Code provides that professionals are to receive an appropriate or reasonable (angemessen) compensation for their services, § 71, as currently written, requires that the insurance funds and the corporate institutions representing the providers must comply with the requirement of premium stability. The German Supreme Social Court (Bundessozialgericht, or BSG) has recently held that the language of the code requires that the principle of premium stability take precedence over the principle of adequate compensation.[70]

German doctors, like their American counterparts, can be paid for any service that they deliver, provided that it has a corresponding billing code.[71] Procedures are approved for listing in the procedure code list, the Einheitlicher Berwertungsmaßstab für ärztliche Leistungen (EBM), by a joint commission of the social insurance funds and the insurance doctor associations, the Bundesausschuß der Ärzte und Krankenkassen, of which more will be said presently.[72] A separate joint committee at the federal level, the Bewertungsausschuß, assigns a value to the various points.[73] The EBM lists basic services that may be ordered by any physician, as well as specialist procedures, and describes the preconditions that must be met for claiming under any particular code.[74] The weight of EBM codes for particular services or specialties is further modified by each regional insurance doctor association using its own Honorverteilungsmaßstab (HVM) (which gives the association the opportunity to adjust the codes for disparities among various doctors or services) to determine reimbursement in each region.[75]

Individual doctors bill for their services using the codes provided by their regional associations. They total up their points and bill them on a quarterly basis. Bills submitted by doctors are screened in several different ways before they are reimbursed. First, they are screened for calculation errors and for "plausibility" in terms of the doctor's specialty of the patient's condition.[76] Second, bills are subjected to economic monitoring—utilization review—to identify doctors whose claims seem excessive. (This process is described further later in this chapter). Third, since 1997, the number of reimbursable points per individual patient for some services have been limited by patient-specific budgets, Praxisbudgets, which vary among specialties and regions.[77]

Once the billable points of each doctor in a region have been identified, these point numbers are summed to yield a total number of points for all services billed during the quarter by all physicians in the region. This total is then divided into the quarterly budget to yield a point value,[78] which is then multiplied by the number of billable points submitted by each doctor to determine the amount each particular doctor is paid.

Hospitals are also paid on the basis of budgets negotiated with the social health insurance funds.[79] Operating costs are currently paid for in part through diagnosis-determined per-case (Fallpauschal) and procedure-specific (Sonderentgelt) payments, with per diem payments covering expenses not covered by these specific payments.[80] The classification scheme for these payments is established through negotiations between the hospitals and regional health insurance fund associations at the national level, while the payment level is based on regional health insurance fund/hospital association negotiations.[81] As noted, recent legislation has endorsed a move toward reimbursement totally based on diagnosis-related groups (DRGs). At the hospital level, however, payments are currently subject to flexible budgets that are negotiated between the individual hospitals and the health insurance funds.[82] The budgets do not operate as absolute limits on hospital expenditures, as payments are ultimately based on services provided. Budgets do, however, rein in health fund expenditures, as per-service payments are sharply reduced once budgetary limits are exceeded.

Germany has also attempted to control pharmaceutical expenditures through fixed budgets (in combination with other strategies like cost sharing by patients and reference prices to encourage the use of lower price drugs).[83] Between 1992 and 1997, spending caps were imposed on drug expenditures on a regional basis, with the regional physician associations liable for expenditures in excess of the spending caps. The idea that grounded this scheme was that doctors can control drug spending through their prescribing, and would be more cost conscious if they were collectively—and ultimately individually—responsible for drug cost overruns. Though this approach seemed to limit drug costs quite effectively in the early years, by the mid-1990s the spending caps were being routinely exceeded, while attempts by the insurance funds to recover overpayments from the doctor's associations were resisted and ultimately proved largely unsuccessful. The Second Social Health Insurance Restructuring Act abolished the regional spending caps effective in 1998, replacing them with practice-specific spending targets and other limitations. But the subsequent 1998 Act to Strengthen Solidarity imposed limited liability on the physician's associations (up to 105% of the budgets), while waiving liability for earlier overbudget prescribing.[84]

The German system of budgeted payments contrasts sharply with the American system of entitlements. As described in Chapter 3 in this volume, the budgetary commitment for entitlement programs in the United States is open-ended. If a covered service is provided to a covered beneficiary by an eligible provider, the program must pay for it. The risk of program expenditures, therefore, rests squarely with the government.

In recent years in the United States, this risk has been shared to some extent with providers. The goal of prospective payment systems (PPS), beginning with the diagnosis-related group hospital prospective payment and continuing on to the PPS systems established for skilled nursing facilities, home health, rehabilitation hospitals, and outpatient treatment by the 1997 Balanced Budget Act, has been to shift to providers some of the risk of treating particular patients. Similarly, a primary reason for the establishment of managed care in Medicaid and under Medicare+Choice has been to shift some of the risk of the cost of care for Medicare beneficiaries and Medicaid recipients to managed-care organizations. Finally, Medicare deductibles, copayments, and coinsurance also shift some of the risk to program beneficiaries.

But there are limits to these strategies. Prospective payment formulas only shift some of the risk of a particular episode of care for a particular patient to a particular provider. Although managed care shifts risk more globally, managed-care payment formulas, at least for Medicare, are risk-adjusted, so that much of the risk remains with the federal government. Further, the vast majority of Medicare beneficiaries, as well as most of Medicaid disabled and elderly patients (who are by far the most costly to care for), are currently not enrolled in managed care.[85]

In Germany, some of the risk of health-care costs is also passed on to insureds through cost-sharing obligations, just as it is under the Medicare program and private insurance in the United States.[86] Reliance on cost sharing in Germany has varied from government to government, but cost-sharing obligations are currently in place with respect to prescription drugs, hospital services, medical supplies, physical and other therapies, medical equipment, dental services, and rehabilitation services. Copayments are very low by U.S. standards, however: 9 euros per day for hospital care, and 4 to 5 euros per package of prescription drugs.[87]

But, to return to the main point, the risk of health-care costs in Germany is borne to a much greater degree by providers—individually or collectively through their corporate institutions—rather than by the insurer or by insureds.

This reduced exposure of the insurer to risk, in turn, diminishes conflict over entitlements between the insurer and insured for most categories of services. It has heightened conflict between providers and the social health insurance funds, however, and among providers and provider groups.

This conflict has become sharply exacerbated in the past few years. The 1988 and 1992 Health Structure Reform Acts imposed restrictions on the number of physicians who could participate as ambulatory physicians in any particular locality. These statutes delayed the effective date of the restrictions until the mid-1990s, causing a large number of doctors to move from hospital practice to the ambulatory sector to avoid being shut out by the restrictions. The number of doctors increased from 88,811 in 1990 to 112,683 in 1998[88] and contributed to an increase in the number of services billed—26% between 1992 and 1995—causing a 10% decrease in the value of points billed.[89] The situation deteriorated further during 1996 and 1997, as physicians billed more and more points, trying to maintain some stability of their income, but collectively driving down the per point value—a situation called in Germany the "hamster wheel effect." This led to the imposition in 1997 of "praxisbudgets," limiting the number of points that could be billed for any particular patient in a quarter, as well as to other limits. Physicians were also successful in getting a provision included in the Second Social Health Insurance Restructuring Act of 1997 committing the social insurance system to return to fixed point values— real fee for service—but the 1998 Act to Strengthen Solidarity in the Social Health Insurance, adopted after a change of government, reinstated fixed budgets for the ambulatory sector, thus retaining floating point values.[90] Germany is currently attempting to implement a system of fixed point values tied to fixed volumes for services.

Although fixed budgets have led to heightened tensions among specialists, who must split up a shrinking pie, and between the funds and participating doctors, as doctors continually push to get out from under the budgets and return to fixed point values, they have not yet led to widespread reports of denial of services to patients. Indeed, the German Bundessozialgericht (BSG) has decided that doctors who contract with the insurance funds must provide services to their patients whether or not they are adequately paid by the funds for particular services.[91] In separate decisions, the court also held that doctors cannot charge socially insured patients extra for covered services beyond authorized copayments,[92] nor may they provide covered services only privately.[93]

The fact that provider budgets are managed at the level of corporate institutions rather than at the level of the individual provider tends to militate against patient-specific rationing. In fact, the system imposes on individual doctors and dentists incentives to do more rather than less for their patients, even though it also presents them with a prisoner's dilemma, for if all doctors and dentists respond in this way to the incentives, all will be worse off.[94]

The important point, however, is that the economic incentives that face individual German physicians are more or less aligned with the legal entitlements of patients to maximize the availability of services to any particular patient. This is in contrast to the United States, where economic incentives and legal entitlements often work at cross purposes, potentially limiting the care received by any particular patient.

## The Social Courts and Coverage Claims

Another important characteristic of the German health-care system is the legal forum that is available to resolve conflicts that do arise among the participants in the system. Legal entitlements are primarily of rhetorical value unless there is some forum in which they can be asserted. In the United States, as discussed in Chapter 3, access to the courts has been limited in the Medicare program by rigorously enforced statutory requirements of exhaustion of remedies and in the Medicaid programs by the indigence of beneficiaries and by the limited scope of justiciable issues. Even insured employees, who receive private insurance subsidized by tax deductions and exclusions, have only limited rights under ERISA and are often barred by ERISA from pursuing state court remedies.

The German health insurance system is actively supervised by a system of special courts, the Sozialgerichte, or social courts. When individuals are denied access to goods or services in the health-care system (durable medical equipment or experimental treatments, for example), or when providers receive less money than they believe themselves to be entitled, they can appeal to the social courts.[95] The courts also supervise the relationships between the social insurance funds and the corporate provider associations, and between the provider associations and their members.

Some 69 trial-level social courts are located throughout Germany.[96] Appeals from decisions of these courts can be made to the Landessozialgerichte, which exist in each of the 16 states.[97] In some instances, appeals from the Landessozialgerichte can be taken to the BSG, which sits in Kassell.[98] In 2001, 96 of the 556 appeals resolved by the BSG involved sickness insurance claims and another 64 of the claims were from insurance doctors, making health insurance issues the largest category of cases decided by the BSG.[99]

Germany is a civil law country, and court decisions do not have precisely the same precedential weight and effect that they have in the United States. Nevertheless, the decisions of the social courts, and of the BSG in particular, are taken very seriously and have a major role in defining the contours and boundaries of German health insurance law. This is especially true because the defendants—the social insurance funds or physician associations—reappear in the cases again and again, and there is therefore a certain res judicata effect of decisions against them.

Social courts are presided over by a panel of judges. In the courts of the first instance, there are usually three judges—a professional judge and two lay judges.[100] In disputes regarding insurance coverage, one of the lay judges represents insureds, the other employers.[101] In matters concerning the relationship between health insurance companies and insurance doctors, one of the lay judges represents the insurance companies, the other the doctors; in matters involving the internal relationships of insurance doctors, both represent the doctors.[102] At the state and national social court levels, the panel consists of three professional judges and two lay judges.[103] The BSG is divided into a number of panels of judges, called senates, each of which has jurisdiction over a particular body of cases. The Sixth Senate, for example, hears disputes involving insurance doctors; the First and Third Senates hear different kinds of coverage disputes.

The courts hold oral proceedings in which the parties are often, though not necessarily or always, represented by attorneys. The judges take an active role in the proceedings, interrogating the parties and their attorneys. In fact, the judges have an obligation to investigate the facts thoroughly and to assist the parties in effectively presenting their cases.[104] Traditionally, there has been no filing fee for filing a complaint in the social courts (though public law entities such as insurance companies must pay a fee), and the victorious claimant has the possibility of receiving his litigation costs from the losing insurance company.[105] Thus, disputes involving social insurance programs end up in court with great frequency.

As noted, most decisions as to whether or not to offer treatment in a particular situation are made implicitly by the treating physician, and not by the insurance funds, and thus treatment decisions escape judicial review (expect perhaps through malpractice cases). Coverage claims come before the social courts only in those cases where an insured must make a claim directly to a fund, as with medical equipment, or where a patient or provider is appealing the general coverage exclusion of a particular procedure or product, usually when experimental or alternative health-care services or products are at issue.

Historically, when the social courts have been presented with claims, they have tended to interpret health-care entitlements expansively. An example of this is the traditional treatment by the BSG of experimental and alternative medicine. On their face, the sections of title 5 the German Social Code (SGB V) dealing with health insurance would appear to strictly limit the services for which the health insurance funds are required to pay. Section 2, which defines the scope of services, provides that services must be provided effectively and economically, and only to the extent necessary,[106] further specifying that quality and efficiency of services must comply with the general state of medical knowledge.[107] Section 12 states even more emphatically that providers may not provide, insureds may not request, and insurers may not pay for services that are unnecessary or that are not economically provided, a directive repeated in §§ 70 and 72.[108] Section 28 again obligates doctors to provide services according to the standards of medical practice, while § 34 excludes payment for ineffective medications.[109] Finally, § 135 provides that new diagnostic and treatment methods may not be ordered at the cost of the social health insurance funds until the Bundesausschuß der Ärzte und Krankenkassen (Federal Commission of Insurance Doctors and Health Insurance Funds), at the request of an insurance doctor's association or the federal organization of health insurance funds, has made recommendations regarding the recognition of the new procedure and qualifications for doctors who may deliver it.[110] Under 1997 amendments to the SGB V, these recommendations must consider the medical necessity and efficiency of the procedure, as well as its effectiveness.[111]

As long as an EBM code exists for a service, a doctor can provide it and be paid for it, subject only to retrospective review for excessive provision of care under the Wirtschaftlichkeitsprüfung process, described below.[112] The EBM applies primarily to traditional medicine, however, and only covers new and experimental treatments only to the extent they have been reviewed under the § 135 new diagnostic and treatment procedure approval process.

Where services are either experimental or nontraditional, and thus not yet recognized in the EBM, coverage policy has been more controversial.[113] Until the late 1990s, the Third Senate of the BSG, which decides issues of coverage policy, had recognized the extension of coverage to alternative or experimental treatment methods in cases of severe illness of unknown origin where traditional treatment methods are ineffective or where recognized treatments are not appropriate for the particular case.[114] In either case, the court required a plausible case to be made that the treatment could be effective.[115] But the court was willing to order the sickness fund to indemnify the patient where a disputed treatment proved, in fact, to be effective.[116]

Arguments that the Social Code should be interpreted to cover alternative and experimental treatments not yet evaluated under the § 135 procedures were based in part on the structure of the Social Code. The SGB V governs both the relationships between insurers and their insureds and between insurers and providers. It was argued that provisions like § 135 might limit payment of providers to particular procedures, but did not limit the independent and superior right of insureds to receive other procedures where those procedures were otherwise covered by the SGB V.[117] Even though providers could not bill directly for services not covered by the EBM, it was argued, patients could receive such services and then claim indemnification from their insurer.[118] In short, the academic commentators argued that the direct payment principle was subordinate to the principle of comprehensive coverage.

Further, some academic commentators argued that the German Constitution would be violated if the SGB V were interpreted to permit decisions of a commission of doctors and insurers to establish rules that would limit the rights of insureds.[119] The delegation doctrine is much more robust in Germany than in the United States, and the German Constitution limits the entities to which authority for making generally binding rules can be delegated and the forms such rules can take. It was argued that the commission that reviews experimental procedures is not an agency that can constitutionally limit the rights of insureds.[120] It was also argued that a total ban on coverage of services not listed in the EBM would violate the constitutional right of doctors to professional freedom,[121] and the constitutional right of self-determination and personal integrity of persons who are required by law to be insured.[122]

In a series of recent decisions, however, the BSG, led by its First Senate, has concluded that in most instances services can be covered by the health insurance funds only once they are approved by the Bundesausschuß. Where new services have not yet been approved by the Bundesausschuß, payment will only be available if the Bundesausschuß has not acted promptly enough, and where the service otherwise has been scientifically validated.

A decision from March 28, 2000, involved a claim for a particular form of experimental therapy to stimulate the immune system of a patient suffering from kidney cancer.[123] The Bundesausschuß had not yet reached a decision regarding coverage for the therapy. The BSG acknowledged that in some instances a social court could review a claim for therapy that the Bundesausschuß had not yet acted upon, but the court could only approve a therapy in those circumstances where the therapy was scientifically established through clinical trials. Even if the disease could prove fatal, and there were no established cures available, the social insurance funds nevertheless had no obligation under the law, or under the Constitution, to pay for a treatment whose effectiveness was not scientifically established.

A pair of BSG decisions decided on April 3, 2001, further strengthened the role of the Bundesausschuß. Both cases involved ICSI, a form of in vitro fertilization in which the sperm is injected directly into the egg. In both cases, the patient had paid for the service directly because there was no approved code under which the doctor could directly bill the service, and in both the patient sought reimbursement from the social insurance fund. In both cases, payment had been denied.

In the first case, the service was received before the 1997 decision of the Bundesausschuß had addressed the question of coverage.[124] The BSG held that, because the service was not yet approved, it was not covered. The court recognized that if the Bundesausschuß had arbitrarily delayed a decision on coverage, the social courts might have been able to intervene, but held that there had not been unreasonable delay in the case at hand. In the second case, the service was received after the Bundesausschuß coverage decision, which had in fact been negative. The BSG proceeded, however, to review the Bundesausschuß decision. Finding that ICSI was similar to conventional in vitro fertilization (already approved for payment) and no more likely to present risks or less likely to succeed, the court held that the Bundesausschuß decision was contrary to the law and permitted the insured to collect the cost of the service.[125] Although the decision turned in part on a special provision of the SGB V that dealt with assisted reproduction, it indicates the direction that the BSG seems to be going in coverage decisions—deferring in the first instance to the corporate institutions, but ultimately subjecting their decisions to reasonableness review.

The tendency of these decisions is to curtail the liberality that previously characterized the German social insurance system. Coverage of services, though still generous, must be based on evidence. In the first instance, it is the job of the corporate institutions, acting through the Bundesausschuß to evaluate the scientific evidence. If the Bundesausschuß fails to do so in a timely manner, or if it does so improperly, the BSG can review its decision, but its review is limited in scope.

On the whole, however, the social courts have been quite protective of the rights of insureds, and probably less deferential to public insurers than have the American courts.[126] The courts also seem to focus more on the substance of coverage disputes and less on procedural issues than American courts do. The German social courts are also far more accessible to insureds than are the American federal courts. The absence of filing fees, the fact that attorneys are not necessary (and that attorney's fees can be paid to prevailing parties), and the less-formal nature of judicial proceedings all combine to make the courts more friendly to insureds than American courts are. Given the responsibility of physicians for providing health-care services under German law, it is also important that the courts are very open to physicians as well, as will be discussed momentarily. Finally, the fact that hearing panels contain lay representatives makes them at least potentially more understanding of the claims of insureds. Therefore, the German social courts provide a model of the role that judicial institutions can play in protecting health-care entitlements.

## Social Court Review of Physician Compensation and Utilization Review

The role of the corporatist institutions in the German health insurance system, the operation of sectoral budgets, and the work of the social courts is also illustrated by BSG oversight of ambulatory physician payment allocation and utilization review in Germany. As noted earlier, physicians in Germany in most instances determine independently what services their patients need. They are paid on a fee-for-service basis and thus face incentives to provide care generously for their patients. The German sense of entitlement, moreover, reinforces the demand for generous provision of services. But, physicians look to their corporate associations for payment, and these associations are paid, in turn, by the social health insurance funds on a negotiated budget basis, as described in this chapter. The associations use both the various screens and budgets described, along with utilization review, to ensure that all of their members are treated fairly and have equal access to their budget. This process is ultimately subject to judicial review in the social courts.[127]

The German utilization review process is known as Wirtschaftlichkeitsprüfung, or economic monitoring, and is established by § 106 of the SGB V.[128] Utilization review does not address the claims of particular individuals to coverage for particular types of services but, rather, analyzes the aggregate provision or ordering of services for patients by particular doctors. It is a process through which doctors and dentists who perform unnecessary procedures or who order unnecessary drugs or therapy are first warned and then, if they persist, have their payments reduced or are subjected to fines.[129] These penalties are assessed by committees composed of representatives of the social health insurance funds and the physician associations and are subject to appeal to the social courts.[130] It is not uncommon for decisions to be appealed and to be reversed by the social courts or settled after appeal.

Doctors (and dentists) have an obligation under the Social Code to provide services sufficiently, effectively, and economically, in no greater volume than necessary.[131] Section 106 of SGB V, and the extensive body of case law interpreting § 106 and earlier provisions of the Reichsversicherungsordnung that preceded it, provide a variety of methods that the physician and health insurance associations may use to ensure that services are economically provided.

The favored approach to economic monitoring for billing for doctors' services is currently statistical review.[132] The key variable in this review is cost per patient, or the average amount the doctor bills per patient.[133] A doctor's claims are reviewed to determine how many points the doctor has billed for each patient. Claims by particular doctors are then compared to average utilization by other doctors.[134] Claims are usually compared by patient group, specifically considering separately older, retired patients, and younger patients.[135] For comparison purposes, doctors are grouped by specialty and locality.[136] The group must be, on the one hand, sufficiently homogenous but, on the other hand, sufficiently large to permit meaningful statistical comparison.[137] Doctors prescribing practices can also be reviewed, comparing them to prescribing guidelines.[138]

The statistical comparison usually encompasses a doctors' total claims, but it can be limited to particular services or categories of services.[139] Doctors' claims are only challenged if they lie well beyond the mean—at least 40% beyond before an "obvious disproportionality" can be found.[140] Where prescribing guidelines are used for comparison, however, a deviation of 15% can result in sanctions.

A doctor who is found to be a statistical outlier has two primary lines of defense. First, and most important, the doctor may argue that there are exceptional circumstances respecting his or her practice that justify the deviation, such as the fact that a doctor is just beginning a practice and must perform an exceptional number of initial interviews and examinations, or that the doctor practices in a particular subspecialty or with a particular method that results in the treatment of more expensive patients.[141] Second, doctors may claim that the high use of certain services is compensated for by low usage in other areas.[142] Doctors may argue, for example, that they gave a high number of injections because they prescribed fewer oral medications.[143]

The individual cases of doctors may also be subjected to review on a case-by-case basis. For a time, the BSG held up individual case review as the preferred form of economic review,[144] but it became obvious that individual review was generally not practical. The court decided quite early that for an individual review to be truly accurate and reliable, the review would have to go beyond the doctor's records, perhaps including an actual examination of the individual patient to determine the patient's actual condition.[145] Moreover, the examination would have to focus not on the patient's condition at the time of the review but, rather, on the patient's condition at the time of the treatment. Since the utilization review commissions do not have the resources to perform such examinations, and have no means to require patients to submit to them, individual review is difficult and rarely done.[146] Only in the dental area, where review can readily be performed on the basis of X-rays, does individual review play a major role.[147]

As described earlier, in the past few years, various forms of budgets and billing limitations—most notably the per patient praxisbudgets—have been imposed to supplement utilization review in controlling physician billing.[148] Application of these budgetary limitations has also been challenged in the social courts. Just as the courts have been more reticent in recent years to order the insurance funds to cover new services, so have they been reluctant to interfere in the setting of payment levels.

In a recent case challenging the praxisbudgets for general practitioners, for example, the BSG held that, even though the budget setting process was in the end subject to judicial review, the process involved establishing norms rather than adjudicating facts, and, therefore, the Bewertungsausschuß had to be accorded considerable discretion.[149] The court upheld the decision of the Bewertungsausschuß for the second quarter of 1998 which was under challenge, but also observed that if the Bewertungsausschuß did not update its methodology by the end of 2002 to take account of new data, its allocation of budgets would no longer be supportable.

In another case from 2000, the BSG upheld the legality of the use of payments for bundled services (Teilbudgets), but stuck down the practice of one of the associations to presume that a doctor was billing fraudulently when the number of claims for a particular service exceeded by 10% the highest number of claims for the same service presented in any quarter in the previous year.[150]

The functioning and judicial review of budgeting and economic review illustrates each of the issues raised by this chapter. First, in contrast to utilization review in the United States, which often takes the form of preauthorization of services, the individual's entitlement to health-care services in Germany is not directly threatened or encumbered by the operation of the economic review system, which looks at practices in aggregate. Second, budgeting of payments and economic review do not result in a direct conflict between providers and insurers but, rather, take place primarily in the context of the relationship between physicians and their own corporate institutions. Third, allocation of budgets and economic review has to date helped to make possible the continuation of fixed sectoral budgets, which limit the risk of insurers and insureds, while at the same time preserving a fee-for-service system that encourages generous provision of health-care services and discourages stinting. Finally, the social courts play a constructive role that is missing in the United States, ensuring that patients and providers are treated fairly, while at the same time taking into consideration the need for cost containment.

## Limitations of the German Social Health Insurance System

Although the German social health insurance system has much to offer as a model for health-care entitlements, it also has significant failings. These have made it increasingly difficult for the system to continue to afford its members generous coverage while at the same time holding down costs.

Perhaps the most important problem facing the system is the limitation of its financing mechanism. The fact that the program is financed out of wage-related contributions (essentially payroll taxes) has several important benefits. First, it creates a certain distance between health insurance and the public budget. The fact that the government decides to spend more on education, or roads, or defense, or prisons has no immediate effect on expenditures for health care. Health care is not forced to compete with other budget priorities for scarce tax dollars. More important, health-care expenditures are not tied directly to levels of taxation. Rising expenditures for health care does not require increases in the levels of income taxation, property tax, or value-added tax.

Second, the contribution approach is less regressive than private insurance-based systems (though not as progressive as taxation-based systems).[151] Premium contributions are strictly proportionate to wages and are not risk-adjusted in any way. The same rate is also charged for family coverage as for individual coverage. Although each fund determines its own premium rates, Germany's risk-equalization system moves money from funds that have older and poorer populations to those that have younger and wealthier populations, thus diminishing incentives for cherry picking. The fact that the wealthy can opt for private insurance, however, and that health insurance contributions are capped results in a system that is more regressive than that of other countries that rely on social insurance.[152]

Germany's use of wage-based contributions to finance the social insurance system has also created significant problems. First, the high level of premiums (averaging 14% of wages in 2002), particularly when added to other social insurance premiums and bargained-for benefits, makes job creation in Germany very difficult. In 2002, total payroll taxes imposed on employers equaled 41.1% of gross wages.[153] These rates make Germany's current high unemployment rates understandable.

Second, because those whose incomes exceed the mandatory insurance level are not obligated to participate in the social insurance funds, the program tends to be funded by those with lower incomes, with little help from the wealthiest members of society. Many of those who participate in the program—pensioners, the unemployed, and those on welfare (whose premiums are paid by the local governments)—contribute relatively little to the funds, though they may require costly care.[154] Part-time employees who earn less than a minimum amount per year are allowed to participate without paying premiums themselves, though their employers must pay premiums at the 10% level.[155] Even those who are allowed to opt out of the system, and who yet participate voluntarily, are in general those who are better off financially by doing so because they are in poor health or have large families, thus the funds suffer from a degree of adverse selection.[156]

Third, the contributions of those who participate in the program are based only on their wages.[157] Other sources of income—for example, investment income, rents, profits, and royalties—are not considered. As an increasing share of national income consists of these forms of income rather than wages, the statutory insurance funds have access to a decreasing share of the national income for support. Between 1980 and 2001, for example, the percentage of GDP spent on health care in Germany increased from 8% to a little over 10%, but wages as a percentage of the GDP product dropped from 74% to 65%, thus the contribution rate as a percentage of wages grew from 11.4% to 14%.[158] This development, as much as the increasing costs of health care, has contributed to the increasing difficulty that social health insurance funds experience in making ends meet.[159]

The German social insurance system, moreover, faces not only problems of inadequate financing, but also of increasing costs. In particular, limiting pharmaceutical costs has proved increasingly difficult in Germany as elsewhere. Germany has tried virtually every approach tried elsewhere, including three-tiered copayments, reference prices, negative formularies, and positive formularies. It has also tried to penalize doctors for overprescribing. Pharmaceutical costs continue to grow largely unabated, however, threatening the financial stability of the system, while patients strongly resist any further limitations on prescribing.

When one turns from the social insurance system to the broader health-care system, further problems become visible. Some of the problems faced by the German system, like the problem of technology assessment[160] or dealing with high-cost diseases[161] are common to all developed health-care systems. Others, such as the strict separation between the ambulatory, inpatient hospital, and long-term care sectors, are more peculiarly German problems.[162] Yet other problems, such as the obligation to pay for services provided elsewhere in Europe or the potential restrictive application of European competition law, are general European problems.

In general, the system seems increasingly driven by cost concerns, which seem to be limiting on the one hand the generous provision of services that Germans have long expected and received and on the other the reasonably liberal payment for services enjoyed by health-care providers. These tendencies are visible in German BSG decisions upholding denials of coverage for experimental services and upholding new approaches to limiting payment for services, like praxisbudgets.

Despite its problems, however, Germany, the first country to recognize public health-care entitlements, still has much to offer as a model for designing health-care entitlements. In fact, Germany has succeeded in providing technologically advanced health-care services to all its residents at a relatively reasonable cost, and has done so under the reasonably exercised oversight of legal institutions that have supported the goal of cost control while respecting the rights of insureds and providers.

# Notes

1. See Detlev Zöllner, "Germany," in *The Evolution of Social Insurance, 1881–1981,* edited by Peter A. Köhler and Hans F. Zacher (London: Frances Pinter, 1982), 13.

2. Ibid., 28–29. This sum equaled about three times the average worker's income in 1882 and resulted in 4.3 million workers being insured by 1885, which was about 40% of persons employed and 10% of the population.

3. Deborah A. Stone, *The Limits of Professional Power: National Health Care in the Federal Republic of Germany* (Cambridge, Mass.: MIT Press, 1980), 78.

4. European Observatory on Health Care Systems, *Health Care Systems in Transition, Germany* (Copenhagen: European Observatory on Health Care Systems, 2000), 39.

5. Ibid., 39.

6. Reinhard Busse, "Germany," in *Observatory, Health Care Systems and Challenges in Eight Countries: Trends and Challenges* (Copenhagen: European Observatory on Health Care Systems, 2002).

7. European Observatory, *Health Care Systems in Transition*, 39.

8. Privately insured patients get a private room and are guaranteed treatment by department chiefs in the hospital. It is also generally believed that they get faster appointments and more solicitous care from ambulatory physicians, who are paid more than twice as much for privately insured patients than for publicly insured. The care they receive is not radically different from those covered by social insurance, however, as is witnessed by the fact that most persons who could purchase private insurance purchase social insurance instead. See Reinhard Busse, Chris Howarth, and Friedrich Schwarz, "The Future Development of the Rights-Based Approach to Health Care in Germany: More Rights or Fewer," in *Hard Choices in Health Care*, edited by Jo Lenahan (London: BMJ British Publishing Group, 1997), 28–30; Richard A. Knox, *Germany: One Nation with Health Care for All* (New York: Faulkner and Gray, 1993), 76–77.

9. "Deutliche Mehrheit für das Solidarprinzip der gesetzlichen Krankenversicherung," available at http://www.aok.de/bv/bundesvb/presse/tab/gesund/691841655802822656.html (June 2000). Full address does not work, but www.aok.de will take you where you need to go.

10. "Höheres Risiko—höherer Beitrag? Ja und nein!" *Ärzte Zeitung*, available at http://www.aerztezeitung.de/docs/1999/10/22/192a0602.asp (October 22, 1999).

11. "Das Solidarprinzip hat oberste Priorität," *Ärtze Zeitung*, available at http://www.aerztezeitung.de/docs/1999/10/18/188a0602.asp (October 18, 1999).

12. See, tracing history, Knox, *Germany*, 25–40, 241–276.

13. See, European Observatory, *Health Care Systems in Transition*, 107–116 (summarizing recent health care reforms).

14. AOK, G&G Blickpunkt (Feb. 2002), 4.

15. Ibid.

16. Karl H. Brückner, "Versicherte sind bereit, mehr Eigenverantwortung zu übernehmen," *Ärzte Zeitung*, available at http://www.aerztezeitung.de/docs/2000/10/06/178a0901.asp (October 6, 2000).

17. "Sparen in der Medizin? Die Deutschen sind skeptisch," *Ärzte Zeitung*, available at http://www.aerztezeitung.de/docs/1999/10/01/177a0102.asp (October 1, 1999).

18. Reinhard Busse, "Priority-Setting and Rationing in German Health Care," *Health Policy* 50 (1999): 71, 84.

19. See Rudolf Klein, *The New Politics of the NHS*, 4th ed. (Harlow, England: Pearson Education, 2001), 4–5.

20. Some 94% of Germans polled support the principle of free choice of physician. Busse, "Priority-Setting and Rationing in German Health Care," 87.

21. Grundgesetz, art. 79, § 3.

22. Detlef Merten, "Verfassungsrechtliche Grundlagen," in *Handbuch des Socialversicherungsrechts: Krankenversicherungsrecht*, edited by Bertram Schulin II (Munich: C. H. Beck, 1994), 152–154.

23. Ibid., 156–157.

24. Bertram Shulin, "Rechtliche Grundprinzipien der gesetzlichen Krankenver-

sicherung und ihre Probleme", in *Handbuch des Socialversicherungsrechts: Kranken-versicherungsrecht* edited by Bertram Schulin (Munich: C. H. Beck, 1994), 187–199.

25. The Social Code was codified in 1969, replacing chapters of the earlier Re-ichsversicherungsordnung. Rolf-Ulrich Schlenker, "Geschichte und Reformperspek-tiven der gesetzlichen Krankenkassen," in *Handbuch des Socialversicherungsrechts: Krankenversicherungsrecht*, edited by Bertram Shulin (Munich: C. H. Beck, 1994), 22.

26. The German system is literally a sickness insurance (Krankenversicherung) rather than a health insurance (Gesundheitsversicherung) program. The insurance funds are called the Krankenkassen, sickness funds. This denomination reflects the historical role of the funds in providing sick pay and in insuring against the costs of illness, and is, in fact, an accurate description of what health insurance does. After all, a healthy person does not need insurance, and insurance can do little to insure health. Rather, it is the costs of sickness that insurance covers. In deference to American custom, however, I will refer to the German insurance as "social health insurance."

27. Christa Altenstetter, "Health Care in Germany," available at http://web.gc.cuny.edu/EUSC/activities/Paper/altenstetter2.htm (cited June 21, 2001).

28. See Peter Rosenberg, "The Origins and Development of Compulsory Health In-surance in Germany," in *Political Values and Health Care: The German Experience* (Cambridge, Mass.: MIT Press, 1986), 105–112; Stone, *The Limits of Professional Power*, 23.

29. Knox, *Germany*, 28.

30. Ibid, 65–66.

31. European Observatory, *Health Care Systems in Transition, Germany*, 110.

32. Busse, "Germany," 52.

33. European Observatory, *Health Care Systems in Transition, Germany*, 40.

34. Reinhard Busse, "Risk Structure Compensation in Germany's Statutory Health Insurance," *European Journal of Public Health* 11 (2001): 174–177.

35. Ibid.

36. Busse, "Germany," 52.

37. Busse, *Observatory, Health Care Systems and Challenges*; Charles Normand and Reinhard Busse, "Social Health Insurance Financing," in *Funding Health Care: Op-tions for Europe*, edited by Elias Mossialos (Buckingham: Open University Press, 2002).

38. *Sozialgesetzbuch* (hereafter SGB), V, § 11.

39. SGB V, § 12, subsection 1.

40. SGB V, § 13, subsection 1.

41. Federal Health Ministry, "Ausgabenanteile im Jahr 2000 Bund," available at http://www.bmgesundheit.de/presse/2001/2001/89.htm (June 26, 2001).

42. See Ingwer Ebsen, "Der Behandlungsanspruch des Versicherten in der ge-setzlichen Krankenversicherung und das Leistungserbringungsrecht," in *Festschrift für Otto Ernst Krasney* (Munich: Beck Verlag, 1997), 81–107.

43. The families of participants are beneficiaries of fund benefits, but not formally members of the fund, in that they do not participate in its governance.

44. These benefits were offered by the funds from 1989 until 1996, when they were abandoned by the Second Health Restructuring Act, but they have been partially rein-troduced by the 2000 Health Reform Act. SGB V, § 20.

45. SGB V, § 10. This is only true to the extent that the family member is not free from the insurance obligation and is not self-employed or self-supporting.

46. European Observatory, *Health Care Systems in Transition*, 26.

47. Ibid.

48. Ibid.

49. This is the *Sachleistungsprinzip*, established by SGB V, § 2, Abs. 2. Private insurance functions on an indemnification basis with respect to ambulatory doctors, but pays hospitals directly, based on contract. See European Observatory, *Health Care Systems in Transition*, 50; Knox, *Germany*, 76–77. Private patients are charged considerably more for services than the funds are charged for services to their patients.

50. European Observatory, *Health Care Systems in Transition*, 59; SGB V, § 76.

51. SGB V, § 76, ¶ 3.

52. European Observatory, *Health Care Systems in Transition*, 59.

53. Ibid., 61.

54. If the patient needs to be admitted to a hospital, of course, a referral from a physician is required under SGB V, § 73; hospitalization can only be ordered when ambulatory care is insufficient. Prescriptions from physicians are also necessary for drugs, home health care, durable medical equipment, sociotherapy, and other services.

55. SGB V, § 76, ¶ 4; Erwin Deutsch, *Medizinrecht* (Heidelberg: Springer Verlag, 1997), 37–39.

56. Deutsch, *Medizinrecht*, 49.

57. "Corporatism" is a model of governance defined by one of its foremost students as "a system of interest representation in which the constituent units are organized into a limited number of singular, compulsory, noncompetitive, hierarchically ordered and functionally differentiated categories, recognized or licensed (if not created) by the state and granted a deliberate representational monopoly within their respective categories in exchange for observing certain controls on their selection of leaders and articulation of demands and supports." Philippe C. Schmitter, "Still the Century for Corporatism?" in *Trends toward Corporatist Intermediation*, edited by Philippe C. Schmitter and Gerhard Lehmbruch (London: Sage Pub., 1979), 7, 13. See also Wolfgang Streeck and Philippe C. Schmitter, "Community, Market, State—and Associations? The Prospective Contribution of Interest Governance to Social Order," in *Private Interest Government: Beyond Market and State*, edited by Wolfgang Streeck and Philippe C. Schmitter (London: Sage, 1985), 1.

58. European Observatory, *Health Care Systems in Transition*, 25. These are basically organized at the *Land* level, but there are 23 of them, as three of the *Länder* have more than one association.

59. European Observatory, *Health Care Systems in Transition*, 102–103; SGB V, §§ 82–83 (the doctors negotiate separate contracts with the regular funds and the substitute funds). See, describing the history of the budgetary process, Friedrich Wilhelm Schwartz and Reinhard Busse, "Fixed Budgets in the Ambulatory Care Sector: The German Experience," in *Fixing Health Budgets: Experience from Europe and North America*, edited by Friedrich Wilhelm Schwartz, Howard Glennerster, and Richard B. Saltman (Chichester: John Wiley, 1996).

60. SGB V, § 72.

61. BSG, B 6 KA 54/00 R (March 14, 2001).

62. Busse, "Germany"; European Observatory, *Health Care Systems in Transition*, 100–101.

63. European Observatory, *Health Care Systems in Transition*, 96–99.

64. Only claims for a few services, like preventive spa treatments, rehabilitative services, and short-term nursing care at home need prior approval. European Observatory, *Health Care Systems in Transition*, 32.

65. Timothy Stoltzfus Jost, "Health Care Rationing in the Courts: A Comparative Study," *Hastings International and Comparative Law Review* 21 (spring 1998): 639.

66. Knox, *Germany*, 88–107; Schwartz and Busse, "Fixed Budgets in the Ambulatory Care Sector," 93–108; European Observatory, *Health Care Systems in Transition*, 102–106.

67. Schwartz and Busse, "Fixed Budgets in the Ambulatory Care Sector," 96–100.

68. European Observatory, *Health Care Systems in Transition*, 17. This goal has been an essential part of the German system since 1977.

69. European Observatory, *Health Care Systems in Transition*, 97; SGB V, § 87.

70. BSG, B 6 KA 20/99 R (May 10, 2000).

71. European Observatory, *Health Care Systems in Transition*, 88–91.

72. SGB V, § 87. See also Winifred Funk, "Vertragarztrecht," in *Handbuch des Sozialversicherungsrechts: Krankenversicherungsrecht*, edited by Bertram Shulin (Munich: C. H. Beck, 1994), 852, 888–890.

73. Raimund Wimmer, "Die sozialgerichtliche Kontrolldichte des Einheitliche Bewertungsmaßstabes," *Neue Zeitschrift für Sozialrecht* (June 2001): 287–293.

74. European Observatory, *Health Care Systems in Transition*, 103.

75. Ibid., 104. Each regional doctor's association establishes its own HVM for dividing up its own budget, and in some regions separate subbudgets are established for various specialties, resulting in different specialists receiving more or less points billed than others. See Günther Schneider, *Handbuch des Kassenarztrechts* (Cologne: Heymann's Verlag, 1994), 435–441.

76. Udo Sydow, *Die vertragärztlichen Abbrechnung: Einschließlich die Fremdkassenzahlungen und der Honorarverteilung* (Cologne: Kassenarztlichen Bundesvereinigung, 2001).

77. See European Observatory, *Health Care Systems in Transition*, 104.

78. Klaus-Dirk Henke, Margaret Murray, and Claudia Ade, "Global Budgeting in Germany: Lessons for the United States," *Health Affairs* 13 (fall 1994): 7–21. In the recent past, moreover, attempts have been made to improve compensation for primary care physicians and to decrease payment for technical services. There has also been a movement toward grouping some services that are billed together into a lump sum.

79. A brief English description of the program is found in U.S. General Accounting Office, *1993 German Health Reforms* (Washington, D.C.: GAO, 1993), 32–34, 45–46. For an exhaustive description of the system, see Karl Heinz Tuschen and Michael Quaas, *Bundespflegesatzverordnung* (Stuttgart: Kohlhammer, 1996).

80. See Tuschen and Quaas, *Bundespflegesatzverordnung*, 72.

81. Ibid.

82. Ibid., 73–75.

83. European Observatory, *Health Care Systems in Transition*, 80–83.

84. Ibid., 83.

85. These issues are discussed in greater detail in Chapter 5 in this volume.

86. Under Medicaid, cost sharing is for the obvious reason of the poverty of the recipients largely excluded. Under Medicare it takes the form of deductibles and coinsurance. Under private insurance cost sharing takes the form of deductibles, coinsurance, and copayments. In Germany, cost sharing is primarily in the form of copayments.

87. Federal Ministry of Health Press Release, http://www.bmgesundheit.de/presse/2001/2001/141.htm (cited June 28, 2002).

88. European Observatory, *Health Care Systems in Transition*, 105; Karl-Heinz Möller, "Verknappung von Vertragsarztsitzen," *Medizinrecht* 12 (2000): 555–559.

89. European Observatory, *Health Care Systems in Transition*, 105.

90. Ibid., 105, 112–114.

91. BSG, B 6 KA 54/00 R (March 14, 2001).

92. BSG, B 6 KA 36/00 R (March 14, 2001).

93. BSG, B 6 KA 67/00 R (March 14, 2001).

94. Schwartz, "Fixed Budgets in the Ambulatory Care Sector," 102.

95. See Peter Kummer, "Das sozialgerichtliche Verfahren," in *Sozialrechtshandbuch*, edited by Brend Baron von Mayell and Franz Ruland (Neuwied: Luchterhand, 1996), 603. Germany has a number of systems of special courts, in addition to its general jurisdiction civil and criminal courts (headed by the Bundesgerichtshof) and its constitutional court (the Bundesverfassungsgericht). These courts have jurisdiction over tax law, employment law, administrative law, and social law.

96. Kummer, "Das sozialgerichtliche Verfahren," 609–611.

97. Ibid., 611–613.

98. Ibid., 613–615.

99. Bundessozialgericht (BSG), *Die Tätigkeit des Bundessozialgerichts im Jahre 2001: Eine Übersicht* (Kassel: BSG, 2001), 29.

100. SGG (Sozialgerichtgesetz), § 12(1).

101. SGG, § 12(2).

102. SGG, § 12(3).

103. SGG, §§ 33 and 40.

104. Kummer, "Das sozialgerichtliche Verfahren," 657–659.

105. Ibid., 695–700.

106. SGB V, § 2(4).

107. SGB V, § 2(1).

108. SGB V, §§ 12(1), 70(10, and 72(2).

109. SGB V, §§ 28(1) and 34(2).

110. SGB V, § 135(1). See Andreas Schmidt-Rögnitz, *Die Gewährung von alternativen sowie neuen Behandlungs-und Heilmethoden durch die gesetzliche Krankenversicherung* (Berlin: Dunker and Humblot, 1996), 92–93, 96–97. On the emerging importance of the Bundesausschuß, see Hans-Jürgen Urban, *Der Bundesausschuß der Ärzte und Krankenkassen und die gesundheitspolitische Wende* (Berlin: Wissenschaftzentrum Berlin für Sozialforschung, 2001).

111. Horst Dieter Schirmer, "Das Kassenarztrecht im 2. GKV-Neuordnungsgesetz: BGBl. 1997 I S. 1520," *Medizinrecht* 15 (1997): 431, 447.

112. See Bertram Schulin, "Alternativ Medizin in der gesetzlichen Krankenversicherung," *Zeitschrift für Sozialreform* 40 (1994): 546, 553.

113. See generally, Schmidt-Rögnitz, *Die Gewährung von alternativen sowie neuen Behandlungs-und Heilmethoden*, 134.

114. Ibid., 98–99, 107; Rolf-Ulrich Schlenker, "Die Außenseitermedizin und das System der gesetzlichen Krankenversicherung," *Die Sozialgerichtsbarkeit* 39, no. 12 (1992): 530; Matthias von Wulffen, "Besondere Therapiemethoden in der Rechtsprechung des Bundessozialgerichts," *Die Sozialgerichtsbarkeit* 43, no. 6 (1996): 250.

115. Schmidt-Rögnitz, *Die Gewährung von alternativen sowie neuen Behandlungs-und Heilmethoden*, 100–101.

116. Stephan von Biehl and Heinz Ortwein, "Sind Außenseitermethoden Maßnahmen außerhalb des Leistungskataloges der gesetzlichen Krankenversicherung (GKV)?" *Sozialgerichstbarkeit* 38, no. 13 (1991): 529, 531–532.

117. See Schmidt-Rögnitz, *Die Gewährung von alternativen sowie neuen Behandlungs-und Heilmethoden*, 104–106; Schulin, "Alternativ Medizin in der gesetzlichen Krankenversicherung," 558–559.

118. Schmidt-Rögnitz, *Die Gewährung von alternativen sowie neuen Behandlungs-und Heilmethoden*, 101.

119. See, discussing the legality and constitutionality of the Bundesausschuß, Thorsten Koch, "Normsetzung durch Richtlinien des Bundesausschusses der Ärzte und Krankenkassen?" *Sozial Gesetzblatt* (March 2001): 109–116 and (April 2001): 166–174; Wolfgang Gitter and Gabriele Köhler-Fleischmann, "Gedanken zur Notwendigkeit und Wirtschaftlichkeit von Leistungen in der gesetzlichen Krankenversicherung und zur Funktion des Bundesausschusses der Ärzte und Krankenkassen," *Die Sozialgerichtsbarkeit* (January 1999): 1–4; Rolf-Ulrich Schlenker, "Das Entscheidungsmonopol des Bundesausschusses für neue medizinische Verfahren und Außenseitermethoden," *Neue Zeitschrift Socialrecht* (September 1998): 411–417; Thomas Clemens, "Verfassungsrechtliche Anforderungen an untergesetzliche Rechtsnormen," *Medizinische Recht* 14 (1996): 432, 438–439.

120. Raimund Wimmer, "Verfassungsrechtliche Anforderungen an untergesetzliche Rechtsetzung im Vertragsarztrecht," *Medizinrecht* 14 (1996): 425; Horst Dieter Schirmer, "Verfassungsrechtliche Probleme der untergesetzlichen Normsetzung im Kassenarztrecht," *Medizinrecht* 14 (1996): 404.

121. Grundgesetz, F.R.G., art. 12.

122. Grundgesetz, F.R.G., arts. 1 and 2.

123. BSG, B 1 KR 11/98 R (March 28, 2000).

124. BSG, B 1 KR 22/00 R (April 3, 2001).

125. BSG, B 1 KR 40/00 R (April 3, 2001).

126. See discussion of judicial review of Medicare and Medicaid decisions in the United States in Chapter 3 of this volume.

127. See Raimund Wimmer, "Die sozialgerichte Kontrolldicte des einheitlichen Bewertungmaßstabes," *Neue Zeitschrift für Socialrecht* (June 2001): 287–293; Ralf Großbölting, "Vorläufige Rechtsschutz im Vertragarztrecht," *Medizinrecht* (March 2001): 132–139.

128. Jost, "Health Care Rationing in the Courts," 669–677.

129. SGB V, § 106(5). This discussion focuses primarily on the process as it is applied to physicians. The process as it is applied to dentists is in most instances almost identical.

130. Ibid.

131. SGB V, §§ 2(4) and 12.

132. BSG 11/15/95, 6 RKa 43/94, SozR 3-2500, § 106, No. 33.

133. Wolfgang Spellbrink, *Wirtschaftlichkeitsprüfung im Kassenarztrecht nach dem Gesundheitsstrukturgesetz* (Neuwied: Luchterhand, 1994), 195–212.

134. See Wolfgang Engelhard, "Änderungen der Wirtschaftlichkeitsprüfungen im Vertragarztrecht durch das GKV-Gesundheitsreformgesetz 2000," *Neue Zeitschrift für Socialrecht* (March 2001): 123–129.

135. Dieter Raddatz, *Die Wirtschaftlichkeit der kassenärztlichen und kassenzahnärtzlichen Versorgung in der Rechtsprechung* (St. Augustin, Germany: Asgard-Verlag Hippe, 1993), 254–255.

136. Ibid., 212–215.

137. Ibid., 215–216.

138. SGB, §§ 84(3) and 106. See Sydow, *Die vertragärztlichen Abbrechnung.*

139. Spellbrink, *Wirtschaftlichkeitsprüfung im Kassenarztrecht,* 198–203.

140. Engelhard, "Änderungen der Wirtschaftlichkeitsprüfungen," 126.

141. Clemens, "Verfassungsrechtliche Anforderungen an untergesetzliche Rechtsnormen," 437–438; Spellbrink, *Wirtschaftlichkeitsprufung im Kassenartztrecht,* 274, 278–280; Raddatz, *Die Wirtschaftlichkeit der kassenärztlichen und kassenzahnärtzlichen Versorgung,* 374–444.

142. Raddatz, *Die Wirtschaftlichkeit der kassenärztlichen und kassenzahnärtzlichen Versorgung*, 330–373.

143. Clemens, "Verfassungsrechtliche Anforderungen an untergesetzliche Rechtsnormen," 441–442.

144. Raddatz, *Die Wirtschaftlichkeit der kassenärztlichen und kassenzahnärtzlichen Versorgung*, 146.

145. See BSG, 6/2/87, 6 RKa 19/86, SozR 2200 § 368n, No. 54; Hans-Siegmund Danckwerts, "Kassenzahnärztliche Versorgung: Überwachung der Wirtschaftlichkeit durch Einzelfallprüfungen," *Die Ortskrankenkasse* 70 (1988): 458.

146. Spellbrink, *Wirtschaftlichkeitsprüfung im Kassenarztrecht*, 315–316.

147. Ibid., 315.

148. See Sydow, *Die vertragärztlichen Abbrechnung*, describing this process.

149. BSG, B 6 KA 33/01 R (May 15, 2002).

150. BSG, B 6 KA 16/99 R (March 8, 2000).

151. Elias Mossialos and Anna Dixon, "Funding Health Care in Europe: Weighing up the Options," in *Funding Health Care: Options for Europe*, edited by Elias Mossialos (Buckingham: Open University Press, 2002), 275–276.

152. Ibid.

153. Altenstetter, "Health Care in Germany."

154. Premiums for the unemployed are paid by the unemployment compensation funds, but at rates below the average paid by employed persons. Premiums for welfare recipients (who make up only about 2% of fund members) are paid by the localities. Premiums for retirees are paid by the retirement funds and the retirees themselves, based on their pensions, but only cover about half the cost of their coverage. See Knox, *Germany*, 58–59, 60–61.

155. European Observatory, *Health Care Systems in Transition*, 40.

156. Knox, *Germany*, 75.

157. SGB V, § 226.

158. *AOK, G&G Blickpunkt*, February 2002, 4.

159. European Observatory, *Health Care Systems in Transition*, 108.

160. Ibid., 118–119.

161. Sachverständigenrat für die konzertierte Aktion im Gesundheitswesen, *Bedarfsgerechtigkeit und Wirtschaftlichkeit, Gutachten 2000/2001* (Baden-Baden: Konzertierte Aktion im Gesundheitswun, 2002).

162. European Observatory, *Health Care Systems in Transition*, 119.

# 11

# Toward an
# Entitlement-Based
# Health-Care System

<br>

THE American, British, and German health-care entitlement programs reviewed in this book illustrate a range of approaches to structuring legal rights to access to health care. How legal rights in health-care systems are defined and structured matters—obviously in terms of the access that they provide to health care, but also in terms of the cost and quality of health care found in various health-care systems and programs.

Legal health-care entitlements can be categorized usefully for further analysis in a number of ways. They can be described:

- in terms of the conceptual basis of the rights asserted
- in terms of the legal enforceability of those rights
- in terms of the populations that they protect
- in terms of the extent to which they require the participation of others in addition to the government to be effectuated.

This chapter describes these different categories of entitlements and then draws conclusions as to the practical implications of making various choices within these categories.

## Approaches to Categorizing Health-Care Entitlements

The Conceptual Basis of Health-Care Entitlements

Broadly speaking, health-care entitlements worldwide can be can be categorized into three families, in terms of the conceptual basis of the right asserted. First, there are social insurance approaches which grew out of the traditional insurance contract. The fundamental nature of the insurance contract, as described here in Chapter 2, is that an individual, faced with an uncertain risk of loss, pays an insurer a fixed premium to transfer to the insurer all or part of that risk. The insurer, in turn, pools the transferred risk with risks assumed from many other insureds, and through the law of large numbers transforms the contingencies facing all of the insureds into a reasonably manageable risk.

Health insurance was originally provided in Europe and in the United States by guilds and fraternal associations.[1] Later, in the United States, nonprofit Blue Cross and Blue Shield plans, and finally commercial plans, began providing health insurance on a contractual basis.[2] Beginning in the late nineteenth century, however, social insurance programs began to emerge, first in Germany, and then in other European and Latin American nations. Finally, in 1965, the United States initiated its own social health insurance program: Medicare. These social insurance programs are financed through "contributions" from employees and their employers and afford coverage to insured employees or former employees and their dependents.

The insurance contract model (be it private or social insurance) is ultimately based on an exchange relationship. The insured pays a premium (or contribution, or payroll tax) and in turn receives the promise of coverage should a risk eventuate. Because of the skewed distribution of risks discussed in the introduction to this book, some insureds receive far more from their insurance than they pay and some far less, although over a lifetime there is some, though not complete, leveling out of usage.[3] But each insured has the constant security of knowing that the insured risk will be covered, if it eventuates.[4]

Private insurance premiums vary based on exposure to risk, however. Social insurance contributions also vary, but usually based on ability to pay.[5] They are based in most countries on a percentage of income, often subject to an upper limit. Payments are thus mildly progressive, although the wealthier use more of some kinds of health-care services in some countries, thus limiting the progressiveness of social insurance.[6] In any event, the fundamental claim to entitlement is still based on payment of a premium: on value for money.

The second family of entitlement programs—general revenue-financed health systems—are not based on an explicit exchange but are provided gratuitously. Historically, gratuitous programs would have been characterized as charity or relief and were recognized as creating privileges rather than rights—

that is, not as entitlements at all. Beginning in the middle of the twentieth century, however, many nations began to recognize a positive human right of "freedom from want," which could form the basis of a claim against society—and ultimately against the state—for basic services such as health care.[7]

Modern taxation-based national health service programs (as well as means-tested welfare programs like our own Medicaid program) fit into this category of entitlements. While claims under these programs are not based on an explicit exchange, neither are they charity any more. For a time in the United States it was argued that these claims were based on property rights.[8] Even though they resemble property rights in that they are based on status rather than on exchange, it is perhaps more appropriate to view them as rights based on citizenship.[9] Indeed, it is arguable that national health services are not actually based on an individual rights model at all, but rather on an "obligation on the part of public health authorities to make provision for the health of the community at large"[10]—that is, a public health model.

It is important to note, however, that universal national health programs, covering entire populations, function rather differently than means-tested, welfare programs, even though they are similar in the basis of their claims. Programs for the poor are indeed poor programs,[11] and Medicaid has never enjoyed the nationwide support and concern that the British National Health Service enjoys.

A third group of entitlement programs are based on tax subsidies. The United States is the only developed nation that relies primarily on tax subsidies to ensure health care to its citizens, but a number of other countries afford their citizens tax subsidies to encourage the purchase of private insurance to supplement or substitute for public insurance programs.[12] Tax exclusions and deductions have been justified on the theory that (a) an income tax should be based on income defined as "real consumption and accumulation," and (b) money spent on health care (and by extension, health insurance) is not consumption because it does not increase welfare but, rather, is intended to simply restore a baseline state of good health.[13] The driving concept here, therefore, is not exchange, or health security, but simply an understanding of taxable income.

Tax subsidies are politically expedient because they tend to conceal government financing of health care and to minimize government supervision of the health-care system. They are thus attractive to those who oppose an active role for government in health-care systems. Tax subsidies, however, do not actually afford a right to health care, only the opportunity to obtain private health insurance if the person who benefits from the subsidy chooses to purchase it, as discussed in Chapter 8 of this volume. They are thus quite limited in their ability to extend health-care coverage.

## The Legal Enforceability of Health-Care Entitlements

A second approach to categorizing rights focuses not on the basis of the claimed right but on its legal enforceability. Three general approaches can be identified in the programs discussed in this book.

One option is to recognize rights that are rhetorical and political in nature, but are not specifically legally enforceable. Thus, if a British hospital or health authority refuses a service to a patient, the patient has little hope of using litigation to compel the hospital to provide the service. The Canadian courts also have generally treated claims for health services as political in nature and nonjusticiable.[14]

At the other end of the spectrum, a second approach recognizes rights that are absolute and specifically enforceable through the courts or through administrative proceedings. For example, a state or federal court can prospectively order a state Medicaid agency to provide coverage to a person eligible for Medicaid but denied coverage, or to provide screening and treatment services to an eligible child denied such services.[15]

A third option is to recognize a right to a process rather than to a result. Thus, the current Medicaid statute requires states to establish a public process for setting hospital and nursing-home rates, which includes the publication and justification of proposed rates; an opportunity for providers, beneficiaries and their representatives to comment on the proposed rates, methodologies, and justifications; and publication of final rates with methodologies and justifications.[16] The statute does not otherwise impose substantive requirements as to the rates that result.

The latter two possibilities will often fade imperceptibly into each other. As discussed in Chapter 10, for example, a member of a German social health insurance fund can sue in the social courts if denied a service, but in the first instance the court will defer to the decision of the Bundesausschuß der Ärzte und Krankenkassen, the administrative agency delegated responsibility for making coverage decisions, for a determination as to whether the service falls within statutory coverage definitions, and will only impose broad reasonableness standards when reviewing the decisions of the Bundesausschuß.

## The Universality of Coverage of Entitlements

A third approach to categorizing entitlements looks at their scope of coverage of the population. Some entitlement programs, like the British National Health Service and the Canadian Medicare program, cover entire populations. Others cover only those whose income is below a certain level. That level may be set quite high in countries (like Germany and the Netherlands) where the intention is to cover all for whom private insurance would not otherwise be readily affordable;

or quite low in countries (like the United States) where the intention is only to cover those who are truly indigent. Still other entitlement programs are directed at particular groups within the population. It is very common, for example, for countries to have separate health-care programs for the military or civil servants, but some also have distinct programs for children, the elderly, the disabled, and indigent populations. Finally, again, combinations are possible. Thus Ireland's national health program makes hospital care available to all, but only covers primary care for those whose incomes fall below a certain level.[17]

## The Number of Actors Necessary to Effectuate Entitlements

Finally, entitlements to health-care financing can be categorized depending on how many actors other than the state must be engaged before the right can be effectuated. Thus, in a pure system of socialized medicine, the state affords the right to health care directly through hospitals or other institutions that it owns and professionals it employs. Systems approaching this model were found in the communist countries and are currently found in Scandinavia, though even in Sweden and Finland private practitioners exist alongside the public clinics and hospitals.[18]

In taxation-based national health services that have not socialized the delivery of health care (such as the American Medicaid program and the British National Health Service with respect to general practice), the state affords a right to care and the funds to pay for it, but the care is delivered by private practitioners (either under contract or based on their willingness to accept reimbursement).

A third possibility is represented by traditional social insurance programs, where three parties are involved in the delivery of health-care services: the state (which guarantees the right to services and usually collects the contributions that fund the program), the quasi-public social insurance fund (which administers the financing of the program), and the providers (private or public) of the services. Germany exemplifies this possibility, but it adds a further complication by involving corporatist institutions that represent the insurers and the providers. Medicare is also an example of this approach insofar as it uses private intermediaries and carriers and managed-care organizations to pay claims.

Finally, some programs only afford incentives to independent actors who must take action before the intended beneficiary even receives insurance. Thus American tax subsidies for employment-related health insurance benefits only result in actual health care services if an employer decides to offer health benefits and if the insurer or managed-care organization decides to pay for a particular health-care service that a particular health-care institution or professional is willing to provide.

## Lessons for the United States

How nations structure their health-care entitlements in terms of these four dimensions has a dramatic and immediate effect on access to health care. Thus, most obviously, entitlements that only insure part of the population leave the rest uncovered. Second, if entitlements only guarantee tax incentives, they afford neither rights to health care nor even to health insurance. In fact, entitlements to health-care coverage may not guarantee health-care services at all if those rights are not legally enforceable, even if the state provides these services directly, as several patients have learned when they sued the British National Health Service.

The way in which entitlements are structured also seems to have an effect on health-care costs. The British health-care system—one of the least expensive systems among developed nations—offers direct and contracted provision of services and does not afford a judicially enforceable right to particular services. This structure gives it maximum leverage to hold down health-care costs, which it has exercised very effectively. The most expensive health-care system in the world is that of the United States, which affords legally enforceable rights to health care through Medicare and Medicaid but tends to involve multiple levels of actors in its insurance programs, thus diluting budgetary control.

What can we learn from our own experience and from that of other nations about how we should structure our health-care entitlements so as to maximize access and quality and minimize cost? To begin, we should aim for an entitlement program that covers the entire population. It should be clear by now that market-based private insurance cannot cover entire populations, even with tax subsidies. We could attempt to cover only those of average and below-average income, leaving high-income individuals to self-insure or buy private insurance, which is the approach taken by the Netherlands and Germany. This strategy leaves scope for free markets and private arrangements, but it also removes the wealthiest and most politically powerful members of society from a stake in the public health-care system. In the long run, this could pose a threat to the system, particularly in a country like the United States that does not have a strong tradition of social solidarity. Only universal access undergirds the sense of solidarity necessary to sustain health-care entitlement programs in the long term.

A closer question is whether private insurance should continue as an option for those who are publicly insured. In all nations with public insurance systems, private insurance continues to be available. In some nations, as in Canada, private insurance covers services not included in the public program; in others, such as France or Medicare supplement policies in the United States, it covers cost-sharing obligations imposed by the public program; and in still others, like the United Kingdom, private insurance allows insureds to jump queues and receive health services more quickly, or conveniently, or in more comfortable settings than those covered by the public program.[19] Only in some Canadian provinces is it illegal to buy private insurance to cover services that are explicitly covered by the public system.[20]

There is no harm in allowing those who can afford it to purchase private insurance to cover services excluded from the public insurance program, as long as the public program is sufficiently generous.[21] Permitting insurance against cost sharing, however, deprives cost-sharing obligations of their incentive effect—an effect that has arguably driven up the cost of the Medicare program in the United States.[22] Permitting private insurance that covers the same services as the public program is even more problematic, creating a shadow health-care system for the wealthy and undermining the national commitment to high-quality health care for the rest of the population.[23] It is particularly problematic if professionals can work in both systems and face incentives to steer their patients from the public to the private system.

In the end, however, outlawing private insurance is probably too much of a stretch for the United States. Leaving private insurance in place might make it slightly easier to sell a public insurance program politically, since those most committed to private insurance and care could always opt out if they chose to (as is the case now with private elementary and secondary schools in the United States). It might be wise, however, to require professionals who engage in private contracting to withdraw from the public system, as is currently done under the Medicare private contracting provisions.[24] This would minimize the ability of providers to undermine the public system for their own gain, a problem alleged to exist in the United Kingdom.

The second issue is the legal conceptual basis for the public system. Since tax subsidy–based systems cannot achieve comprehensive coverage, the initial choice for a comprehensive system leaves us with the option of an exchange-based system or a citizens' rights-based system. Our experience with Medicare and Medicaid gives us direction here. Medicare was based on the Social Security program—payroll tax–financed, and, therefore, exchange-based. Medicare has enjoyed great political protection because those who have paid payroll taxes over the years expect to receive a return on them. On the other hand, even though Medicaid—a general tax-financed program—has long been recognized legally as an entitlement, it has never possessed the political sanctity that Medicare has enjoyed.

In the end, entitlements are political claims. Politicians can, and do, abandon or weaken welfare programs. Within the past decade the United States has abolished the Aid for Families with Dependent Children program, which had been in place for over six decades, and came within a pen stroke of ending Medicaid as an entitlement program. Ending health insurance programs that insureds have paid for over a lifetime is much more difficult, however, as the experience of American politicians who threaten Medicare demonstrates.

The use of hypothecated taxes also assures that money will be used for health care and not diverted to other purposes. Many surveys have shown stronger support for health-care expenditures than for other uses of taxes, along with support for increased federal spending on health care.[25] International experience also shows less resistance to increasing hypothecated taxes for health care than to general tax increases.[26] Health-care expenditures in the United Kingdom are so low, as compared with expenditures in social insurance–based countries, because health-care expenditures must compete with other public goods, and the public is less open to simply raising taxes generally.

It might not be wise, however, to depend solely on payroll taxes. Systems that are financed only through payroll taxes are at risk as a larger share of the economy moves into returns on capital or other non-wage-based income, and as more persons dependent on payroll-taxed systems participate only partially or intermittently in the labor market.[27] This has become a serious problem in Germany. If the share of wages subject to payroll taxes is capped, moreover, as it now is in Germany and formerly was in the United States, the progressivity of taxation to support the health-care system also drops, and the system imposes even higher burdens on those who are least able to cope with the expense. The best system might be one based on a hypothecated tax that is based on income generally and is not subject to any caps.

An additional argument for not limiting funding to payroll taxes is that a system that draws more widely on taxation of income would include in the revenue base persons who are not currently employed but are financially capable of contributing. In the German system, for example, retired persons pay a modest premium based on their retirement income. This not only increases funds available within the system, but also enhances solidarity (and decreases resentment on the part of younger, employed persons).

With respect to the third issue, the enforceability of rights, a middle course seems advisable. On the one hand, middle-class Americans are unlikely to accept rights that are merely rhetorical and political. One of the primary factors driving the backlash against managed care at the end of the 1990s was a frustration experience by members of managed-care plans who felt that they had no means to challenge plan decisions that they regarded to be arbitrary and irrational. Further, giving unreviewable discretion to a bureaucracy responsible to govern something as important as health care seems very ill-advised.

On the other hand, allowing the courts free rein to make health-care resource allocation decisions is a recipe for disaster. Requiring courts to decide between concrete and present individual claims for resources and the amorphous desire to save money, especially in life-threatening situations, is likely to result in excessive expenditures.[28] The best approach here is likely to be to afford an entitlement to a process—preferably a process that involves health-care experts, representatives of the public, and persons who are legally trained.

The German model, which relies on expert decision making, subject to review by social courts, which are in turn staffed by both professionally trained judges and judges representing the points of view of interested parties, is a useful model to consider. Models currently emerging in our own American system for making coverage decisions, including internal, external, and ultimately judicial review, also provide a balance between the need for transparency, rationality, consistency, and legitimacy, on the one hand, and reasonable consideration of the finitude of resources, on the other.[29]

Finally, we come to the most difficult of the four design choices set before us: How many actors should be involved in effectuating entitlements in the health-care system? A totally socialized system, in which the government delivered all health care, is unimaginable in the United States. It is also probably inadvisable, as it would in all likelihood result in restrictions on health-care resources and a degree of politicization and bureaucratization of health-care delivery unacceptable in the United States, or possibly anywhere. It is probably not an accident that even the Scandinavian systems, which come the closest to pure socialism among developed nations, generally administer their systems at the local or regional level, thus insulating health-care delivery somewhat from national political forces. The British system, which relies on private general practitioners and has been moving toward more independence for hospitals, still endures a level of political interference in the health-care system that is probably unwise.

Alternatively, the system currently in place in the United States for most of the population—under which tax subsidies are used to encourage employers to buy insurance from insurers or managed-care companies, which, in turn, purchase services from professionals and providers for employee/insureds—simply does not work for many Americans. It fails to afford access to health care for 41 million people, on the one hand, while creating the most expensive health-care system in the world, on the other. There are simply no levers in the system to either ensure access or control costs.

It will certainly be necessary to maintain private professionals and providers within the United States, for political reasons if for no other. A harder question is whether there should be a continuing role for insurers or managed-care organizations (MCOs). Since everyone would be covered by public insurance under the system here envisioned, there would be no continuing need for insurers as risk poolers and spreaders, except insofar as they offered marginal coverage for those who chose to seek coverage beyond the public system. MCOs, however, could play a useful role: coordinating care and managing disease for the chronically ill, for example, or helping to manage costs.

The primary question must be, Does participation of private MCOs in the government plan add value commensurate to its cost? It must be remembered that managing care is not cheap, and that integrating MCOs into a health-care system imposes significant administrative costs. If MCOs compete primarily on the basis of risk selections rather than by controlling costs, they detract from, rather than add to, the value of the health-care system. The evidence suggests that the Medicare managed-care program has imposed costs on the Medicare program without bringing commensurate value. Although Medicare MCOs have offered added value to their members, this has been at the expense of the Medicare program, which the MCOs have manipulated (perhaps unintentionally) through risk selection. In the Medicaid program, however, it is possible that MCOs have in some states added value by offering recipients better access to providers or better coordination of care.

The larger question is whether there is a continuing role for market institutions in health care. For much of the past six decades in the United States, public or private insurance paid for health care while professionals and patients controlled demand (and, often, professionals and providers controlled supply). If there is anything we can learn from health economists, it is that when those who determine demand are not burdened with the price of goods and services, they are unlikely to purchase them responsibly. One strategy for controlling costs, therefore, is to visit the full cost, or a large part of the cost, of health care on the consumer—that is, on the patient. The argument of this book, however, is that the price to society of relying wholly on markets to control costs—the exclusion of the poor, chronically ill, and aged from the benefits of health care—is too high to justify the control over cost that markets might give us. Also, in many instances consumers simply lack the information to choose knowledgeably which health-care services to consume and which to forego, thus total consumer sovereignty may not enhance consumer welfare.[30] Therefore, we cannot wholly rely on markets for controlling health-care costs.

The use of economic incentives should not be rejected totally as a cost-control strategy, however. In fact, most of the world's health-care systems now incorporate some form of patient cost sharing, although the poor and chronically ill are often protected from the full brunt of cost sharing obligations, and cost-sharing is often driven as much by the desire to shift costs to consumers as by the desire to control costs.[31] Indeed, it is often providers who are most aggressive in their desire for cost sharing, realizing that it is more likely to enhance than to limit their incomes.[32] But carefully targeted cost sharing might play a useful role in steering consumers from high-cost to lower-cost treatment modalities. Perhaps consumers should pay more for name brand than for generic drugs, or for the use of emergency rooms for primary care (but the poor and chronically ill should be protected from facing levels of cost sharing that would deter them from obtaining effective care). Nevertheless, market forces should remain at the margins of health system organization rather than at the center.

It may be useful to consider both the root cause of the difficulty of controlling health-care costs (which is arguably the failure of markets) and the factors that keep health-care costs high and climbing. The overwhelming consensus is that the leading driver of cost is the continual expansion of medical technology.[33] We are constantly developing new drugs, devices, and procedures for diagnosing and curing diseases; for improving functioning; and for delaying death. This is no accident. As noted in Chapter 6, the public strongly supports research and the development of medical technology, and the American government invests more in support of basic health-care research than any other country (and asks little from the private sector as a return on this investment). Indeed, in the recent past, the federal government has dramatically increased funding for health-care research, just as it has been calling for limiting expenditures on health-care services. This public investment feeds into and is complemented by private investment. Our intellectual property laws and systems of health-care payment, in turn, generously reward private investment. The result is a steady stream of medical innovations. These innovations, however, generally increase, rather than reduce costs.[34] Thus costs keep climbing.

It is important that payments for health-care services remain high enough to support innovation and quality. But as a society we must find some way of deciding how much we are willing to pay for medical technology, and not pay more than that amount. We must also become more effective in recovering public investments in health-care research and in screening out technologies that add cost without adding value.

A second factor driving cost is the fact that health care is labor intensive. Increased productivity in labor-intensive sectors tends to increase, rather than decrease, costs (the Baumol effect).[35] In many other industries, capital can be substituted for labor, driving down costs over time, but this is often not possible in health care. Nor in most health-care settings can labor-intensive production processes simply be moved overseas, where labor is cheaper. The labor that is needed to provide health care, moreover, is often the labor of highly trained professionals—indeed, of licensed professionals who have completed lengthy and onerous educational programs and who are often in limited supply. There is considerable evidence that we are much more generous in paying these professionals in the United States than in other countries, for whatever reason, but there is also evidence that those countries that hold down costs too firmly face labor shortages.[36]

A final factor is the high administrative costs of the American system.[37] First, as has been noted often throughout this book, private insurance imposes high costs for marketing and underwriting that are completely useless in terms of providing health care—the goal of a health-care system. Also, though private managed care has helped some over the past decade to control the prices, and probably to a lesser extent the utilization, of health care, this care-management function has come at a high price in terms of administrative costs.

The countries that have been most successful at controlling costs have been those that, like the United Kingdom, impose universal budgets on the health-care system and then rely on health-care providers to ration supply. Countries with centralized budget controls address all three factors that are driving cost expansion in the United States: they limit the introduction of technology and ration access to it by limiting funding for new technologies; they use their dominant power in the market for health-care labor to hold down labor costs; they avoid the high costs of administering private insurance systems found in the United States, and thus hold down administrative costs.

These constraints can be pressed too far, however. Countries that set their health-care budgets through the general public budgeting process, like the United Kingdom, risk putting too much pressure on health-care costs, resulting in wait lists, late adoption of useful technologies, and heightened public dissatisfaction. Countries that rely on hypothecated taxes, such as payroll taxes, and that draw on multiple levels of government to fund health care, or that provide a role for quasi-independent social insurers in financing the health-care system, have more breathing room to achieve a more appropriate level of health-care expenditures.

In the United States, we have no current tradition of independent social insurance funds to draw on (though at an earlier time the Blue Cross/Blue Shield organizations might have been adaptable to this purpose). We do have a tradition of independent commissions to distance important functions from politics, however. An arrangement where Congress set an overall level of spending growth, but an independent, bipartisan commission managed the actual national social health insurance program, would probably give us our best approximation of a traditional social insurance program.[38] It might also be advisable to permit the states to have programs to supplement a basic federal entitlement to health care, thus allowing for regional variation above a federal floor.

One lesson that we must learn from other nations is that completely open-ended budgets for health-care entitlement programs are not sustainable. Other health-care systems impose ex ante limits on expenditures, either through public budgets (as in the United Kingdom) or through setting limits on the rate of growth of expenditures (as in Germany). America's open-ended entitlements are peculiarly American and have contributed to America's uniquely high levels of health-care expenditures. We must accept limits, and then develop legal institutions that can reasonably allocate resources within those limits.

Once overall levels of expenditures are established and an entity is chosen to manage the program, some sort of flexible process is necessary for allocating funds among health-care sectors and then for rationing services within those sectors. There are real risks in separating budgets among sectors too sharply in terms of distorting allocations and stifling innovation. A better approach is to rely on gatekeeper primary care physicians or physician groups to take the

lead in allocating resources through their referral decisions. There are also difficult issues involved in determining how to pay professionals and providers.
Fee-for-service, obviously, encourages overuse; capitation and prospective
payment create risks of stinting. Probably some mix, and probably a mix that
changes over time, will come closer to optimal results than exclusive reliance
on one or the other. Both the British and German systems pay primary care
providers using a mixed payment system.

Although a single-payer system would exclude the possibility of multiple,
competing managed-care plans, it need not exclude the possibility of competition. Competition should be at the provider level, however, and should be
based on quality. Sweden has encouraged quality-based competition among
health-care providers with modest success.[39] Primary care providers, for example, could be organized into groups, which could be evaluated based on their
performance: in carrying out preventive care; in patient satisfaction surveys; or
in managing chronic conditions, such as diabetes and asthma. Secondary and
tertiary care providers could also be evaluated based on quality and performance, and they could compete for referrals from primary care groups. Once
competition was focused on quality, rather than on risk avoidance, it could yield
positive results for the patients.

One particular benefit of moving toward a single-payer system is that it would
indeed facilitate long-term relationships between professionals and patients.
Our current system—under which patients change providers on a regular basis when they change jobs, when their employer changes managed-care plans,
or when they gain or lose public insurance—discourages provision of preventive care and long-term management of chronic conditions. Why should a
managed-care company invest in preventive care for a member who is likely
to leave at the end of the year? In other countries, stable financing of health
care makes stable relationships with health-care providers, and thus better primary and preventive care, possible.

It is well beyond the scope of this book to design a complete blueprint for
the reconstruction of our health-care system. The important point is that in designing or evaluating health-care systems it is vital to consider the role of legal
rights. Legal rights obviously play a central role in assuring patients (or insureds
or consumers) access to health-care goods and services. But if resources for
providing health care are not unbounded, rights also cannot be unbounded;
rather, they must be rights to a process that determines in some equitable and
reasonable way where the boundaries should be. Finally, in fact, rights must
be rights to health care, not merely rights to purchase health insurance if one
is wealthy—and healthy—enough.

Of course, this is only one vision of what a health-care system could look
like—a system based on legal entitlements. The alternative vision, which seems
so powerful today, embraces a privatized, individualized, devolved, and largely

market-based health-care system. The argument for this vision is appealing: competition promotes choice, quality, and innovation and brings down cost, in turn extending access. In reality, however, as this book repeatedly demonstrates, competition in unregulated markets for health-care financing focuses on avoiding risks, thus diminishing access. It has also proved largely ineffective in controlling costs. Moreover, although it may be theoretically possible to structure markets for managed-care plans in such a way as to provide access for all and to focus competition on cost rather than on risk, such a market would have to be so highly regulated and subsidized by public tax expenditures that it would only be a "private market" in the sense that private firms were profiting from it. There is no hard evidence, however, that systems organized in such a way could outperform public systems.

In the end, our choice is between entitlement and disentitlement. I have little confidence that we will make the right choice soon. Powerful and well-financed forces are arrayed against expanding entitlements, as the Clintons learned in 1993–1994, and in the American political system money speaks louder than reason. But current trends cannot continue forever. Surveys have long shown that Americans are much less satisfied with their health-care system than are the citizens of other nations. (See Figure 11–1.) If both health-care costs and the numbers of the uninsured keep rising, at some point political leaders of courage and integrity will realize that something has to be done.

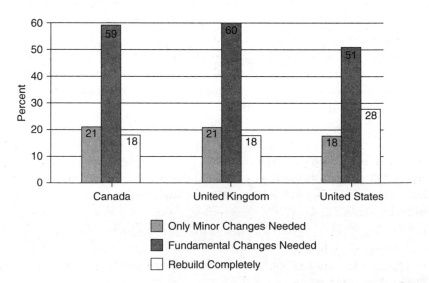

FIGURE 11–1. Citizens' overall views about their health-care systems, 2001. *Source:* Adapted from Robert J. Blendon et al., "Inequities in Health Care: A Five-Country Survey," *Health Affairs* 21 (May/June 2002), 182, 183, based on Commonwealth Fund/Harvard/Harris 2001 International Health Policy Survey.

The market solutions described in this book will not do the job—they cannot expand access and are unlikely to restrain cost. Americans, too, will have to look to international experience and to some form of health-care entitlement. One can only hope that, in the end, entitlement will triumph over disentitlement.

# Notes

1. Timothy Stoltzfus Jost, "Private or Public Approaches to Insuring the Uninsured: Lessons from International Experience with Private Insurance," *New York University Law Review* 76 (2001): 419, 437.

2. Institute of Medicine, *Employment and Health Policy: A Connection at Risk* (Washington, D.C.: National Academy Press, 1993), 65–73.

3. Marian Gornick, Alma McMillan, and James Lubitz, "A Longitudinal Perspective on Patterns of Medicare Payments," *Health Affairs* 12 (summer 1993): 140–150.

4. Karl Hinrichs, *Health Care Policy in the German Social Insurance State: From Solidarity to Privatization?* (Bremen: Centre for Social Policy Studies, 1999).

5. Adam Wagstaff and Eddy van Doorslaer, "Equity in Health Care Finance and Delivery," in *Handbook of Health Economics*, vol 1B, (Amsterdam: Elsevier, 2000) 1817–1818.

6. Ibid., 1824–1828, 1833–1846; but see Jay Bhattacharya and Darius Lakdawalla, *Does Medicare Benefit the Poor? New Answers to an Old Question* (October 2, 2002). Concluding that Medicare disproportionately benefits the poor.

7. See Sir William Beveridge, *Social Insurance and Allied Services* (New York: Macmillan, 1942), 6–9.

8. See Charles Reich, "The New Property," *Yale Law Journal* 73 (1964): 733.

9. See James W. Fox Jr., "Liberalism, Democratic Citizenship, and Welfare Reform: The Troubling Case for Workfare," *Washington University Law Quarterly* 74 (1996): 103, 123–129, 138–145.

10. Rudolph Klein, *The New Politics of the NHS*, 4th ed. (Harlow: Prentice Hall, 2001), 4–5.

11. This aphorism is generally attributed to Wilbur Cohen.

12. Elias Mossialos and Sarah Thomson, "Voluntary Health Insurance," in *Funding Health Care: Options for Europe*, edited by Elias Mossialos et al. (Buckingham: Open University Press, 2002), 133–135.

13. William D. Andrews, "Personal Deductions and an Ideal Income Tax," *Harvard Law Review* 86 (1972): 309. See also, critiquing Andrews' position, Jay A. Soled, "Taxation of Employer-Provided Health Coverage: Inclusion, Timing, and Policy Issues," *Virginia Tax Review* 15 (1996): 447–487; Bradley W. Joondeph, "Tax Policy and Health Care Reform: Rethinking the Tax Treatment of Employer-Sponsored Health Insurance," 1995 *Brigham Young University Law Review* (1995): 1229–1261.

14. Sujit Choudry, "The Enforcement of the Canada Health Act," *McGill Law Journal* 41 (1996): 461–508.

15. See *Westside Mothers v. Haveman*, 289 F. 3d 852 (6th Cir. 2002) (reaffirming the ability of the federal courts to order state officials to conform to federal law), and *John B. v. Menke*, 176 F. Supp. 2d 786 (M.D. Tenn. 2001) (ordering the state of Tennessee to conform Tennessee's Medicaid EPSDT program to law).

16. 42 U.S.C. § 1396a(13)(A).

17. Jenny Hughes, "Health Expenditure and Cost Containment in Ireland," in *Health Care and Cost Containment in the European Union*, edited by Elias Mossialos and Julian Le Grand (Brookefield, Vt.: Ashgate, 1999), 483–487.

18. Unto Häkkinen, "Cost Containment in Finnish Health Care," in *Health Care and Cost Containment in the European Union*, edited by Elias Mossialos and Julian Le Grand (Brookefield, Vt.: Ashgate, 1999), 661–699; Anders Anell and Patrick Svarvar, "Health Care Reforms and Cost Containment in Sweden," in ibid., 701–723.

19. Jost, "Public or Private Approaches," 419; Mossialos and Thomson, "Voluntary Health Insurance," 129–131.

20. Colleen Flood, "The Structure and Dynamics of Canada's Health Care System," in *Canadian Health Law and Policy*, edited by Jocelyn Downie and Timothy Caulfield (Toronto: Butterworths, 1999), 29.

21. There has been some concern in Canada that current attempts to "delist," services—that is, to declare them not medically necessary—will result in some important services being covered only for those who are privately insured. See Carolyn Hughes Tuohy, "The Costs of Constraint and Prospects for Health Care Reform in Canada," *Health Affairs* 21, no. 3 (2002): 42–43.

22. Congressional Budget Office, *Long-Term Budgetary Pressures and Policy Options: Report to the Senate and House Committees on Budget* (Washington, D.C.: CBO, 1998); Physician Payment Review Commission (PPRC), *Private Supplemental Insurance for Medicare Beneficiaries* (Washington, D.C.: PPRC, 1997), 13.

23. This argument convinced a Canadian court to uphold Quebec's ban on private insurance; see *Chaoulli v. Quebec*, No. 500-50-035610-9798 (Que. Super Ct. Feb. 25, 2000). See also Jeremiah Hurley et al., *Parallel Private Health Insurance in Australia: A Cautionary Tale and Lessons for Canada* (Canberra: Australian National University Centre for Economic Policy Research, 2002).

24. See 42 U.S.C. § 1395a(b).

25. See, e.g., Ruy Teixiera, "Washington's Deaf Ear," *Economic Policy Institute Issue Briefs*, no. 135, available at www.epinet.org/Issuebriefs (cited September 23, 1999).

26. Elias Mossialos and Anna Dixon, "Funding Health Care: An Introduction," in *Funding Health Care: Options for Europe*, edited by Elias Mossialos et al. (Buckingham: Open University Press, 2002), 16–17.

27. Charles Normand and Reinhard Busse, "Social Health Insurance Financing," in *Funding Health Care: Options for Europe*, edited by Elias Mossialos et al. (Buckingham: Open University Press, 2002), 73.

28. See Mark A. Hall and Gerald F. Anderson, "Health Insurers Assessment of Medical Necessity," *University of Pennsylvania Law Review* 140 (1992): 1637.

29. See Eleanor Kinney, *Protecting Health Care Consumers* (Durham, N.C.: Duke University Press, 2002); Norman Daniels and James Sabin, "Fair Procedures, Democratic Deliberation, and the Legitimacy Problem for Insurers," *Philosophy and Public Affairs* 26, no. 4 (1997): 303–350.

30. See Thomas Rice, *The Economics of Health Reconsidered* (Chicago: Health Administration Press, 1998), 64–80; James C. Robinson, "The End of Managed Care," *Journal of the American Medical Association*, 285 (May 23–30, 2001): 2622, 2626.

31. Ray Robinson, "User Charges in Health Care," in *Funding Health Care: Options for Europe*, edited by Elias Mossialos et al. (Buckingham: Open University Press, 2002), 161, 178.

32. See Robert G. Evans, "Going for the Gold: The Redistributive Agenda behind

Market-Based Health Care Reform," *Journal of Health Politics, Policy, and Law* 22 (1997): 427–460.

33. Penny E. Mohr et al., *The Impact of Medical Technology on Future Health Care Costs: Final Report* (Bethesda, Md.: Project Hope, 2001).

34. Michael Moran, *Governing the Health Care State* (Manchester: Manchester University Press, 1999).

35. Named after American economist, William J. Baumol, who first identified it. *Penguin Dictionary of Economics* (1998), available at www.xrefer.com/entry/444673 (cited July 4, 2002).

36. Average physician income in 1996, the most recent year for which data are available, averaged $199,000 compared to an OECD median of $70,324. The ratio of average physician income to average worker income was 5.5 in the United States, compared to 3.4 in Germany and 1.4 in the United Kingdom. Uwe Reinhardt, Peter S. Hussey, and Gerard F. Anderson, "Cross-National Comparisons of Health Systems using OECD Data, 1999," *Health Affairs* 21, no. 3 (May/June 2002): 169–180.

37. Reinhardt et al., "Cross-National Comparisons," 171.

38. See National Academy of Social Insurance, *Improving Medicare's Governance and Management* (Washington, D.C.: NASI, 2002): 61–64.

39. Michael I. Harrison, "Health Professionals and the Right to Health Care," in *The Right to Health Care in Several European Countries*, edited by Anadré den Exeter and Herbert Hermans (The Hague: Kluwer, 1999), 81, 91–93.

# INDEX